Positive Relationships

Sue Roffey

Editor

Positive Relationships

Evidence Based Practice across the World

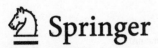 Springer

Editor
Sue Roffey
School of Education
University of Western Sydney
Sydney, Australia

Department of Clinical,
Educational and Health Psychology
University College
London, UK
sue@sueroffey.com

ISBN 978-94-007-2146-3 (hardcover)   e-ISBN 978-94-007-2147-0
ISBN 978-94-007-5658-8 (softcover)
DOI 10.1007/978-94-007-2147-0
Springer Dordrecht Heidelberg London New York

Library of Congress Control Number: 2011938235

Printed on acid-free paper

Springer is part of Springer Science+Business Media (www.springer.com)

For Dz – of course.

Foreword

The past decade has seen a seismic shift within psychology and allied sciences towards an increasing emphasis on what makes life go well. Positive Psychology has played a central role in rebalancing the previous obsession with problems, pathology and dysfunction. The happiness and wellbeing of individuals has been at the core of this new science, and we have learned much about the value of positive emotions, the characteristics of happy people, and ways to promote individual happiness and wellbeing. However, the foundation of what makes lives go well is not the individual, but the quality of our relationships – the development of trust, the giving and receiving of love and support, and the myriad ways in which relationships can be life enhancing.

In this seminal book, Sue Roffey and a team of international experts move beyond a focus on the individual, putting relationships at the heart of life going well. In doing so, this book follows a fine tradition which goes back to Darwin, who recognised that the extraordinary complexity of human behaviour, including thinking, language, the diversity and subtlety of emotions, and our ability to envisage the future, are all derived from our evolution as social animals, and are manifestations of our social brain. Neuroscience has shown that the human brain has evolved the capacity to sense what other people are thinking and feeling. It is 'mirror' cells in the human brain that are activated when we feel empathy or compassion allowing us to share another persons joy or pain. Other brain regions have become specialised to allow us to 'mind read' or understand what other people are thinking, hoping and planning. Social relationships have not only shaped human evolution, but they play a profoundly important role in human development. From the moment of birth (and even in utero), children enter a world of relationships to which they respond and through which they learn to navigate. Research has shown that the quality of these early relationships can have lifelong effects on mental health, cognitive capability, lifestyle behaviours and, of course, later relationships. But formative as these early years are, research has also shown that they are not deterministic, and later social influences can alter these trajectories for better or for worse.

The rich variety and depth of the research presented in the 17 chapters of this book explores both what is known about the development of positive relationships, and the wide range of approaches which have been employed to enhance the quality of relationships. Recognising the fundamental importance of the type and quality of our early relationships, many chapters are devoted to relationships with family. Effective parenting and positive parent-child interactions are dynamic processes requiring constant adaptation as the child develops through infancy and the primary years to adolescence and young adulthood. The dynamics of this process and the skills required for positive relationships at each stage are clearly described in this volume. The brilliant body of research by John Gottman on couples and the qualities associated with positive couple relationships is described, and this volume also considers what happens for children when a couple's relationship breaks down beyond repair. We learn about the importance of listening to children's voices and maximising their wellbeing in the context of family breakdown, and ways in which this can be achieved. The seminal role of the child-teacher relationship and the quality of relationships with peers, particularly the nature of friendship are addressed in depth. An understanding is provided both of what makes for positive relationships in this context and a critical evaluation of approaches employed to improve such relationships. Strong evidence is presented for the importance of a whole school approach to relationship quality and its impact on learning and wellbeing.

A good deal of attention is given to inter-personal relationships in the workplace where a growing body of evidence shows that positive relationships can improve productivity and financial success. However, positive relationships at work are of value in their own right quite apart from benefits to the 'bottom line'. Positive relationships at work can in turn feed into more positive relationships with family, friends and community members. Much has been written about the importance of leadership in the workplace, and it is now recognised that the ability to foster positive relationships is at the heart of good leadership. Inspiration and innovation are not enough – true leaders also need emotional and social intelligence to engage workers in co-creating their vision. Mentorship is widely regarded as a valuable function in the workplace, although there can be wide variations in style and quality. The role of professional consultants is also at heart a relational matter, and we need a better understanding of the factors which make consultations more effective. These and numerous other facets of positive relationships in the workplace are engagingly and insightfully explored in this volume.

The book goes beyond inter-personal relationships to investigate positive community relationships, which is an area of positive psychology much in need of further development. Schools, workplaces and other organisations are analysed at the level of communities, and innovative approaches to enhancing positive community relationships are presented. A particular strength of the book is the cultural awareness that it brings to all the topics covered, including a variety of approaches to building positive community relationships where there are major differences in ethnicity, culture or beliefs. Building harmonious and peaceful relationships in families, institutions and communities is eloquently addressed in a number of chapters, including the idea of healthy conflict and the power of restorative justice to strengthen understanding, relationships and wellbeing.

As the book's editor, Sue Roffey has created a first rate, comprehensive account
of the wealth of relationships which impinge on our daily lives, characterising their
positive attributes across a wide range of life stages and contexts, and providing
valuable information about how to make relationships more positive. I have learned
a great deal from this informative volume on evidence-based practice and the
enhancement of positive relationships. I believe it will have a lasting impact on the
field of positive psychology, and encourage further research, theorising and application, which goes beyond the individual to the multitude of ways we can be positively
connected with others.

Professor Felicia A. Huppert
Director of the Well-being Institute
University of Cambridge

Acknowledgments

I would like to thank the following individuals for their involvement in the completion of this volume.

Esther Otten of Springer whose initiative, positive energy and strong support not only made the project possible in the first place but helped bring it to fruition.

All of the authors who probably wondered what they had let themselves in for when working on their nth draft. I am immensely grateful for their efforts, patience and responsiveness in shaping the final version..

Geoffrey Abbott, Angelika Anderson, Ed Baines, Gawaian Bodkin-Andrews, Joshua Brown, Bill Bumberry, Tim Corcoran, Helena Cornelius, Joanna Finkelstein, Michael Flood, Bill Hansberry, Betty Holmes, Belinda Hopkins, Suzy Green, Bridget Grenville-Cleave, Tamera Linseisen, Jan Long, Emma Marshall, Christina Michaelson, Wendy Moran, Yin Paradies, Gail Parfitt, Jennifer Smith, Scott Smith, Alison Soutter, Greta Sykes, Marilyn Tew, Marg Thorsbourne, Julie-Anne Tooth, Judith Trowell, Dianne Vella-Brodrick, Arlene Vetere, Patsy Wagner, Roz Walker and Di Yerbury all gave their time generously to read and comment on the developing chapters.

Without the efforts of those whose work is cited here, psychology would not have raised its game in discovering what makes a real difference in promoting the quality of people's lives and relationships. Thanks to you all.

My partner David checked references, formatted all the chapters and kept me sane when we had major computer glitches – and was often able to fix them. He is my friend (sometimes critical friend!), husband, supporter, comforter, challenger, technical advisor and the major source of my wellbeing, I could not have done this without him.

Contents

Chapter 1
Introduction to Positive Relationships: Evidence-Based Practice Across the World

Sue Roffey

1.1 A Foundation for Wellbeing

The human race has developed technology almost beyond comprehension. We can perform what a century ago would have been in the realms of magic and fantasy. The Internet, air travel and the genome project are just a few examples of the way knowledge and its application has expanded to change our lives – especially for those in the privileged, 'developed' world.

And yet we have progressed much less in matters of wisdom and living well. Conflicts continue to rage across the globe, family breakdown is rife, parenting skills often lacking, antisocial behaviour, intolerance and addictions are all increasingly a concern. Many individuals and communities are 'languishing' rather than 'flourishing' (Keyes and Haidt 2003).

There is a disconnect between people that is partly framed by economics and the dominance of the individual. The world is increasingly focused on 'the bottom line', which is not about intrinsic value and meaning in our lives but about extrinsic monetary worth. We are living in times when the quality of relationships often matters less than our bank balance, profit margins and having the latest and best of everything.

The media – and often politicians – regularly feed us a diet of how *not* to get on well with people: fostering fear, revenge and contempt rather than understanding and compassion. We are encouraged to laugh at the downfall of others and immediately feel better about ourselves by comparison. Politicians are sometimes congratulated for how 'cleverly' they put others down and do not make the connection between this

S. Roffey (✉)
School of Education, University of Western Sydney, Sydney, Australia

Department of Clinical, Educational and Health Psychology, University College, London, UK
e-mail: sue@sueroffey.com

S. Roffey (ed.), *Positive Relationships: Evidence Based Practice across the World*,
DOI 10.1007/978-94-007-2147-0_1, © Springer Science+Business Media B.V. 2012

behaviour and the level of bullying in our schools. Our competitive world encourages us to believe that being more successful, rich, famous, beautiful or popular than those around us will bring us happiness. Positive psychology research is increasingly providing evidence that authentic and sustainable wellbeing lies elsewhere – confirming what many of us know already.

Human beings are social animals. We need each other. At the deepest level, we want to feel that we belong, that we are connected with others, and most of us seek relationships that nurture our mind, body and spirit. Reis and Gable (2003) consider that relationships may be the most important source of life satisfaction and wellbeing. From the fundamental importance of early attachment in infancy, through learning to make friends as children and belonging to teenage groups, onto romantic, sexual relationships and becoming parents and workers, relationships are threaded through every stage of life and are intrinsic to many things we do. We therefore need to know how to connect well in all the different relationships in our lives, at home, at work, at school and at play.

1.2   The Project

This volume on positive relationships is, to say the least, an ambitious project – some might say a foolhardy one. How can a handful of authors, however knowledgeable, encapsulate one of the most central and dynamic issues of all time – how we relate to each other in the diverse roles of our lives? Surely this has been done to death? Well, yes and no. There are certainly plenty of books – and journals – on parenting, conflict, work relationships, couple relationships and just about every other chapter here, but not, to my knowledge, on relationships as a theme across multiple dimensions and written primarily from a positive perspective: what we know about what is effective, builds the best between people, has a strengths and solution focus and aims not just to explore problems but enhance both individual and community wellbeing.

When I was asked to edit this book, I thought it was a great opportunity to disseminate important knowledge, but underestimated the extent of the endeavour I was taking on. It has been a demanding but also a fascinating and stimulating task. Every chapter has been doubly peer reviewed and re-crafted, often several times, to reflect current knowledge across the world. Undoubtedly significant evidence will have been omitted, and some researchers do not get the credit they deserve. Steve Duck springs to mind. His book *Friends for Life* (1983) inspired me when I first started being interested in these issues and his work since has been prolific. If this volume stimulates you to explore further, perhaps start with the (4th) revised edition of *Human Relationships* (Duck 2007). Further chapters around specific relational themes could have been included here but in the end decisions have to be made on what to include and what to leave out. What I have chosen are relationships and aspects of relationships that most people experience in a personal capacity.

There is a strong focus throughout the book on children and young people; education around relational issues is implicit or explicit in many of the chapters. Perhaps an emphasis on the next generation is more hopeful and optimistic. If we can support a better understanding of positive relationships, and the values and skills to develop these, with those who will become the citizens, workers, parents and leaders of the future, then maybe our world will become a safer and more civilised place to be.

The authors are a mix of practitioners and academics – some both – from Europe, Australasia, North America and Asia. The depth and breadth of knowledge gained by working in the field is often not given sufficient acknowledgement or credence, so we have deliberately encapsulated not only evidence-based practice but also practice-based evidence to explore what is healthy, sustaining and has the best outcomes. This evidence is both quantitative and qualitative – measuring what is effective and understanding the meaning and processes of how things work.

All authors were responsive to numerous editorial demands and dedicated to the task in hand. I am grateful to them for their patience and hard work, especially as many were also occupied with their own projects and on-going work commitments. Without exception, in the yearlong process of putting this volume together, they personified the qualities of positive relationships.

1.3 Positive Psychology

The science of positive psychology has transformed the direction of thinking. Rather than investigate problems in human functioning, researchers have focused on ways to achieve maximum wellbeing and 'authentic happiness'. This has led to some surprising findings, but also confirmed some of the basic wisdoms for living life well, many of which are encapsulated in these chapters.

The three pillars of authentic happiness, first identified by Seligman (2002) and widely extended by others, are:

- The pleasant life – positive feelings and experiences
- The engaged life – being absorbed by something you find deeply interesting
- The meaningful life – what is over and above the self – relationships, service to others and spirituality

Although the first is of great importance, it does not lead to sustainable wellbeing on its own. It is based in what is known as hedonic wellbeing: feelings of pleasure. These are gained in such experiences as a wedding, passing a test, having a new car or enjoying a meal with friends – all wonderful but temporary. Fredrickson (2009) has studied the value and benefit of positive feelings in optimising aspects of wellbeing, such as creativity and problem solving, but acknowledges that we also need to have sad or otherwise negative feelings from time to time to experience life fully. Meaning and engagement are based in 'eudaimonic' wellbeing, which comprises an approach towards life and a way of being that is deeper and more sustainable (Ryan and Deci 2001).

Seligman's most recent model for wellbeing goes by the acronym of PERMA: Positive emotions, Engagement, Relationships, Meaning and Accomplishment/ achievement (Seligman 2011). Relationships may therefore have a higher profile in positive psychology in the future.

Critics of positive psychology sometimes say that it focuses too strongly on subjective wellbeing and risks people being blamed (or blaming themselves) for their situations – the tyranny of the positive (Held 2008). There is a related concern, particularly amongst community psychologists, that the discourse of wellbeing will undermine social efforts to improve the plight of the disadvantaged. As several authors demonstrate, positive psychology is linked more with social justice than might at first be apparent.

There is also at least one alternative theory for this lack of empathy in society: Belief in a Just World (Lerner 1980) is the theory or mindset that says everyone gets what they deserve. For instance, if you work hard at school you will be successful and get a good job – if you are lazy you won't. There is of course a reality to this statement – but it is far from the whole story. It is not surprising that young people get depressed or disengaged when they try their best but don't do as well as expected, or find they can never succeed in comparison to others, or that events outside school curtail their concentration or motivation. It also means that people who have terrible things happen to them – such as being a refugee, homeless or in a tsunami – are not seen as being in the wrong place at the wrong time but somehow responsible for their plight. The Belief in a Just World is the basis of the American dream – that everyone can make it – and faulty because it does not take account of chance events, including where and to whom you were born. Yes, we can do things personally to change our lives for the better, both in actions and attitudes; yes, other people are often involved in our life events for better or worse, but things also happen by accident or as a result of interactive dynamics – there isn't always someone to blame.

Positive psychology helps people understand not only what they can do to make a difference for their individual wellbeing but also that this is also intricately connected to our relationships with others. Taking that on board in various ways not only enhances our own happiness but also the wellbeing of the communities and societies in which we live. One simple example is that science has shown that performing acts of kindness has several outcomes that benefit the giver as well as the recipient (Lyubermirsky 2007). Increasingly researchers are finding that individual authentic wellbeing cannot be separated from what is best for all of us. The Prilleltenskys (2006) have made strong connections between individual, organisational and community wellbeing; Gardner and his colleagues (2001) consider the elements of what can be considered '*Good Work*', maintaining ethical relational values alongside a focus on excellence; Huppert (2005) is concerned with provision for whole populations in respect of positive mental health.

1.4   Politics, Power and Equality

Money does increase our wellbeing, especially if we are short of it, but above a certain (surprisingly) low level, it does not make much sustainable difference. Whilst some people with many material advantages do *not* flourish, others who live in relatively disadvantaged circumstances perceive themselves as having high levels of wellbeing (Huppert and So 2009). Even the boost to happiness that lottery winners experience decreases after a few months to their basic 'set point' for happiness (Brickman et al. 1978). Sonja Lyubirmirsky (2007) refers to this as 'hedonic adaptation', and it occurs in both positive and negative directions. What does matter in regards to money, however, exists in our relationship with others – if someone in a similar situation to us is getting a lot more than we are, we feel the inequality and it is this that affects our wellbeing. There appears to be an acceptance of bonuses for bosses, but when that becomes disproportionate – from several times as much as the average pay in an organisation to hundreds of times more – then anger and resentment surface. Fairness is a fundamental need for a healthy relationship – and a healthy society. Wilkinson and Pickett (2010) summarise research around the world that demonstrates this in many areas, including physical and mental health, criminality, violence and our 'social inheritance' – how we connect with others. The more equal the society, the more able we are to share, support and collaborate.

This book has not gone into depth on issues of power in relationships although this is often addressed by implication. It is apparent throughout that you cannot have a healthy relationship if you are only self-serving. It is imperative to consider the needs and perspectives of others as well as yourself. Where one person, community, company or nation tries to dominate a relationship for their own ends, not only does it impair the wellbeing of the weaker and infringe their basic human rights but it does not bring *authentic* wellbeing to the stronger either.

For me, the personal is political. If you hold the values of fairness, empathy and respect for others and believe that ethical behaviour matters, you will not only attempt to live by these principles in your own life but also aim to create a world in which they are fostered and will seek their representation in all aspects of government. The hard-line economists tell us that this not what really matters – the evidence in this book says otherwise.

1.5   Human (and Animal!) Nature

There are those who say that it is human nature to be acquisitive, aggressive and competitive, and it would be foolish to deny that these are powerful determinants of human behaviour. Our thoughts, attitudes and actions are, however, also socially constructed and even emotions are determined by how issues are discussed and cultural norms developed. We all learn what to do and how to be by listening to these 'dominant discourses', watching and copying others. This is true of the youngster who feels angry that someone has said something negative about his family in school and therefore 'duty bound' to punch the person who said it – to political rallies where people are led to feel that certain races are so unacceptable that their humanity can be dismissed and whole communities brutalised. Indigenous Australians were not fully classified as citizens of their own country and not counted in the census until the 1960s when cultural norms changed sufficiently to give them the vote.

A recent study of baboons also shows that aggressive behaviours in primates are not inevitable (Sapolski and Share 2004). During the mid 1980s, half of all males in a baboon troupe died of TB. The disease was transmitted through raiding human garbage, so it was the aggressive (alpha) males who ate more of the contaminated food and died – leaving a cohort of atypically unaggressive male survivors. A unique and more harmonious culture developed with more social grooming, affiliation with females, a relaxed dominance hierarchy and less stress among low ranking males. Sexual behaviours remained the same. A decade later, these behavioural patterns persisted, with young males joining the troop adopting the less aggressive behaviours.

Healthy relationships, and positive emotions within these, are essential for survival. Although the basic emotions of fear and anger in the face of threat get maximum attention, we also have other basic emotions of affection, interest and empathy that enable us to collaborate and support each other in times of need. Children are born egocentric for their own survival – they need to grow into being cooperative for the survival of the species (Roffey 2006). Crocker and her colleagues (2005) talk about the need to shift the paradigm in inter-group processes from an 'ego-system' motivation concerned with personal rights, self preservation and individual gain to one which explores what is supportive for everyone and is focused on the 'eco-system'. Egocentric emotions dominate our society. Threats are no longer just about physical survival but about preserving a positive sense of self that can be undermined in countless ways. Threats can be real but also conjured up, imagined or exaggerated. They all lead to behaviours that are about getting the better of others in order to protect the self. Eco-centric emotions – those that foster collaboration and understanding – are equally important, and their active development across all levels in society would perhaps be a sign of maturity.

1.6   The Content

1.6.1   Section One: The Power of Positive Relationships and How We Learn These

There are five sections to the book. The first explores two major reasons why positive relationships are so significant for both individual and community wellbeing, and then goes on to detail how relationships are learnt. In Chap. 2, Toni Noble and Helen McGrath summarise the wealth of research that highlights the centrality of healthy connection with others for resilience and dealing with adversity. I know from my own work that vulnerable children, who are dealing with difficult situations and often presenting with challenging behaviour, can have their futures 'rescued' by sensitive and caring teachers who make them feel worthwhile, focus on their strengths and foster a sense of belonging in the classroom.

Violence is endemic in many societies and communities – particularly where inequality thrives. Aggressive and coercive behaviour in interpersonal relationships is not, however, inevitable, despite TV soap dramas that often suggest that it is! It is possible for individuals to modify their responses in situations and become more aware of the benefits of cooperation, negotiation and mutual respect. As Wolfe et al. (1999) found, empowering people to develop healthy relationships provides an alternative to violence. Robyn Hromek and Angela Walsh are practitioners who have been involved in two different aspects of improving relationships to prevent violence. Their case studies in Chap. 3 provide vivid illustrations of what can be achieved. Robyn recounts her experiences in a school where efforts were made to reduce bullying and other aggressive student behaviour by 'planting the peace virus'. Angela writes about the Love Bites project that helps young people think through issues of gender relationships to reduce sexual and family violence.

Chapter 4 in this section details what is required from infancy onwards in learning what is involved in a healthy and sustaining relationship and what helps someone grow to choose pro-social behaviours. Gretchen Brion-Meisels and Stephanie Jones outline the 'stage-salient' tasks required at different ages for children to become confident and empathic in their interactions with others. The authors also summarise innovative programmes in schools in the US and in Colombia that are helping young people to learn and develop positive relationships.

1.6.2   Section Two: Close Relationships

The second section deals with our most intimate relationships. In Chap. 5, Vagdevi Meunier and Wayne Baker refer, amongst others, to John Gottman's seminal work on couple relationships and the factors that contribute to a happy marriage or romantic/sexual partnership. The ways in which individuals deal with differences amongst them appears to be crucial in whether or not relationships flourish.

Kimberley O'Brien, a child and family psychologist, and Jane Mosco, an educational psychologist, work extensively with children, young people, their parents and carers. In their chapter on parent–child relationships, these authors explore different parenting 'styles' and their outcomes for children. Baumrind's authoritative style (1989) (also referred to as facilitative by later commentators) enables children to grow up to be independent, self-controlled, persistent and caring. The authors give examples of how this style might be incorporated into different life stages for these positive outcomes.

Breakdown in family relationships is now sadly commonplace in most of the Western world. Separation and divorce, however, do not stop people being parents. In Chap. 7, Emilia Dowling and Di Elliott, who work in mediation and family therapy, summarise what supports children in these situations of loss and change and what adults need to take into account. The rights of the child are paramount.

Friendship is important to most of us. We often experience positive feelings in interactions with friends that boost our resilience, confidence and a positive sense of self. Our friends may also provide the stable, positive alliance that families do not always manage. Friendship is therefore critical for our psychological health. In Chap. 8, Karen Majors outlines the functions of friendship and the ways in which positive reciprocal relationships with peers enhance wellbeing. She emphasises the importance of children learning the skills that enable them to establish a threshold for friendship.

1.6.3   Section Three: Relationships at School and at Work

The third section moves away from the most intimate but includes important relationships that sustain wellbeing in different areas of life. Relationships in school are having an increasingly high profile, not only for wellbeing but also for an effective learning environment (Hattie 2009). Relationships in one part of the school system impact on others, so schools are either building a healthy environment with high levels of social capital and relational quality or maintaining one that is full of anxiety and of benefit only to those who can be 'successful' in tightly defined ways. I outline the ecology of positive relationships in schools in Chap. 9.

The advent of positive organisational psychology is an exciting development with an increasing evidence base of what makes a difference. Sue Langley works with organisations across the world to bring higher levels of emotional intelligence into the workplace. In Chap. 10, she explores what promotes a cooperative, effective and flourishing working environment. She also identifies the strengths and qualities of relationships that increase motivation, commitment and build social capital in an organisation. This not only enables people to achieve fulfilment in their work but also leads to more creative and effective outputs.

Chapter 11 is also about relationships at work but from a different perspective. Elizabeth Gillies writes about positive professional relationships and what is required in a relationship between client and a provider of services in order to gain the best outcome. This can be for artisans such as builders through to therapeutic services. This chapter explores solution-focused and strengths-based approaches for effective engagement with others along with a consultation model for interaction.

Ann Brewer, in Chap. 12, writes about how a mentoring relationship can nurture potential by contributing to life learning, enhancing perspectives of thinking and values as well as improving outcomes for both individuals and organisations. She explores the bi-directional influence within mentoring relationships and what is needed to ensure they work well. She also identifies different ways of conducting a mentoring relationship.

The final chapter in this section, Chap. 13, addresses leadership and what positive psychology offers for a new paradigm. Hilary Armstrong makes the point that leadership skills often focus on measureable technical knowledge rather than the relationship skills that make the most difference. She refers to a specific study on organisational coaching to illustrate the importance and effectiveness of social intelligence in leadership.

1.6.4   Section Four: Relationships in the Wider World

This section goes beyond the interpersonal to the wider community. I first experienced a small shift in community relationships at a street party in London. The little terraced houses were 100 years old that year, and my neighbours and I thought this was worth a celebration. In the 40 or so houses in the street were representatives from Ireland, Scotland, Poland, Cyprus, the Caribbean, India and England. The 6 months of meetings to discuss and plan what we would do on midsummer's day led to greater connection and understanding between people. Even families who were not much involved in the planning 'came to the party' on the day and joined in with decorating the street, dressing up, cooking and dancing. The street was closed to traffic and everyone brought out tables and chairs onto the pavement and shared food. The sun obligingly shone! From that time onwards we knew who our neighbours were, could greet them with a smile and sometimes stop for a chat on the way to the shops. The more we knew about each other, the less we could prejudge on the basis of stereotypes and assumptions. Barriers came down as we shared a common goal, and the benefits lasted long afterwards.

In Chap. 14, Margaret Vickers and Florence McCarthy have written about the complexities of community relationships in rural Australia. They present a case study that illustrates how positive community relations can be created, overcoming complex real and symbolic boundaries. As in the example above, this also occurred through the development of joint activities bringing disparate groups together. In this case, these included school staff and students, university students, community organisations, a non-government organisation and indigenous elders with the common goal of promoting the teaching and learning of indigenous languages. The authors conclude that community wellbeing can only grow out of reconstructed relationships replacing marginalisation and discrimination with respect and inclusion.

Zalman Kastel is also concerned with promoting positive interactions between people of different cultures, although his focus is specifically the difference in religious beliefs. He initiated the organisation now known as Together for Humanity where adults of different faiths (Jewish, Muslim and Christian) work with young people in schools and communities around Australia to enhance interfaith understanding and tolerance. As Chap. 15 illustrates this is a far from straightforward task, but there is evidence that concerted, sensitive and thoughtful efforts do make a difference to how people perceive each other.

1.6.5   Section Five: Responding Positively to Challenges in Relationships

In my experience, many people are skilled at establishing and maintaining positive relationships but get lost when dealing with direct challenges or situations that create tension. They put their head in the sand and pretend it isn't happening, duck out of confrontation and agree with everything for a quiet life or explode with frustration and anger. This final section is therefore as important as all those that have gone before in exploring how we use a positive approach in potentially negative situations.

Lois Edmund, in Chap. 16, explores how healthy conflict can strengthen a relationship and ways in which to mitigate negative outcomes of conflict. She makes the link between the science of positive psychology and the study of conflict resolution.

Finally, Chap. 17 looks at how relationships might be repaired after they have been damaged. Peta Blood gives an account of the practice and value of restorative approaches to reconnect individuals and communities and importantly to encourage offenders to take authentic responsibility for their behaviour. These approaches are increasingly being seen to have value in various spheres from the justice system to schools. Not only are they more likely to rebuild healthy communities but also reduce the potential for further harm.

1.7   Threads and Connections Between Chapters

One of the challenges of putting together a book on a single theme is to make each chapter discrete and offer some specific and unique insights. The authors have, by and large, achieved this. Inevitably, however, there are commonalities that run through many chapters. This also has benefits in showing how certain principles and ways of thinking are relevant to many different interpersonal situations and circumstances.

As well as positive psychology, several authors refer to other theoretical approaches that they have found useful and congruent. Purists may be dismissive, but many applied psychologists are eclectic in their thinking and employ what they find helpful. The following themes are mentioned throughout the book, although not in every chapter.

1.7.1   Ecological (Systems) Theory

There is rarely linear causation in matters of human behaviour. Outcomes at any one time are the result of bi-directional, circular and accumulative causation. This assertion by Urie Bronfenbrenner (1979) on ecological systems theory is reflected in many chapters. This theory, originally on child development, says that we all live in nested systems, and there is bi-directional influence between them. The most influential is the micro system, comprising the day-to-day experiences with those in our immediate circle. For young children, this is the interaction with their families and carers. What happens here, however, is affected by other systems, from the resources provided by the local neighbourhood to the expectations in workplaces and schools to socio-political dimensions of the whole culture and the dominant values expressed there. Bronfenbrenner later added the chronosystem – an acknowledgement that ecologies do not remain static but change over time.

1.7.2 Social Constructionist Theory

This theory emphasises the importance of meaning and how individuals and groups have different 'realities' based in how people around them – including in the media – talk about things – often referred to as 'dominant discourses'. Several chapters touch on how language matters in the creation of the world we live in, our priorities, perspectives and behaviour. It is useful to reflect on how these discourses come about in society and in whose interest they might be. Sir Ken Robinson (2010) has some interesting things to say about this in relation to education and creativity.

1.7.3 Connection and Resilience

Although Chap. 2 deals with this directly, the importance of feeling you belong somewhere and that at least one significant person believes that you are worthwhile is referred to several times in other chapters. Emily Werner and her colleagues began their longitudinal study in 1955 in Hawaii with babies born in circumstances of multiple disadvantages which put them at risk of negative outcomes. They followed up the life trajectory of nearly 700 children into adolescence and adulthood and found that certain factors made the difference to their ability to overcome adversity. Of these, one of the most powerful is positive connection with others (Werner and Smith 2001). This begins, but doesn't end, with attachment; the early experiences in infancy where parent/carer responsiveness and emotional nurturing have such a powerful impact on how we feel about ourselves and our place in the world and therefore our future relationships (Bowlby 1969). There is also evidence that the quality of attachment affects the development of the brain (Gerhardt 2004).

1.7.4 Emotional and Social Intelligence/Literacy and Learning

Although still open to academic debate, emotional intelligence (intrapersonal knowledge and skills) and social intelligence (interpersonal skills) have become widely recognised as the symbiotic abilities that underpin both positive functioning and healthy social interactions (Ciarrochi and Scott 2006; Schutte et al. 2001; Goleman 2006). First given prominence by Howard Gardner in his early work on multiple intelligences (1983) and later widely publicised by Daniel Goleman (1995, 2006) with extended research by Peter Salovey, John Mayer (1990) and others, emotional and social intelligence has become part of the twenty-first century zeitgeist.

Many authors refer to the need for children to learn to become socially and emotionally literate – to be able to understand and manage their feelings, construct positive interactions with others and cope well with adversity. The work of CASEL (The Collaborative for Academic, Social and Emotional Learning) in the US and Antidote in the UK have resulted in both countries putting SEL high on the educational agenda. Other countries are following this lead. Skills include emotional recognition, regulation and expression, empathy and concern for others, positive communication, responsible decision-making and goal setting. Social skills alone, however, can be self-serving and manipulative. To ensure that relationships develop in healthy and reciprocal ways, they need to be embedded in relational values and be learnt in congruent contexts (Roffey 2010). The relational value mentioned most often here is respect. This is not the respect that comes from deference to authority, but from being willing to listen to someone else even if you don't agree with them (Roffey 2005). It means treating someone as worthy, not putting them down or making them feel inferior. Pro-social behaviour puts this into practice by acts of inclusion, kindness, interest, generosity and acceptance. For all but the most hardened individuals, this meets a basic psychological need for feeling valued and connected.

1.7.5 A Strengths and Solution Focus

Traditional psychology addresses problems and deficits. Positive psychology has moved away from this focus into exploring what is going well and how to get more of it. This includes personal qualities, the strengths of organisations and the positives within any situation.

Positive relationships are more likely if people seek to identify not only their own strengths and use these to reach goals but also do the same with others. Self-concepts and the resulting behaviours are influenced by how significant others describe individuals. A child who is told she is helpful will begin to see herself that way; a young man who is told he is lazy will have nothing to live up to.

Many authors refer to a strengths approach. Although there are many versions of these, the VIA inventory (Values in Action) devised by Chris Peterson and Martin Seligman (2004) identifies 24 specific strengths classified under the six virtues of wisdom, courage, humanity, justice, temperance and transcendence.

Rather than deconstruct a problem into its component parts, asking questions such as 'what went wrong?', a solution focus explores what people want and the extent to which they are already there (Greene and Grant 2006). This is not only optimistic and future-focused but also ensures that energies are utilised in constructive action rather than negative rumination.

There are strengths to celebrate in the field of positive relationships and these are that we look to build on. There are couples in supportive, loving partnerships, and when these work well, they may meet the needs of both parties possibly better than ever before. I look around at some of my friends' long-lasting marriages and see equality, companionship and mutual support. Many families are aware of good parenting practices, and children grow to be strong, independent and caring of others. Although it still exists, racism is less acceptable in society than it once was, and workplaces in the civilised world are no longer workhouses where employees live in fear of the unrestrained power of the bosses. There is much to be learnt from these developments, to hold on to and to evolve.

1.7.6 Social Capital

Physical capital comprises hardware resources such as buildings and equipment and human capital comprises knowledge and skills. Social capital here refers to the quality of relationships within an organisation or community and the social cohesion they promote. Although basically a term originating in sociology, social capital is increasingly recognised by psychologists working in organisational and group settings and can be found here in several chapters. Although there is still debate over the precise definition, the concept continues to gain ground as a useful way of describing and analysing the relational quality of organisations and communities. High levels of social capital are developed by positive everyday interactions between people. These are marked by mutual trust, reciprocity and shared responsibility towards meeting agreed goals that put the common good over self-interest. Toxic environments, marked by cliques, negative communications and interactions, where power is wielded for the benefit of a few, have low social capital. For most people, they are uncomfortable places to work, live or learn. Where there is goodwill towards others in the norm, life becomes not only more pleasant but also more productive. Helliwell and Putnam (2004) have found from large samples of data from several countries that social capital, as measured by the strength of family, neighbourhood, religious and community ties, supports both physical health and subjective wellbeing.

1.8 Summary

This book is not presented as a panacea but as a search for the possible. Positive relationships are what people really do seem to want in their lives – at home, at work and in their communities. Nearly everyone wants to feel valued, connected and supported. A baby learning to smile at only 6 weeks shows just how deeply embedded this need for social connection is in our biology as well as across cultures. Despite the complexities of establishing and maintaining positive relationships, this book demonstrates what might be involved across different contexts in doing just that. Most of this isn't rocket science – at one level we have always known it – now we have the evidence to prove it. Perhaps we need to reflect on whether or not, individually and collectively, we will take note of this evidence and put it into practice – choose what works. Like going on a diet to lose weight, good intentions do not always translate into sustained action. You are more likely to succeed when you take up the challenge with others – the more we talk about it together, the more likely we are to believe that this is achievable and take action to make it happen.

> We are bound together by the common thread of humanity; when this is broken we are all undone.

Perhaps only when we recognise this can we all achieve authentic, sustainable wellbeing.

References

Baumrind, D. (1989). Rearing competent children. In M. Damon (Ed.), *Child development today and tomorrow* (pp. 349–378). San Francisco: Jossey-Bass.

Bowlby, J. (1969). *Attachment: Attachment and loss* (Vol. I). London: Hogarth.

Brickman, P., Coates, D., & Janoff-Bulman, R. (1978). Lottery winners and accident victims: Is happiness relative? *Journal of Personality and Social Psychology, 36*, 917–927.

Bronfenbrenner, U. (1979). *The ecology of human development: Experiments by nature and design.* Cambridge: Harvard University Press.

Ciarrochi, J., & Scott, G. (2006). The link between emotional competence and well-being: A longitudinal study. *British Journal of Guidance and Counselling, 34*, 231–244.

Crocker, J., Garcia, J. A., & Nuer, N. (2005, July). *From egosystem to ecosystem in intergroup interactions: Implications for intergroup reconciliation.* University of Michigan. Paper presented at Self Concept Conference, Ann Arbor, MI.

Duck, S. (1983). *Friends for life: The psychology of close relationships.* Brighton: Harvester Press.

Duck, S. (2007). *Human relationships* (4th ed.). London: Sage Publications.

Fredrickson, B. (2009). *Positivity.* New York: Crown Publishers.

Gardner, H. (1983). *Frames of mind: The theory of multiple intelligences.* London: Fontana.

Gardner, H., Cziksenmihaly, M., & Damon, W. (2001). *Good work: When excellence and ethics meet.* New York: Basic Books.

Gerhardt, S. (2004). *Why love matters: How affection shapes a Baby's brain.* Hove/New York: Brunner Routledge.

Goleman, D. (1995). *Emotional intelligence.* New York: Bantam Books.

Goleman, D. (2006). *Social intelligence: The new science of human relationships.* New York: Bantam Books.

Greene, J., & Grant, A. M. (2006). *Solution focused coaching: Managing people in a complex world.* Harlow: Pearson Education.

Hattie, J. (2009). *Visible learning, a synthesis of over 800 meta-analyses relating to achievement.* London: Routledge.

Held, B. S. (2008). Combating the tyranny of the positive attitude. In J. Allison & D. Gediman (Eds.), *This I believe II: More personal philosophies of remarkable men and women* (pp. 106–108). New York: Henry Holt.

Helliwell, J. F., & Putnam, R. D. (2004). The social context of wellbeing. *Philosophical Transactions of the Royal Society of London Series B, 359*, 1435–1446.

Huppert, F. A. (2005). Positive mental health in individuals and populations. In F. A. Huppert, N. Baylis, & B. Keverne (Eds.), *The science of wellbeing* (pp. 308–340). Oxford: Oxford University Press.

Huppert, F. A., & So, T. (2009, July 23/24). *What percentage of people in Europe are flourishing and what characterises them?* Briefing document for OECD/ISQOLS meeting "Measuring subjective well-being: an opportunity for NSOs?", Florence. http://www.isqols2009.istitutode-glinnocenti.it/Content_en/Huppert.pdf

Keyes, C. L. M., & Haidt, J. (Eds.). (2003). *Flourishing: Positive psychology and the life well lived*. Washington, DC: American Psychological Association.

Lerner, M. (1980). *The belief in a just world*. New York: Plenum Press.

Lyubermirsky, S. (2007). *The how of happiness*. London: Sphere Books.

Peterson, C., & Seligman, M. E. P. (2004). *Character strengths and virtues: A handbook and classification*. New York: Oxford University Press.

Prilleltensky, I., & Prilleltensky, O. (2006). *Promoting well-being: Linking personal, organizational, and community change*. Hoboken: Wiley.

Reis, H. T., & Gable, S. L. (2003). Toward a positive psychology of relationships. In C. L. M. Keyes & J. Haidt (Eds.), *Flourishing: Positive psychology and the life well lived* (pp. 129–159). Washington, DC: American Psychological Association.

Robinson, K. (2010). *Changing paradigms in education*. Accessed January 3, 2011, from RSA Animate. http://www.youtube.com/watch?v=zDZFcDGpL4U

Roffey, S. (2005). *'Respect' in practice – the challenge of emotional literacy in education'*. Australian Association for Research in Education. Available at http://www.aare.edu.au/05pap/rof05356.pdf

Roffey, S. (2006). *Helping with behaviour in the early years: Promoting the positive and dealing with the difficult*. London: Routledge.

Roffey, S. (2010). Content and context for learning relationships: A cohesive framework for individual and whole school development. *Educational and Child Psychology, 27*(1), 156–167.

Ryan, R. M., & Deci, E. L. (2001). On happiness and human potential: A review of research on hedonic and eudaimonic wellbeing. *Annual Review of Psychology, 52*, 141–166.

Salovey, P., & Mayer, J. D. (1990). Emotional intelligence. *Imagination, Cognition and Personality, 9*(3), 185–211.

Sapolski, R. M., & Share, L. J. (2004). A pacific culture among wild baboons: Its emergence and transmission. *Public Library of Science: Biology, 2*(4), e106. doi:10.371/journal.pbio.0020106.

Schutte, N. S., Malouff, J. M., Bobik, C., Coston, T. D., Greeson, C., Jedlicka, C., Rhodes, E., & Wendorf, G. (2001). Emotional intelligence and interpersonal relations. *Journal of Social Psychology, 141*(4), 523–36.

Seligman, M. E. P. (2002). *Authentic happiness: Using the new positive psychology to realize your potential for lasting fulfilment*. New York: Free Press.

Seligman, M. E. P. (2011). *Flourish: A visionary new understanding of happiness and wellbeing*. New York: Free Press.

Werner, E. E., & Smith, R. S. (2001). *Journeys from childhood to midlife: Risk, resilience, and recovery*. Ithaca: Cornell University Press.

Wilkinson, R., & Pickett, K. (2010). *The spirit level: Why equality is better for everyone*. London: Penguin.

Wolfe, D. A., Wekerle, C., & Scott, K. (1999). *Alternatives to violence: Empowering youth to develop healthy relationships*. Thousand Oaks: Sage Publications.

Sue Roffey is an educational psychologist, Adjunct Associate Professor at the School of Education, University of Western Sydney and an Honorary Lecturer at University College, London. She is a prolific author on behavioural and relational issues, works internationally as an educational consultant, and is a founder member of the Wellbeing Australia network. Sue is on the editorial board of *Educational and Child Psychology* and *a Fellow of the Royal Society of Arts*.

Contact: sue@sueroffey.com

Chapter 2
Wellbeing and Resilience in Young People and the Role of Positive Relationships

Toni Noble and Helen McGrath

2.1 Introduction

Over the last 10 years, there has been a gradual shift in both research and community and school practices away from the concept of youth welfare, with its focus on supporting young people in distress, and towards the concept of youth wellbeing and resilience. This trend towards wellbeing and resilience is consistent with a positive psychology approach (Seligman 2011) and more recently the positive psychology/positive education approach (Noble and McGrath 2008). Positive psychology focuses primarily on the empirical study of human wellbeing, strengths and resilience to negative life events and the conditions that allow individuals, groups and organisations to flourish.

2.2 What Is Wellbeing?

Wellbeing is an overarching term that encapsulates an individual's quality of life, happiness, satisfaction with life and experience of good mental and physical health. A comprehensive and systematic review by Noble et al. (2008) of the research literature on 'wellbeing' was undertaken to identify the common features in definitions of wellbeing. The most common components identified included: positive

T. Noble (✉)
School of Educational Leadership, Australian Catholic University, Sydney, Australia
e-mail: toni.noble@acu.edu.au

H. McGrath
Faculty of Education, Deakin University, Melbourne, Australia

RMIT University, Melbourne, Australia
e-mail: helenmc@deakin.edu.au

S. Roffey (ed.), *Positive Relationships: Evidence Based Practice across the World*,
DOI 10.1007/978-94-007-2147-0_2, © Springer Science+Business Media B.V. 2012

affect (an emotional component), resilience (a coping component), perceived satisfaction with relationships and other dimensions of one's life (a cognitive component) and effective functioning and/or the maximising of one's potential (a performance component).

Sustainable psychological wellbeing has been described as the perception that one's life is going well (Huppert and So 2009). These authors equate wellbeing with the concept of 'flourishing', which is a combination of feeling good and functioning effectively. Researchers such as Diener and Seligman (2004) and Layard (2005) have argued that people's subjective perceptions of satisfaction with their lives are a better indicator of wellbeing than the more traditional indicators such as their level of physical health, their wealth, their quality of housing and the level of safety in their community. Stanley (2003) has noted that Australia's economic prosperity and technological progress have not delivered a better life for a significant proportion of its population of children, young people and their families and that this seemingly paradoxical pattern has also been observed in many other similarly developed nations. Huppert and So (2009) point out that some people in very favourable objective circumstances do *not* flourish, whilst others who live in relatively harsh circumstances have high levels of wellbeing.

People who have a high level of psychological wellbeing (i.e. satisfaction with the quality of their life experiences) are likely to learn more effectively and work more productively and have lower levels of absenteeism at school and in the workplace; they also tend to have more satisfying and successful relationships with others, make a greater contribution to their community and have fewer health problems (Diener et al. 2009; Huppert 2009).

Whilst most educators and psychologists support the importance of 'student wellbeing' (i.e. children and young people's wellbeing at school) for their academic achievement and social–emotional adjustment, there is very little consensus on what student wellbeing actually is (Fraillon 2004). Only three definitions were identified in the literature search mentioned above (Noble et al. 2008): Engels et al. (2004) define student wellbeing as a positive emotional state resulting from a harmony between the sum of specific context factors and the personal needs and expectations towards the school; De Fraine et al. (2005:297) more simply define it as the degree to which a student feels good in the school environment; Fraillon (2004:24) defines wellbeing in terms of the degree to which a student is functioning effectively in the school community.

A clearer, more specific and robust definition of student wellbeing could serve to more effectively guide educational policy and school practices to enhance the wellbeing and resilience of young people. In a scoping study by Noble et al. (2008), a modified Delphi methodology was used to seek clarification and agreement on the characteristics of a draft definition of student wellbeing. The draft was developed from a synthesis of the common components of previous definitions of student wellbeing and of general wellbeing applied to a school context. The first stage of the Delphi process involved contacting 30 worldwide experts in the area of general wellbeing and/or student wellbeing – researchers, theorists and/or writers around the world who had made substantial and relatively recent published contributions to the field of 'wellbeing' – and inviting them to participate in the process. Twenty-six of the invited experts participated, representing a range of countries including Australia, Denmark, the UK, Italy, New Zealand, Portugal and the USA.

In stage 1, they were asked to indicate their level of agreement (in an online survey) with the draft definition as well as each component in the definition and to make additional comments and suggestions. The experts' responses were collated, and the key findings were summarised and returned to them in stage 2 for further comments and to seek consensus. There was a very significant (but not total) agreement amongst the experts on each component and on the wording in the final definition, which was:

> Optimal student wellbeing is a sustainable emotional state characterised by (predominantly) positive mood, attitude and relationships at school, resilience, self-optimisation and a high level of satisfaction with learning experiences.

Optimal student wellbeing is the desirable level of wellbeing for all students.

A sustainable state is a relatively consistent mental or emotional condition that is pervasive and maintained over time despite minor variations triggered by life events.

Predominantly positive mood, attitude and relationships at school implies mainly positive feelings and an optimistic approach to school, plus high-quality and prosocial relationships with peers and teachers at school that engender social satisfaction and support.

Self-optimisation is a realistic awareness of (and predominantly positive judgement about) one's own strengths and a willingness to strive to build and use them in meaningful ways.

Satisfaction with learning experiences at school describes a student's satisfaction with the nature, quality and relevance of their learning experiences at school.

The constructs of wellbeing and resilience are closely linked. Most definitions of wellbeing incorporate some reference, either explicit or implied, to the capacity of the individual to be resilient. Developing a capacity for resilience can enhance mental health and wellbeing (Raphael 2000). Both constructs represent a shift in perspective from a deficit model of young people 'at risk' to a model that focuses on the personal strengths and environmental factors that help young people withstand high levels of 'risk' and, in many cases, flourish. Many researchers and advocates (e.g. Battistich 2001; Cefai 2004; Levine 2003; Martin 2002; Stanley 2003) have argued for a stronger emphasis on preventative action, or, as Knight (2007) has described it, the broadening of the construct of resilience, as an effective way of protecting and promoting the wellbeing of all children.

2.3   What Is Resilience?

The construct of resilience emerged from the work of researchers who undertook longitudinal developmental studies of 'at-risk' children. For example, Werner and Smith (1992) followed a cohort of nearly 700 boys and girls from birth until they were 40-year-old adults. These children lived in a community in Kauai (Hawaii) where there were high levels of poverty, unemployment and parents with alcoholism and mental illnesses. Vaillant (2003) followed two very large cohorts of adolescent males for 50 years, including one cohort who had grown up in neighbourhoods that were characterised by crime and poverty. These research studies found that, despite encountering these life stressors as they grew up, a significant number of young people (30–50%) not only survived but even thrived and flourished (Silva and Stanton 1996; Werner and Smith 2001).

Further support for the construct of resilience comes from studies of children and young people who have socially and psychologically recovered from natural disasters such as hurricanes or man-made disasters such as wars. The International Resilience Research Project collected ongoing data on 1,225 children (aged 3–11 years) and their families who had experienced natural or man-made disasters across 27 sites in 22 countries between 1993 and 1997. The results (Grotberg 2001) showed that one-third of the children developed resilience, that socioeconomic status had very little impact on whether or not a child responded resiliently and that girls used more interpersonal skills in dealing with the adversities that affected them whereas boys used more pragmatic problem solving skills. Ratrin Hestyanti (2006) studied fifty young people (aged 11–15 years) who survived the Tsunami in Aceh, Indonesia in 2004. Six of them were identified as resilient. Among the personal skills that these six resilient young people demonstrated were: willingness to talk to other people about their experiences, a sense of humour, strong motivation to recover from the trauma, behaviour that reflected kindness to others and self-efficacy. They also benefited from external factors such as: emotional support from others, opportunities to participate in familiar religious and cultural ceremonies and a chance to play in and enjoy natural recreational resources such as a nearby river.

There are many different definitions of resilience but all refer to the capacity of the individual to demonstrate the personal strengths needed to cope with some kind of challenge, hardship or adversity. Benard (2004) suggests resilience is a set of qualities or protective mechanisms that give rise to successful adaptation despite high risk factors during the course of development. The International Resilience Project provides a broader definition that focuses on the universal capacity that enables a person, group or community to prevent, minimise or overcome the damaging effects of adversity (Grotberg 1997:7). Grotberg (1993) has described a resilient child as one who bounces back, persists and functions effectively under great odds and tends to become a competent adult. McGrath and Noble (2003, 2011) define resilience as the capacity to cope and bounce back after encountering negative events, difficult situations or adversity and to return to almost the same level of emotional wellbeing.

Resilience in young people is also linked to long-term occupational and life success, as well as the prevention of substance abuse, violence and suicide (Fuller 2001). Children and young people can also apply the attitudes and skills of 'bouncing back' to everyday challenges, e.g. not giving up on a difficult task, adapting to a step-family situation, resolving a fallout with a friend, coping with not getting into a team or moving to a new house or school. Being resilient also involves seeking new experiences and opportunities and taking risks. Risk taking is likely to mean some setbacks and rejections, but it also creates more opportunities for successes and greater self-confidence.

Protective factors are those personal and environmental factors that lead to resilience, buffer the negative impact of hardship and trauma and minimise the likelihood of psychological difficulties in the face of adverse risk factors (Werner 1996).

2.4 Protective Personal Factors That Contribute to Resilience and Wellbeing

The following skills, attitudes and behaviours have been identified as contributing to higher levels of coping and resilient behaviour.

Social skills: Social skills that enhance cooperation and underpin positive relationships appear to be especially important for resilience and wellbeing (Bornstein et al. 2003; Cove et al. 2005; National Crime Prevention 1999; Zins et al. 2004).

Behaviour that reflects empathy and prosocial values such as kindness, fairness and altruism: Resilient students and those with optimal levels of wellbeing are more likely to demonstrate prosocial behaviour and empathy for others (Gilman 2001; Vandiver 2001; Werner and Smith 1992).

Emotional regulation: Managing one's emotions requires skills for regulating strong feelings such as anxiety, fear and anger (Masten 2004).

Optimistic thinking: In their review of the construct of optimism, MacLeod and Moore (2000) concluded that an optimistic way of interpreting and adjusting to negative life events is an essential component of coping. Students with high levels of resilience and hence wellbeing are more likely to use more optimistic thinking (Ben-Zur 2003; Seligman et al. 1995). There are four components to optimism:

1. Positivity: finding the positives in negative situations, however small
2. Mastery: feeling some sense of competence and control over one's life
3. Having a disposition or tendency to expect things to work out, to be forward looking and proactive and to have the confidence to persevere when faced with adversity
4. Having an optimistic explanatory style which involves believing that bad situations are temporary, acknowledging that bad situations are usually not all your fault, and believing that bad situations are specific and don't affect everything else or necessarily flow over into all aspects of your life (Gillham and Reivich 2004; Seligman 1992; Seligman et al. 1995)

Optimistic thinking also includes believing that failures and setbacks will happen but that things will get better and you can try again (Benard 1997).

Helpful thinking skills: Helpful thinking is both rational (i.e. reflects how things really are rather than how they should be or how an individual would like them to be) and helps an individual to feel more emotionally in control and more able to solve problems (Werner and Smith 1992; Ellis 1997). It is also based on the assumption that negative emotions, although powerful, can be managed. Helpful and rational thinking derives from the original Cognitive Behaviour Therapy (CBT) model, based on the understanding that how you think affects how you feel, which in turn influences how you behave. In particular, rational thinking is drawn from Rational Emotive Therapy (RET), developed from the original CBT model by Albert Ellis (Ellis 1997; Ellis and Dryden 1987).

Adaptive distancing: This involves a range of behaviours such as: detaching from negative influences; withdrawing from family members who are enmeshed in antisocial or dysfunctional behaviour (Werner and Smith 1992); and emotionally distancing oneself from distressing and unalterable situations rather than immersing oneself in the situation and thinking about the negative situation.

A sense of humour: Individuals are less likely to succumb to feelings of depression and helplessness if they are able to find something funny, even if small, in an adverse situation (Benard 2004). Lefcourt (2001) has argued that humour enables individuals to live in what are often unbearable circumstances. Humour is also a form of optimism that helps to keep things in perspective.

Goal-setting skills: These are underpinned by a drive to change and recover and succeed. They include: willingness to delay short-term gratification in order to achieve longer-term outcomes (Masten and Obradović 2008; Vaillant 2003; Werner and Smith 1992); time management, organisational and planning skills; and preparedness to work hard towards a goal (Werner and Smith 1992). Other behaviours such as showing initiative, problem solving skills and being resourceful are also related to successful goal setting and hence resilience (Werner 1993).

A sense of autonomy, self-efficacy and an awareness of one's strengths: Personal competence is linked to knowing one's strengths and limitations and using this self knowledge to be able to set realistic and meaningful goals. Goals are seen to be more meaningful if a person is using their strengths in the service of others (Masten 2004; Vaillant 2003).

A sense of meaning and purpose: This may be gained through different kinds of endeavour such as working towards academic achievement or participating in community service. Cove et al. (2005) found that resilient children and young people in their study had many positive experiences with activities that involved care and responsibility, such as minding younger siblings, mentoring younger children and camp counselling.

Spiritual connectedness: Religious beliefs and practices may mobilise emotional self-regulation – e.g. through prayer or meditation – or social support – e.g. through rituals, ceremonies and a set of guidelines for living (Haglund et al. 2007; Masten and Obradović 2008).

2.5 Protective External Factors That Contribute to Resilience and Wellbeing

The external factor that appears to make the largest contribution to children and young people's wellbeing and resilience is their experience of positive relationships. In a review of research studies, Luthar (2006) has concluded that resilience for children and young people is fundamentally built on the foundation of relationships.

2.5.1 Parent–Child Relationships

Children and young people who have positive relationships with their parents are more likely to be resilient and have optimal levels of wellbeing than are those without close parental ties. Positive parent–child relationships are characterised by warmth, emotional support and an authoritative parenting style (demanding, warm and encouraging of children's independent striving) as opposed to authoritarian (controlling and detached) or permissive (warm but non-demanding) parenting styles (Baumrind 1989). Two specific dimensions of positive parent–child relationships have been linked to children's academic achievement and competence in the classroom (Grolnick and Ryan 1989): *parental involvement* (a high level of awareness of their child's whereabouts and time spent with and enjoyment of their child) and *autonomy support* (inclusion of the child in family decision making and decisions using reasoning as part of managing their child).

Processes in positive parent–child relationships that contribute to resilience include validation and affirmation, availability, listening and emotional support and support for independent behaviour and self-efficacy. However, many families living with poverty, unemployment, high levels of stress, substance abuse or mental health difficulties can find it difficult to provide a supportive relationship-based environment for their children (Muir et al. 2009).

2.5.2 Relationships with a Caring Adult

Children who have a significant emotional bond with an adult, in addition to or instead of a parent, tend to face their challenges more productively and are more likely to experience success (Garmezy 1992; White-Hood 1993). This caring adult may be a family member (e.g. an older sibling, cousin, a grandparent or aunt) or a teacher or an adult involved in the child's sporting club or recreational club. Werner and Smith (1992) noted that resilient young people were more likely to seek support through a relationship with a non-parental adult. Most often, these relationships were with teachers, ministers of religion or neighbours. Having a positive relationship with an adult mentor at school has also been shown to have a positive impact on school success and resilience (e.g. DuBois et al. 2002; Liang et al. 2002; Vance et al. 1998).

Some of the processes in these relationships that contribute to resilience are validation and affirmation, the provision of emotional, material and educational support and the modelling of different types of problem solving.

2.5.3 Peer Relationships

One of the strongest themes in research (e.g. Zins et al. 2004) is the significant contribution of positive peer relationships to young people's wellbeing and resilience. A student's level of social competence and their friendship networks are also predictive of their academic achievement (Asher and Paquette 2003; Ladd and Troop-Gordon 2003). Having at least one mutual friendship in childhood is related to lower levels of loneliness, anxiety and being bullied (Ladd et al. 1996).

Feeling accepted by peers and having positive peer interactions can enhance the confidence of vulnerable students and make it more likely that they will behave in ways that further encourage positive interactions with others. Criss et al. (2002) have demonstrated that peer acceptance and peer friendships can moderate aggressive and acting-out behaviour in young children with family backgrounds characterised by family adversity. Research suggests that having high-quality friendships, or at least one best friend, can also help prevent children and young people from being bullied (Bollmer et al. 2005; Fox and Boulton 2006).

The number of friendships that a child has is not as important as the quality of those friendships. Werner and Smith (1992) identified that resilient young people, although not necessarily popular, tended to develop a small number of friendships with people who stuck with them, sometimes from primary school to middle age. High-quality friendships are characterised by this kind of loyalty and support as well as a willingness to stand up for their friend (Bollmer et al. 2005). Poor-quality friendships feature negative qualities such as conflict or betrayal and have been linked with emotional difficulties (Greco and Morris 2005). In some cases, bullying can occur within low-quality friendships (Mishima 2003; Mishna et al. 2008). It is helpful to teach children and young people skills for making and keeping friends and also skills for monitoring the quality of one's friendships.

Friendships at school can provide a buffer for students when they are bullied or having difficulties. Adolescent girls in particular are more likely to seek peer support than family support when they are experiencing difficulties (Fischmann and Cotterell 2000). Friendships provide students with intimacy, a sense of belonging, security, validation and affirmation and social and practical support. They also offer opportunities for students to practise and refine their social skills and discuss moral dilemmas. This assists students in the development of empathy and socio-moral reasoning (Schonert-Reichl 1993; Thoma and Ladewig 1993).

2.5.4 Positive Teacher–Student Relationships

Positive teacher–student relationships play an important role in the development of students' resilience and wellbeing (Brazelton and Greenspan 2000; Nadel and Muir 2005; Raskauskas et al. 2010; Weare 2000). Resnick et al. (1997), for example, found that young people who reported having a close and positive relationship with teachers were less likely to use drugs and alcohol, attempt suicide or self-harm, behave in violent ways or engage in sexual behaviour at an early age. Close, warm and affectionate teacher–student relationships are also associated with children's social competence at both preschool level (Howes and Ritchie 1999) and primary school level (Pianta et al. 2008).

The quality of the teacher–student relationship has also been shown to be one of the most significant factors influencing student-learning outcomes (Cornelius-White 2007; Hattie 2009; Rowe 2001). Many studies have found that children with close, positive teacher–student relationships achieve more highly, have more positive attitudes towards school, are more engaged in the learning that occurs in the classroom and are less likely to repeat a grade (Hamre and Pianta 2001).

Many researchers and educators have argued that relationships with students cannot just be left to chance and that it is a teacher's professional responsibility to ensure that they establish a positive relationship with each student (Krause et al. 2006; Marzano et al. 2003). Both teachers and students believe that fostering positive relationships with students is a core aspect of what effective teachers do (Good and Brophy 2000; Larrivee 2005). When evaluating whether or not their teacher is a 'good teacher', students tend to focus most on the interpersonal quality of their relationship with them (Rowe 2004; Slade and Trent 2000; Werner 2002).

Meta-analytical research undertaken by Marzano (2003) strongly suggests that positive teacher–student relationships are also the foundation of effective classroom management. He found that, on average, teachers who had high-quality relationships with their students had 31% fewer discipline and related problems in a given year than did teachers who did not have this type of relationship with their students.

As with peer relationships, the *quality* of a teacher–student relationship is also important. High-quality relationships are characterised by involvement, emotional safety, understanding, warmth, closeness, trust, respect, care and support (Brazelton and Greenspan 2000; Good and Brophy 2000; Krause et al. 2006; Larrivee 2005).

Pianta and Nimetz (1991) note that a high-quality teacher–student relationship in early childhood and lower primary settings is one that is 'secure' rather than 'dependent'. A secure relationship is characterised by trust, a sense of safety and ease in seeking help if needed. A dependent relationship is more likely to be characterised by constant seeking of help or reassurance and difficulties with separation. Secure relationships are more likely to develop when teachers show sensitivity towards and have frequent positive interactions with students (Howes and Hamilton 1992; Kontos et al. 1995).

Teachers who have positive relationships with their students are more likely to behave towards them in the following ways:

- They acknowledge them, greet them by name and with a smile and notice when they are absent (Benard 1997; Stipek 2006).
- They respond to misbehaviour with explanations rather than with punishment or coercion (Bergin and Bergin 2009; Stipek 2006).
- They take a personal interest in them as individuals and get to know them (Marzano et al. 2003; Stipek 2006); they also endeavour to know and understand them as individuals with a life outside school (Slade and Trent 2000).
- They are available and approachable (Pianta 1999; Weissberg et al. 1991).
- They are fair and respectful (Stipek 2006). Keddie and Churchill (2004) found that, when asked what they liked about the good relationships they had with certain teachers, adolescent boys most frequently referred to the fair and respectful way in which their teachers treated them.
- They have fun with their students and let students get to know them through some degree of self-disclosure and being 'real' with them (Davis 2003). In this way, common interests and experiences can be identified.
- They support their students in the development of autonomy, e.g. by offering choice and opportunities for students to be involved in decision making (Gurland and Grolnick 2003).
- They listen to them when they have concerns or worries and offer emotional support (Benard 1997).

High-quality teacher–student relationships lead to feelings of security that empower children to interact confidently with their environment and encourage them to adopt the behaviour and values modelled by the teacher (Bergin and Bergin 2009). Children's behaviour will be influenced by the behaviour of people around them that they trust or who function as a secure base within a relationship (Masten and Obradović 2008). Feelings of security also promote self-reliance and independence (Bretherton and Munholland 1999). Students who believe that their teachers care about them are more motivated to try hard, pay attention in class and do well and are therefore more likely to achieve and stay in school rather than drop out (Benard 2004; Pianta 1999; Sztejnberg et al. 2004). Students who experience good relationships with their teachers are more likely to be open and responsive to their directives and advice (Gregory et al. 2010) and more reluctant to disappoint them by failing to complete assignments, being absent from school or engaging in antisocial behaviour (Stipek 2006).

2.6 Curriculum Programmes for Developing Student Wellbeing and Resilience

If teachers (or other community members) are to assist children and young people to be resilient and have optimal levels of wellbeing, then they need to have the capacity to be resilient and promote their *own* wellbeing too (Ungar 2008). Teaching a curriculum programme designed to foster coping skills and relationship skills and having a positive relationship with each of their students also contribute to teacher wellbeing and job satisfaction (Axford et al. 2010; Goldstein and Lake 2000).

Curriculum programmes that teach social and emotional skills for coping, self-management and establishing and maintaining positive relationships have been described as among the most successful interventions ever offered to school-aged young people (Payton et al. 2008). Many research studies have demonstrated the positive effects of school-based prevention programmes on developing student wellbeing and creating protective factors and resilience (Anderson and Doyle 2005). Several guiding principles about effective curriculum programmes of this type have emerged. These include:

- It is important to start teaching these programmes when children are very young (Greenberg et al. 2003; O'Shaughnessy et al. 2002).
- A whole-school programme works best: i.e. the programme is not just an 'add-on' but is embedded in the curriculum and general life of the classroom and school and involves the whole school, families and community (Scheckner et al. 2002; Wells et al. 2003).
- The programme should be delivered by teachers and integrated with academic learning (Durlak et al. 2011; Weissberg and O'Brien 2004).
- A universal programme, taught to all students and not just those who are identified as 'at risk', is more effective (Greenberg et al. 2003; Durlak et al. 2011).
- Long-term, multilevel and multi-strategic approaches are more likely to produce enduring benefits and are more sustainable especially when taught across year levels (Durlak et al. 2011).
- The programme should include a significant component of skills derived from cognitive behaviour approaches (Andrews et al. 2001, 2002; Scheckner et al. 2002).

2.6.1   Examples of Programmes and Initiatives That Foster Student Wellbeing, Resilience and Positive Relationships

The 'PATHS curriculum' for Years K-5 (Kusché and Greenberg 2004) is a programme from the USA that focuses on developing young people's social and emotional competence in order to build protective factors and decrease the risk of behavioural and social problems. Topics covered include: relationships, emotions, self-management and social problem-solving skills. *PATHS* is a flexible programme that allows the implementation of the 131 lessons over a 5-year period.

The 'Primary SEAL (Social and Emotional Aspects of Learning) programme' is a nationwide social and emotional whole-school programme from the UK for K-6 students taught by classroom teachers. It focuses on social and emotional skills in order to enhance student relationships, attendance, behaviour, learning and emotional wellbeing (Department for Education and Skills 2005). It has been adopted in 80% of British schools (Humphrey et al. 2008). It includes options for early intervention with small group learning for students who are deemed to need extra support, and follow up and individual interventions with those students who do not appear to have benefited from either the whole-class programme or the small group early interventions (DfES 2005).

KidsMatter is an Australian Primary Schools Mental Health Initiative. An evaluation of the effectiveness of the KidsMatter initiative in 100 schools indicated that there were significant and positive changes in the schools, teachers, parents/caregivers and students over the 2-year trial. In particular, there were statistically and practically significant improvements in students' measured mental health in terms of both reduced mental health difficulties and increased mental health strengths. The impact of KidsMatter was especially apparent for students who were rated as having higher levels of mental health difficulties at the start of the trial (Dix et al. 2009).

'Bounce Back! A Classroom Wellbeing and Resilience Program' (McGrath and Noble 2003, 2011) is an Australian preventative whole-school multi-year social and emotional learning curriculum programme (for Years K-8) that is built on the principles of Cognitive Behaviour Therapy and Positive Psychology. It was selected by 64% of the KidsMatter schools that chose to implement a specific programme as their preferred social and emotional learning programme. Topics covered include: core values, skills for 'bouncing back', finding courage, optimistic thinking, managing emotions, relationships skills, using humour, no bullying and successful goal setting. All topics and sub-topics are introduced through a variety of picture books and junior novels. The programme also focuses on strategies for developing learning environments that foster positive peer relationships and teacher–student relationships.

2.7 Conclusion

If we are able to help young people develop a sense of wellbeing and resilience, then we need a clear understanding of what these constructs mean. We also need a strong evidence base for the protective factors that are most likely to facilitate the development of their wellbeing and resilience. Wellbeing is an overarching construct that encapsulates one's quality of life. Teaching the personal skills of wellbeing and resilience and providing environments based on positive relationships offer hope that those responsible for parenting, relating or working with young people can make a significant difference in terms of their health and wellbeing.

References

Anderson, S., & Doyle, M. (2005). Intervention and prevention programs to support student mental health: Literature and examples from the MindMatters plus initiative. *Australian Journal of Guidance and Counselling, 15*(2), 220–227.

Andrews, G., Szabó, M., & Burns, J. (2001). *Avertable risk factors for depression.* Beyondblue, The Australian National Depression Initiative.

Andrews, G., Szabó, M., & Burns, J. (2002). Preventing major depression in young people. *The British Journal of Psychiatry, 2002*(181), 460–462.

Asher, S. R., & Paquette, J. A. (2003). Loneliness and peer relations in childhood. *Current Directions in Psychological Sciences, 12*(3), 75–78.

Axford, S., Blythe, K. & Schepens, R. (2010). *Can we help children learn coping skills for life?* Perth and Kinross Council Publication, Scotland.

Battistich, V. (2001). Effects of elementary school intervention on students' connectedness to school and social adjustment during middle school. In J. Brown (Ed.), *Resilience education: Theoretical, interactive and empirical applications*. Symposium at Annual Meeting of American Educational Research Association, Seattle.

Baumrind, D. (1989). Rearing competent children. In M. Damon (Ed.), *Child development today and tomorrow* (pp. 349–378). San Francisco: Jossey-Bass.

Benard, B. (1997). How to be a turnaround teacher/mentor. *Reaching Today's Youth, 2*(3), 31–35.

Benard, B. (2004). *Resiliency: What we have learned*. San Francisco: WestEd.

Ben-Zur, H. (2003). Happy adolescents: The link between subjective wellbeing, internal resources and parental factors. *Journal of Youth and Adolescence, 32*, 67–79.

Bergin, C., & Bergin, D. (2009). Attachment in the classroom. *Education Psychology Review, 21*(2), 141–170.

Bollmer, J. M., Milich, R., Harris, M. J., & Maras, M. (2005). A friend in need: Friendship quality, internalizing/externalizing behavior, and peer victimization. *Journal of Interpersonal Violence, 20*, 701–712.

Bornstein, M. H., Davidson, L., Keyes, C. L. M., & Moore, K. A. (2003). *Well-being positive development across the life course*. Mahwah: Lawrence Erlbaum.

Brazelton, T., & Greenspan, S. (2000). *The irreducible needs of children: What every child must have to grow, learn, and flourish*. Cambridge: Perseus Publishing.

Bretherton, I., & Munholland, K. (1999). Internal working models in attachment relationships: A construct revisited. In J. Cassidy & P. Shaver (Eds.), *Handbook of attachment: Theory, research, and clinical applications* (pp. 89–111). New York: Guilford.

Cefai, C. (2004). Pupil resilience in the classroom: A teacher's framework. *Emotional and Behavioural Difficulties, 9*(3), 149–170.

Cornelius-White, J. (2007). Learner-centered teacher–student relationships are effective: A meta-analysis. *Review of Educational Research, 77*(1), 113–143.

Cove, E., Eiseman, M., & Popkin, S. J. (2005). *Resilient children: literature review and evidence from the HOPE VI panel study*. Urban Institute. http://www.urban.org/uploadedpdf/411255_resilient_children.pdf. Accessed June, 3, 2010.

Criss, M. M., Pettit, G. S., Bates, J. E., Dodge, K. A., & Lapp, A. L. (2002). Family adversity, positive peer relationships, and children's externalizing behaviour: A longitudinal perspective on risk and resilience. *Child Development, 73*, 1220–1237.

Davis, H. (2003). Conceptualizing the role and influence of student-teacher relationships on children's social and cognitive development. *Educational Psychologist, 38*(4), 207–234.

De Fraine, B., Van Landeghem, G., & Van Damme, J. (2005). An analysis of well-being in secondary school with multilevel growth curve models and multilevel multivariate models. *Quality and Quantity, 39*, 297–316.

Department for Education and Skills. (2005). *Social and emotional aspects of learning (SEAL)*. http://nationalstrategies.standards.dcsf.gov.uk/node/87009. Accessed June, 23, 2010.

Diener, E., & Seligman, M. E. P. (2004). Beyond money: Toward an economy of well-being. *Psychological Science in the Public Interest, 5*(1), 1–31.

Diener, E., Lucas, E. R., Schimmack, U., & Helliwell, J. F. (2009). *Wellbeing for public policy*. Oxford: Oxford University Press.

Dix, K. L., Owens, S., & Spears, B. (2009). *KidsMatter evaluation executive summary*. http://www.kidsmatter.edu.au/wp/wp-content/uploads/2009/10/kidsmatter-executive-summary. Accessed January 7, 2010

DuBois, D. L., Holloway, B. E., Valentine, J. C., & Cooper, H. (2002). Effectiveness of mentoring programs for youth: A meta-analytic review. *American Journal of Community Psychology, 30*, 157–198.

Durlak, J. A., Weissberg, R. P., Dymnicki, A. B., Taylor, R. D., & Schellinger, K. D., (2011). The impact of enhancing students' social and emotional learning: A meta-analysis of school-based universal interventions. *Child Development, 82*(1), 405–432.

Ellis, A. (1997). *Stress counselling: A rational emotive behaviour approach.* London: Cassell.

Ellis, A., & Dryden, W. A. (1987). *The practice of rational emotive therapy.* New York: Springer.

Engels, N., Aelterman, A., Van Petegem, K., & Schepens, A. (2004). Factors which influence the well- being of pupils in Flemish secondary schools. *Educational Studies, 30*(2), 127–143.

Fischmann, S., & Cotterell, J. L. (2000). Coping styles and support sources of at-risk students. *Australian Educational and Developmental Psychologist, 17*(2), 58–69.

Fox, C. L., & Boulton, M. J. (2006). Friendship as a moderator of the relationship between social skills problems and peer victimisation. *Aggressive Behavior, 32*(2), 110–121.

Fraillon, J. (2004). *Measuring student wellbeing in the context of Australian schooling.* http://www.mceetya.edu.au/verve/resources. Accessed February 6, 2010.

Fuller, A. (2001). A blueprint for building social competencies in children and young people and adolescents. *Australian Journal of Middle Schooling 1*(1), 40–48.

Garmezy, N. (1992). Resiliency and vulnerability to adverse developmental outcomes associated with poverty. In T. Thompson & S. C. Hupp (Eds.), *Saving children at-risk: Poverty and disabilities* (pp. 45–60). Newbury Park: Sage.

Gillham, J., & Reivich, K. (2004). Cultivating optimism in childhood and adolescence. *The Annals of the American Academy of Political and Social Science, 591,* 146–163.

Gilman, R. (2001). The relationship between life satisfaction, social interest and frequency of extracurricular activities among adolescent students. *Journal of Youth and Adolescence, 20,* 749–767.

Goldstein, L., & Lake, V. (2000). Love, love, and more love for children: Exploring preservice teachers' understandings of caring. *Teaching and Teacher Education, 16*(8), 861–872.

Good, T., & Brophy, J. (2000). *Looking in classrooms.* New York: Longman.

Greco, L. A., & Morris, T. L. (2005). Factors linking social anxiety to peer acceptance: Contributions of social skills and close friendships. *Behavior Therapy, 36,* 197–205.

Greenberg, M., Weissberg, R., O'Brien, M. U., Zins, J. E., Fredericks, L., Resnik, H., & Elias, M. (2003). Enhancing school-based prevention and youth development through coordinated social, emotional, and academic learning. *American Psychologist, 58,* 466–474.

Gregory, A., Cornell, D., Fan, X., Sheras, P., Shih, T., & Huang, F. (2010). Authoritative school discipline: High school practices associated with lower student bullying and victimization. *Journal of Educational Psychology, 102*(2), 483–496.

Grolnick, W. S., & Ryan, R. M. (1989). Parent styles associated with children's self-regulation and competence in school. *Journal of Educational Psychology, 81,* 143–154.

Grotberg, E. (1993). *Promoting resilience in children: A new approach.* Birmingham: University of Alabama at Birmingham, Civitan International Research Center.

Grotberg, E. (1997). *A guide to promoting resilience in children: Strengthening the human spirit.* Hague: Bernard van Leer Foundation.

Grotberg, E. (2001). Resilience programs for children in disaster. *Ambulatory Child Health, 7,* 75–83.

Gurland, S., & Grolnick, W. (2003). Children's expectancies and perceptions of adults: Effects on rapport. *Child Development, 74*(4), 1212–1224.

Haglund, M. E. M., Nestadt, P. S., Cooper, N. S., Southwick, S. M., & Charney, D. S. (2007). Psychobiological mechanisms of resilience: Relevance to prevention and treatment of stress-related psychopathy. *Development and Psychopathology, 19*(3), 889–920.

Hamre, B. K., & Pianta, R. C. (2001). Early teacher-child relationships and the trajectory of children's school outcomes through eighth grade. *Child Development, 72*(2), 625–638.

Hattie, J. (2009). *Visible learning: A synthesis of over 800 meta-analyses relating to achievement.* London: Routledge.

Howes, C., & Hamilton, C. E. (1992). Children's relationships with caregivers: Mothers and child care teachers. *Child Development, 63,* 859–866.

Howes, C., & Ritchie, S. (1999). Attachment organizations in children with difficult life circumstances. *Development and Psychopathology, 11,* 251–268.

Humphrey, A., Kalambouka, A., Bolton, J., Lendrum, A., Wigelsworth, M., Lennie, C., & Farrell, P. (2008). *Primary Social and Emotional Aspects of Learning (SEAL) – Evaluation of small group work.* http://www.dcsf.gov.uk/research/data/uploadfiles/DCSF-RB064.pdf. Accessed February 19, 2010

Huppert, F. A. (2009). Psychological well-being: Evidence regarding its causes and consequences. *Applied Psychology: Health and Well-being, 1*(2), 137–164.

Huppert, F. A., & So, T. (2009, July 23/24). *What percentage of people in Europe are flourishing and what characterises them?* Briefing document for OECD/ISQOLS meeting "Measuring subjective well-being: an opportunity for NSOs?" Florence. http://www.isqols2009.istitutode-glinnocenti.it/Content_en/Huppert.pdf

Keddie, A., & Churchill, R. (2004). Power, control and authority: Issues at the centre of boys' relationships with their teachers. *Queensland Journal of Teacher Education, 19*(1), 13–27.

Knight, C. (2007). A resilience framework for educators. *Health Education, 107*(6), 543–555.

Kontos, S., Howes, C., Shinn, B., & Galinsky, E. (1995). *Quality in family childcare and relative care.* New York: Teachers College Press.

Krause, K., Bochner, S., & Duchesne, S. (2006). *Educational psychology for learning and teaching.* Southbank: Nelson Australia.

Kusché, C., & Greenberg, M. (2004). *The PATHS curriculum.* http://www.prevention.psu.edu/projects/PATHS.htm

Ladd, G. W., & Troop-Gordon, W. (2003). The role of chronic peer difficulties in the development of children's psychological adjustment problems. *Child Development, 74*(5), 1344–1367.

Ladd, G. W., Kochenderfer, B. J., & Coleman, C. C. (1996). Friendship quality as a predictor of young children's early school adjustment. *Child Development, 67*(3), 1103–1118.

Larrivee, B. (2005). *Authentic classroom management: Creating a learning community and building reflective practice.* Boston: Pearson Education.

Layard, R. (2005). *Happiness: Lessons from a new science.* London: Allen Lane.

Lefcourt, H. M. (2001). *Humor: The psychology of living buoyantly.* New York: Plenum.

Levine, D. (2003). *Building classroom communities.* Bloomington: National Educational Service.

Liang, B., Tracy, A. J., Taylor, C. A., & Williams, L. M. (2002). Mentoring college-age women: A relational approach. *American Journal of Community Psychology, 30*, 271–288.

Luthar, S. S. (2006). Resilience in development: A synthesis of research across five decades. In D. Cicchetti & D. J. Cohen (Eds.), *Developmental psychopathology* (Risk, disorder, and adaptation, Vol. 3, pp. 739–795). Hoboken: Wiley.

MacLeod, A. K., & Moore, R. (2000). Positive thinking revisited: Positive cognitions, well-being and mental health. *Clinical Psychology & Psychotherapy, 7*, 1–10.

Martin, A. (2002). Motivation and academic resilience: Developing a model for student enhancement. *Australian Journal of Education, 46*(1), 34–49.

Marzano, R., Marzano, J., & Pickering, D. (2003). *Classroom management that works: Research-based strategies for every teacher.* Alexandria: Association for Supervision and Curriculum Development.

Masten, A. S. (2004). Regulatory processes, risk and resilience in adolescent development. *Annals of the New York Academy of Sciences, 1021*, 310–319.

Masten, A. S., & Obradović, J. (2008). Disaster preparation and recovery: Lessons from research on resilience in human development. *Ecology and Society, 13*(1), 9.

McGrath, H., & Noble, T. (2003, 2011). *Bounceback! A wellbeing and resiliency program.* Melbourne: Pearson Education.

Mishima, K. (2003). Bullying amongst close friends in elementary school. *Japanese Journal of Social Psychology, 19*, 41–50.

Mishna, F., Weiner, J., & Pepler, D. (2008). Some of my best friends: Experiences of bullying within friendships. *School Psychology International, 29*, 549–573.

Muir, K., Mullan, K., Powell, A., Flaxman, S., Thompson, D., & Griffiths, M. (2009). *State of Australia's Young People: A report on the social, economic, health and family lives of young people.* Canberra: Department of Education, Employment and Workplace Relations.

Nadel, J., & Muir, D. (2005). *Emotional development: Recent research advances.* Oxford: Oxford University Press.

National Crime Prevention. (1999). *Pathways to prevention: Developmental and early intervention approaches to crime in Australia.* Canberra: Attorney-General's Department.

Noble, T., & McGrath, H. (2008). The positive educational practices framework: A tool for facilitating the work of educational psychologists in promoting pupil wellbeing. *Educational and Child Psychology, 25*(2), 119–134.

Noble, T., McGrath, H., Roffey, S., & Rowling, L. (2008). *A scoping study on student wellbeing.* Canberra: Department of Education, Employment and Workplace Relations.

O'Shaughnessy, T. E., Lane, K. L., & Gresham, F. M. (2002). Students with or at risk for learning and emotional-behavioral difficulties: An integrated system of prevention and intervention. In K. L. Lane, F. M. Gresham, & T. E. O'Shaughnessy (Eds.), *Interventions for students with or at-risk for emotional and behavioral disorders.* Boston: Allyn and Bacon.

Payton, J., Weissberg, R. P., Durlak, J. A., Dymnicki, A. B., Taylor, R. D., Schellinger, K. B., & Pachan, M. (2008). *The positive impact of social and emotional learning for kindergarten to eighth-grade students: Findings from three scientific reviews.* Chicago: Collaborative for Academic, Social, and Emotional Learning. http://www.casel.org/downloads/PackardTR.pdf. Accessed June 11, 2010

Pianta, R. (1999). *Enhancing relationships between children and teachers.* Washington, DC: American Psychological Association.

Pianta, R. C., & Nimetz, S. (1991). Relationship between children and teachers: Associations with classroom and home behavior. *Journal of Applied Developmental Psychology, 12*, 379–393.

Pianta, R. C., Belsky, J., Vandergrift, N., Houts, R. M., & Morrison, F. J. (2008). Classroom effects on children's achievement trajectories in elementary school. *American Educational Research Journal, 45*(2), 365–397.

Raphael, B. (2000). *Promoting the mental health and wellbeing of children and young people, discussion paper: Key principles and directions.* Canberra: Department of Health and Aged Care. http://www.health.gov.au/internet/main/publishing.nsf/Content/48F5C63B02F2CE07C A2572450013F488/$File/promdisc.pdf. Accessed May 3, 2010.

Raskauskas, J. L., Gregory, J., Harvey, S. T., Rifshana, F., & Evans, I. M. (2010). Bullying among primary school children in New Zealand: Relationships with prosocial behaviour and classroom climate. *Educational Research, 52*(1), 1–13.

Ratrin Hestyanti, Y. (2006). Children survivors of the 2004 tsunami in Aceh, Indonesia: A study of resiliency. *Annals of the New York Academy of Sciences, 1094*, 303–307.

Resnick, M. D., Bearman, P. S., Blum, R. W., Bauman, K. E., Harris, K. M., Jones, J., Tabor, J., Beuhring, T., Sieving, R. E., Shew, M., Ireland, M., Bearinger, L. H., & Udry, J. R. (1997). Protecting adolescents from harm: Findings from the national longitudinal study on adolescent health. *Journal of the American Medical Association, 278*, 823–832.

Rowe, K. (2001). *Keynote address.* In Symposium titled Educating Boys in the Middle Years of Schooling. Sydney: St Ignatius School, Riverview.

Rowe, K. (2004). In good hands? The importance of teacher quality. *Educare, 149*, 4–14.

Scheckner, S., Rollin, S. A., Kaiser-Ulrey, C., & Wagner, R. (2002). School violence in children and adolescents: A meta-analysis of the effectiveness of current interventions. *Journal of School Violence, 1*(2), 5–32.

Schonert-Reichl, K. A. (1993). Empathy and social relationships in adolescents with behavioral disorders. *Behavioral Disorders, 18*, 189–204.

Seligman, M. E. P. (1992). *Learned optimism.* New York: Random House.

Seligman, M. E. P. (2011). *Flourish.* Simon & Schuster. *Using the new positive psychology to realize your potential for lasting fulfillment.* New York: Free Press.

Seligman, M. E. P., Reivich, K., Jaycox, L., & Gillham, J. (1995). *The optimistic child.* New York: Houghton Mifflin.

Silva, P., & Stanton, W. (Eds.). (1996). *From child to adult: The Dunedin multidisciplinary health and development study.* Auckland: Oxford University Press.

Slade, M., & Trent, F. (2000). What the boys are saying: An examination of the views of boys about declining rates of achievement and retention. *International Journal of Education, 1*(3), 201–229.

Stanley, F. (2003). The real brain drain: Why putting children first is so important for Australia. *Newsletter of the Australian Cerebral Palsy Association, 8*(2).

Stipek, D. (2006). Relationships matter. *Educational Leadership, 64*(1), 46–49.

Sztejnberg, A., den Brok, P., & Hurek, J. (2004). Preferred teacher-student interpersonal behaviour: Differences between polish primary and higher education students' perceptions. *Journal of Classroom Interaction, 39*(2), 32–40.

Thoma, S. J., & Ladewig, B. H. (1993). *Moral judgment development and adjustment in late adolescence*. Paper for American Educational Research Association, Atlanta.

Ungar, M. (2008). Resilience across cultures. *British Journal of Social Work, 38*(2), 218–223.

Vaillant, G. (2003). *Aging well: Surprising guideposts to a happier life from the landmark harvard study of adult development*. New York: Little Brown.

Vance, J. E., Fernandez, G., & Biber, M. (1998). Educational progress in a population of youth with aggression and emotional disturbance: The role of risk and protective factors. *Journal of Emotional and Behavioral Disorders, 6*, 214–221.

Vandiver, T. (2001). Children's social competence, academic competence, and aggressiveness as related to ability to make judgments of fairness. *Psychological Reports, 89*(1), 111–121.

Weare, K. (2000). *Promoting mental, emotional and social health: A whole school approach*. New York: Routledge.

Weissberg, R. P., & O'Brien, M. U. (2004). What works in school-based social and emotional learning programs for positive youth development. *The Annals of the American Academy of Political and Social Science, 591*, 86–97.

Weissberg, R., Caplan, M., & Harwood, R. (1991). Promoting competent young people in competence-enhancing environments: A systems-based perspective on primary prevention. *Journal of Consulting and Clinical Psychology, 59*(6), 830–841.

Wells, J., Barlow, J., & Stewart-Brown, S. (2003). A systematic review of universal approaches to mental health promotion in schools. *Health Education, 103*(4), 197–220.

Werner, E. E. (1993). Risk, resilience and recovery: Perspectives from the Kauai longitudinal study. *Development and Psychopathology, 5*, 503–515.

Werner, E. E. (1996). Risk and resilience in individuals with learning disabilities: Lessons learned from the Kauai longitudinal study. In S. Green (Project Director), *Timely issues in print series: The resilience factor* (pp. 86–92). Greenville: East Carolina University Press.

Werner, E. E. (2002). Looking for trouble in paradise: Some lessons learned from the Kauai Longitudinal Study. In E. Phelps, F. F. Furstenberg, & A. Colby (Eds.), *Looking at lives: American longitudinal studies of the 20th century* (pp. 297–314). New York: Russell Sage.

Werner, E. E., & Smith, R. S. (1992). *Overcoming the odds: High risk children from birth to adulthood*. New York: Adams, Bannister and Cox.

Werner, E. E., & Smith, R. S. (2001). *Journeys from childhood to midlife: Risk, resilience, and recovery*. Ithaca: Cornell University Press.

White-Hood, M. (1993). Taking up the mentoring challenge. *Educational Leadership, 51*(3), 76–78.

Zins, J. E., Bloodworth, M. R., Weissberg, R. P., & Walberg, H. J. (2004). The scientific base linking social and emotional learning to school success. In J. E. Zins, R. P. Weissberg, M. C. Wang, & H. J. Walberg (Eds.), *Building academic success on social and emotional learning: What does the research say?* (pp. 2–22). New York: Teacher College Press.

Toni Noble is an Adjunct Professor in the School of Educational Leadership at ACU National (Australian Catholic University) and is based in Sydney. She is on the advisory board of the Wellbeing Australia network.
Contact: toni.noble@acu.edu.au.

Helen McGrath is a Senior Lecturer in the Faculty of Education at Deakin University and an Adjunct Professor at RMIT University Melbourne, Australia.
Contact: helenmc@deakin.edu.au.

Chapter 3
Peaceful and Compassionate Futures: Positive Relationships as an Antidote to Violence

Robyn Hromek and Angela Walsh

3.1 Introduction

This chapter focuses on two case studies described separately by the two authors to illustrate how building relational values, knowledge and skills in young people might address violence and construct more peaceful communities of the future.

The word 'violence' is open to many definitions and interpretations, including vehemence or intensity of expression. The authors here focus on deliberate acts of physical or psychological aggression with the primary intention to hurt, intimidate or otherwise abuse power.

Western societies expend considerable resources in both trying to control violence and dealing with the aftermath, including retribution for offenders. Although the expression of violence is most commonly seen within the context of relationships (Wolfe et al. 1999), the behaviour of individuals does not stand alone but is embedded in social mores. Interpersonal violence is often linked to who has most power within a culture. Women and children, along with minority groups, are therefore often the recipients of violent acts (WHO 2002).

Reducing violence therefore needs to be addressed at several levels, including organisational and societal. Peaceful and compassionate societies are built on a history of social evolution where liberties have been won and securities assured; where education and employment are sought for all and disadvantage is recompensed. Trust and goodwill can only flourish where fair structures are in place to protect rights and foster responsibilities. There is now extensive evidence that more equal

R. Hromek (✉)
The University of Sydney, Sydney, NSW, Australia
e-mail: Robyn.Hromek@det.nsw.edu.au

A. Walsh
National Association for Prevention of Child Abuse and Neglect, Sydney, NSW, Australia

Women's Health (North Coast Area Health Service), Sydney, NSW, Australia
e-mail: angelalovebites@gmail.com

S. Roffey (ed.), *Positive Relationships: Evidence Based Practice across the World*,
DOI 10.1007/978-94-007-2147-0_3, © Springer Science+Business Media B.V. 2012

societies are better for everyone (Wilkinson and Pickett 2010), including the reduction of violent crime (Dorling 2005).

This utopian vision of social progress and happiness is underpinned by the positive, respectful relationships that grow within a community. At the basis of this is the ability to understand and value both oneself and others. Children and young people learn these skills in their homes, schools and communities. It is within a social milieu that they gain an understanding of who they are and how to manage emotional states. If others model respect and hold positive relational values, then they connect more successfully to others and contribute to social harmony. As societies grow in moral and ethical understanding, the physical, mental, social and spiritual development of individuals is enhanced and the 'brotherhood of man' is more likely to be realised (Gardner et al. 2001).

3.2 Relationships and Resilience Are Learnt in the Complexity of Social Settings

Homes and schools play major roles in creating the sense of belonging that nurtures young people. A social network of respectful, caring relationships can reduce the severity and duration of problems like substance abuse, bullying, violence and mental health problems (Benard 2004; Blum 2000). Resilience is a comprehensive process, not a single programme. Cultures that promote resilience provide opportunities for young people to become competent emotionally, socially and academically (Farmer et al. 2007). They provide opportunities to contribute through leadership roles and humanitarian programmes and to participate in adventure and fun-based programmes which give young people a sense of purpose and enjoyment. These positive interconnections support and build flourishing communities. The seeds of a peaceful and compassionate future are planted in this soil, growing through the generosity of individuals to share knowledge, humour, compassion, creativity, courage, forgiveness, communication, celebration, respect and loyalty (Post and Neimark 2007).

3.3 Case Study One: Planting the Peace Virus in a School Community

3.3.1 Background Information

'Planting the peace virus' (Hromek 2004) is a metaphor for the evolution of a systematic, whole-school approach to conflict that significantly reduced violence and harassment in a large elementary school in New South Wales. There were 600 students aged 5–12 years old in the school in a busy seaside tourist town. Tensions existed between the children of long-standing conservative families and the children of newcomers who brought alternative, colourful ways of living. The project began by establishing a committee of teachers interested in the wellbeing of children. Over several years the school engaged in 'action research' to address student behaviour. They met weekly to discuss issues of violence and harassment and examined ideas for changing the culture in their school. Their first task was to gather data from the playground and classrooms to determine the extent of the problem and to create a baseline on which to evaluate change. An initial survey of the playground found that up to 30 students every lunchtime were sent to the detention room on account of aggressive behaviour. Data collected revealed several incidents of physical violence each day. Teasing and bullying was widespread with one young girl found to have up to 50 harassers calling her names on a regular basis. The school's negative responses to these situations were not changing this behaviour, just managing it. It was clear that something else had to be done.

3.3.2   Taking Action

Ongoing dialogue in staff meetings, classrooms, parent forums and related child services laid the foundation for shared understandings about what was meant by violence, harassment, teasing, conflict and rough play. The values of respect, dignity and fairness emerged, and strategies were found to address conflict and aggression in peaceful ways and to include parents and related child support services as necessary. New ideas began to shape responses by establishing structures to promote clear, positive communications, monitor wellbeing and follow up every incident consistently. Protocols and letters home were developed, with quick-tick checklists to make implementing and monitoring of the programme easy and efficient for teachers. Playtime behaviour was discussed in class and at assemblies and incentives introduced.

An action cycle of adjustment and improvement led to an intervention plan that was tailor-made to the community, with strategies implemented at three levels across the school:

- Universal strategies were broadcast across classrooms and playgrounds to support positive, respectful interactions and to place social and emotional learning in the curriculum.
- A secondary level of targeted interventions was activated when violence or harassment occurred. A hierarchy of staff responses was developed to intervene consistently, with executive staff available immediately when there was physical violence or sustained harassment. Mediation and games-based learning activities were used in small groups to teach social skills with a skilled facilitator.
- Tertiary interventions were initiated if problems persisted. Intense support was sought from specialist teachers and counsellors. Parents and child services were involved.

According to the students, the most effective parts of the programme were the leadership opportunities and the positive, interactive, fun-based elements that made it easy for young people to have a voice and engage.

By the third year, data indicated that conflict levels had dramatically reduced, with physical violence occurring once or twice per week. The strategies and structures that had been put in place became self-sustaining amongst the students as they developed courteous and friendly relationships where conflicts were dealt with in restorative ways. Gradually a cohort of children progressed through the school that taught each other and initiated newcomers into the way things were done at 'our school'. As conflict reduced, much less attention was required from the teachers and the school was able to focus on other priorities. Sustained commitment and effort had paid valuable dividends.

3.3.3   The Research and Ideas that Guided the School on Its Journey

3.3.3.1   New Paradigms

Until the late 1960s, pedagogy relied on competitive systems where experts transferred information to learners using textbooks and lectures. Success was measured by written examination with individual effort paramount. When students did not conform to expectations, there was an over-reliance on punishment and exclusion. This created adversarial environments with negative cycles of resentment and revenge (Donnellan et al. 1988; Mayer and Sulzer-Azaroff 1990).

Evidence suggests that this 'old' paradigm still exists in some school settings and therefore upholds a system that does nothing to reduce violence and may in fact be perpetrating conflict (Skiba et al. 2006). School structures and parenting practices that use intimidation, arbitration and punishment must be challenged in order to engage young people in meaningful dialogue about their lives and what matters to them.

Pedagogy has moved on to broader understandings about the collaborative nature of learning and the pivotal role of social and emotional development. New instructional technologies recognise the value of experience-based learning that is interactive and relational. Simulations, games, role plays, case studies, scenarios, cooperative research and problem-solving and multimedia presentations are effective ways to engage young learners (Hromek and Roffey 2009; Ruben 1999). Research increasingly demonstrates the potential to impact on social and emotional learning to enhance positive relationships through programmes like peer mediation, peer support, restorative practice, circle time and therapeutic games.

3.3.3.2   Adult Leadership

School leaders represent the values of their community and play an important role as agents of educational change (Fullan 2003; Goleman 2000). They work with school staff and families in a respectful and dignified way to identify priorities and develop projects in an ongoing cycle of improvement. A professional educational community is supported in schools by leaders who provide opportunities for:

- Ongoing improvement cycles of assessment, response planning, implementation, evaluation and refocus
- Professional development, reflection and planning, space, release from other duties, teamwork (Maeroff 1993)
- Communication systems, regular meetings, information boards, electronic mail, newsletters, suggestion boxes, questionnaires, monitoring systems
- Curriculum materials, departmental personnel and resources, liaison with other schools, current research, other agencies
- Flexible responses to ongoing feedback
- An opportunity for the voices of all stakeholders to be heard, especially students

3.3.3.3 Modelling Language and Conflict Resolution

Each interaction models a 'response style' to children, whether diplomatic and respectful or authoritarian and aggressive. Young people's interactions are more likely to be positive when the wider social environment models respect, dignity and generosity of spirit. These skills are transmitted as much as taught and are demonstrated in every interaction. Strategies like modelling, coaching, behavioural rehearsal and social reinforcement will enhance positive relationships (Jennings and Greenberg 2009; Hromek 2007; Bandura 1986). Words and language patterns are fundamental to understanding and can scaffold learning, including social and emotional development (Vygotsky 1986). With guidance, children can learn 'scripts' of language that reflect calmness, confidence and control and help develop cooperative, respectful mindsets when resolving conflict.

3.3.3.4 Early Intervention

Early intervention is fundamental to positive life outcomes for young people and is economically efficient when redressing disadvantage in the community (Surgeon General 2001; Karoly et al. 1998; Perry 1996). Children who are 'at risk' often arrive at school having learnt violent responses to issues without any intervention to address these difficulties or support more positive relationships. Schools are well placed to intervene early into the social and emotional wellbeing of students by providing structured learning opportunities in the classroom and playground. Walker and colleagues (1996) re-conceptualise the role of schools in preventing antisocial behaviour through:

- Coordination of schools, families, social service agencies and medical clinics
- Fair policies and practices that are communicated clearly and monitored closely
- Universal approaches that reduce risk factors and enhance protective factors
- Meeting the needs of 'at-risk' children early with remedial programmes rather than exclusion

3.3.3.5 Home, School and Community Collaboration

As the importance of early intervention is recognised, structures are developed to bring together education, social services, health and housing agencies to support young children. Dialogues that encourage perspective-taking and mutual respect increase the potential for repair and growth when difficulties arise. Shared responsibility is encouraged when information is presented in different formats and forums with a range of flexible procedures in place. Problems and deficits become challenges and opportunities as stakeholders collaborate to create solution-focused and strengths-based approaches (Leadbeater et al. 2004; Roffey 2002). Families possess a wide range of characteristics that determine the vulnerability or resilience of young people. Respectful support of families helps develop positive relationships, ultimately producing better outcomes for children (Ungar 2008). Resilience building characteristics within families include:

- Communication – talking, listening
- Togetherness – a sense of belonging
- Shared activity – family rituals, outings, fun, celebrations
- Support – physical and emotional assistance
- Affection – eye contact, touching, hugging
- Acceptance – acknowledging and accepting each other's strengths and weaknesses
- Commitment – being there for each other in all circumstances

3.3.3.6 Universal, Targeted and Tertiary Programmes

Universal approaches to student wellbeing reduce risk factors and enhance protective factors that young people might bring to schools (Noble et al. 2008). Most young people will respond to this level of intervention. Targeted programmes support individual student needs and provide a humane alternative to exclusionary practices. Having a skilled facilitator ensures that social and emotional skills are honed in a systematic and fun-based manner. A small number of children need this intense level of intervention. Tertiary programmes acknowledge that for some children there are significant problems impacting negatively on their development. Children who require this level of support usually have difficulties arising from medical conditions, developmental disorders or child-rearing issues in the family (Walker et al. 1996). Tertiary programmes are the most costly and should be delivered early in a child's life to be effective.

3.3.3.7 Student Leadership Programmes

Young people with well-developed social skills usually enjoy contributing to the school and wider community. Young people have a way of relating to each other that eludes most adults. Students who take on leadership roles gain life-long skills in public speaking, acting confidently, being organised, working in teams, making decisions and taking responsibility (Grose 2004). Leadership roles like peer mediation, peer refereeing, peer mentoring, student councils and fund raising for charities model positive relationships and help the work of teachers. With a little thought, creativity and dedication, this student-based resource can be tapped for the benefit of the school community.

3.3.3.8   Social and Emotional Literacy in the Classroom

Social and emotional literacy not only increases student wellbeing; it also increases the learning capacity of students across the curriculum (Frey et al. 2000; Zins et al. 2004). Social literacy refers to the ability to read other people in social situations and to engage and interact with them to reach common goals (Goldstein et al. 1998). Emotional literacy refers to the ability to read emotions in the self and others and to manage these emotions so that cordial relationships develop. It includes motivation, zeal and persistence (Goleman 1996). Goleman asserts that the emotional habits of children may be shaped if we intervene early. Philosophical discussion in the classroom helps children learn critical thinking skills and how to apply them to social situations where they need to be able to cooperate or stand up for what is right (Cam 2006). Examples of curriculum-based programmes include:

- Circle time – a framework for group interaction based on the principles of democracy, inclusion, respect and safety (Roffey 2006)
- Restorative practice – supports open, transparent, honest and fair ways of relating and resolving conflict (McCold 2002; O'Connell and McCold 2004)
- Skill-streaming social development (Goldstein et al. 1998)
- Bounce Back! (McGrath and Noble 2003)
- Philosophy in the classroom (Cam 2006)

3.3.3.9   Positive Playground Programmes

For many children the playground is the best part of school. This is where they plot, plan, organise and negotiate games, and children need a free environment in which to practise their social skills, relax and 'do their own thing'. Play is the learning vehicle that children naturally adopt, and for the most part they do this well. For some children, however, it is a complete mystery, full of worries or aggression, and these individuals need assistance. Positive playground programmes ensure there is enough fun, freedom, resources and incentives to support children's play and encourage pro-social behaviour with as little interference from adults as possible (Hromek 2004; Blatchford 1998). Following are some ways to provide this:

- Direct teaching of friendly playtime behaviour in the classroom and at assemblies
- Incentive programmes to reinforce positive behaviour – raffles, awards, celebrations

- Student consultation about playground issues – physical layout, play equipment, rosters
- Adequate resources – play equipment, tables, stools, bins, playground markings, passive games
- Events – sports, drama, dance, chess competitions
- A 'playground box' for seeking help and giving suggestions in a formal, confidential way

3.3.3.10 Monitoring and Evaluation

Systematic monitoring and evaluation of programmes helps focus effort and provides the basis of feedback to the wider community. Monitoring also acts as a deterrent. Children who know they are being monitored and are called to account for their behaviour are more motivated to adjust and self-monitor. It ensures that extra attention is paid to those young people who need it and that parents are kept informed of their progress. Simple practical systems for data collection and analysis make it easier for staff to carry out this vital step. The 'playground bag' (Hromek 2004) is a simple tool that provides playground monitors easy access to:

- Data collection sheets
- A behaviour-response hierarchy
- Red emergency disc to summon immediate assistance
- Profiles of special-needs children (medical, emotional, behavioural) – useful for big schools and casual teachers
- Student self-referral sheets
- Peer mediation rosters
- Raffle tickets for the playground incentive programme
- Simple first aid kit – tissues, band-aids, rubber gloves, antiseptic cream
- Pencil, sharpener, pens

3.3.3.11 The Attention Room

The concept of an attention or 'chill out' room is a positive slant on the more traditional detention room. Attention rooms are open at playtimes and function as the main venue for dealing with playground difficulties. This is where teachers are rostered on duty to organise mediation sessions, friendship circles and therapeutic games. Life space interviews assist students in taking responsibility for their actions in a fair and respectful manner and working towards a solution (Wood and Long 1991). Emotional coaching (Hromek 2007) provides ongoing support for the development of self-regulation by working regularly with children to set goals and map progress. When young people are flooding with emotions like anger and sadness, 'emotional first aid' provides time and space to allow them to regain their self-control. Emotional first aid refers to having a drink of water, sitting away from others, saying self-soothing things, taking deep breaths, walking away from situations.

3.3.3.12   Therapeutic Games

Therapeutic games (Hromek 2005) are psycho-educational tools that teach a range of social and emotional skills including friendship skills, handling harassment, self-regulation, managing anxiety, authentic happiness and success at school. Games are highly motivating, making them a great vehicle for targeted programmes and ideal to include in lunchtime programmes.

3.3.4   For the Future

3.3.4.1   Some Words of Caution

Having begun the task of changing a culture of violence and harassment in a school, it is essential to continue, especially if children have been encouraged to confront violence through help-seeking or assertiveness training. Children who ask for help from a teacher must be assisted until the problem is resolved, otherwise violence may go 'underground' where aggressors may make threats to 'get them' after school or 'bash them' if they tell. Physical violence may be extinguished from a child's behavioural repertoire only to be replaced by verbal or emotional abuse.

3.3.4.2   Some Words of Encouragement

The first few months and possibly years of creating peaceful and compassionate school environments can be intense depending on pre-existing levels of student conflict. It helps to see this phase as transitory as it will be followed by a more settled era. When progress seems slow, teachers need to remind themselves that every step taken works towards reducing violence and harassment, especially in the first few years of a child's schooling.

There are many ways to reach the goal of a peaceful and compassionate school environment. School communities first need to believe that violence is neither inevitable nor acceptable and, through appropriate culture development and clear positive relationship education, can be substantially eliminated. Adopting some of the ideas presented here and maintaining other proven, successful programmes will equip the school to meet the specific needs of the community.

3.4   Case Study Two: Preventing Violence Against Women and Children

The prevention of violence against women is not an aspirational goal but, rather, is well within our reach. We now know that practice in prevention of violence against women has an evidence base, sound rationale for action and support for development by government, non-government, philanthropic and corporate sectors (VicHealth 2008: 5).

This part of the chapter talks more specifically about the important role that schools can play in preventing gendered violence and the elimination of violence against women and children through the effective delivery of respectful relationship education. Governments, experts in family violence and academics around the world concur with this. Flood, Fergus and Heenan's report *Respectful Relationships Education – Violence prevention and respectful relationships education in Victorian Schools* (2009), for the Victorian Department of Education and Early Childhood Development, presents a strong rationale for delivering effective primary prevention respectful relationships education programmes in schools. Flood and his colleagues state that '*starting young ... can have a lasting effect on children's and young people's later relationships*' (p. 8) specifically as children and young people are already developing beliefs and attitudes towards violence and many may have already experienced violence in their homes and in their own relationships. They state that schools are important as the main place where children and young people '*learn, negotiate and potentially contest the norms and attitudes that encourage and maintain interpersonal violence*'. Peers in schools heavily influence other children and young people positively, as supports and ethical bystanders, or negatively through involvement in violent behaviours. Flood et al. consider that the school environment can be positive and respectful, one in which children and young people can safely learn about respectful relationship through partnerships with community service providers (Police, Sexual Assault services, Domestic Violence Services, Aboriginal Service), parents and teachers.

3.4.1   The Extent of the Problem

Western societies have been grappling with how to eliminate violence against women and children since feminists placed the issue on the political stage in the 1970s. Although much violence against women and children happens behind closed doors, it is no longer a hidden social phenomenon but recognised as a major issue that demands attention from governments around the world. Violence against women is defined as 'physical and sexual violence, threats, verbal abuse, harassment and stalking, intimidation, emotional, psychological and social abuse, spiritual and cultural abuse and economic deprivation' (Partnerships Against Domestic Violence 2000). Despite the ongoing efforts of many, it remains firmly entrenched in and perpetuated by global societal structures and the gender inequality in societies that promote male power

(Flood 2007). The International Violence Against Women Survey Project commissioned by the United Nations found that violence against women and children is a 'universal phenomenon and occurs in every age and economic group' and 'continues to be frighteningly common and considered as "normal" within too many societies' around the world (WHO 2005). This gender inequality denies women, men, young people and children their right to physical, mental and social wellbeing.

The first comparative research report of the International Violence Against Women Survey data in 11 countries was published jointly by Springer and the European Institute for Crime Prevention and Control affiliated with the United Nations in early 2008. The survey found that between 35% and 60% of women in all the surveyed countries had experienced violence by a man during their lifetime (Johnson et al. 2008). In Australia alone 1.2 million Australian women aged 18 and over have experienced sexual violence or its threat since they were 15 years old (ABS 2006), and around one in three young people have experienced some form of violence in their own relationships (Flood and Fergus 2008). The economic cost of violence against women and their children to the Australian Economy in 2007/2008 was estimated be $13.6 billion, which is higher than the total cost of the Australian Government's stimulus package ($10.4 billion) rolled out to address the Global Financial Crisis in 2009 (Australian Government 2009a).

The World Health Organization (2005) states: 'Violence against women has a far deeper impact of the immediate harm caused. It has devastating consequences for the women who experience it, and a traumatic effect on those who "are exposed" to it, particularly children'. Violence against women also has a devastating effect and high emotional cost for boys and young men who are exposed to and are also victims of gender-based violence, and as possible future perpetrators of violence (Katz 2006). Young men and women need to be given the opportunity to develop healthy and respectful relationships in their lives free from violence and abuse.

3.4.2   An Investment for Change

Motivating communities to eliminate violence against women and children requires an emotional, practical and financial investment and a comprehensive commitment to challenging and changing attitudes and behaviours, not just for children and young people, but on all levels, including individual, interpersonal, community and societal. The World Health Organization (2002) identifies an ecological approach to prevention as there is no single factor that explains why some individuals or communities experience higher rates of violence than others. This ecological model is supported by The Victorian Health Promotion Foundation (VicHealth 2008) in their paper *Preventing Violence Before It Occurs: A Framework and Background Paper to Guide the Primary Prevention of Violence Against Women in Victoria*. This says 'that factors influencing violent behaviours or vulnerability to violence lie at multiple and interacting levels of influence – individual/relationship, community and organisational and societal' (VicHealth 2008: 12).

International organisations and governments are embracing the ecological approach in developing national and international strategies to address family violence. At the time of writing, Scotland, Australia, Brazil, Canada, Ecuador, Germany, Indonesia, New Zealand, Norway, Spain and Switzerland have all developed national plans of action to eliminate violence against women and children (Amnesty International 2008). These plans have common themes including long-term strategies which address the underlying causes of such violence (Australian Government 2009b; Scottish Executive 2003; Amnesty International 2008). These include:

- Promoting gender equality and human rights
- Public awareness raising through multimedia awareness raising campaigns
- Primary prevention respectful relationship education for children
- Individual responsibility for preventing violence against women and children
- Long-term commitment and sustained investment in preventing violence against women
- Promoting multileveled responses from the community, government, services and the NGO sector and society
- Delivering comprehensive services for women and children affected by violence
- Delivering comprehensive services for perpetrators of violence to raise personal responsibility and promote behavioural change
- Legislative reform on violence against women

Respectful relationship education for children and young people is an integral part of this approach. Evaluations of school-based interventions in the United States and Canada demonstrate promising outcomes in relation to changing attitudes and reducing some levels of abuse (Hassall and Hanna 2007; Flood et al. 2009). The Safe Dates Program in North America is showing positive outcomes up to 6 years after the programme (Foshee et al. 2004). Recommendations from these and other evaluations suggest that programmes are more effective if delivered in multiple sessions over time connected to the wider community (specifically students' families) and are backed by institutional and national leadership and a national strategy (WHO 2009a).

These recommendations have been substantiated by recent research in violence prevention (Carmody et al. 2009; Flood et al. 2009). These studies have delivered key criteria and standards for quality violence prevention programmes as follows:

- A clear programme logic and framework that articulates why violence against women and children occurs and effective programming that supports this
- That programmes are based on attitudinal change, behaviour change and skills building
- A whole of school/service approach encompassing high-level support for programming, comprehensive violence prevention school/service policies and procedures, the development of a school/service culture that promotes violence prevention
- Partnerships with community services to assist with delivering programmes and staff training on violence prevention

- Effective curriculum/programme delivery focusing on appropriate programme content and structure
- Relevant, inclusive and culturally sensitive practice
- Impact evaluation framework
- Communities supported with thorough training and professional development of educators

3.4.3   LOVE BiTES – A Programme to Reduce Violence Towards Women and Children

The Love Bites programme was originally developed on the mid north coast of New South Wales, Australia, and was based on the best practice standards recommended by Mulroney in the Australian Domestic and Family Violence Clearing House paper *Australian Prevention Programmes for Young People* (Mulroney 2003). Love Bites is a respectful relationship programme for young people aged 14–16 years that includes a number of 1-day workshops delivered by community service providers, follow-up sessions delivered by teachers and the development of a violence prevention community campaign by the students for their local community. This takes place in partnership with local service providers to connect young people with their community. The Love Bites programme explores the issues of sexual assault and relationship violence including definition, myth deconstruction, consent, ethical bystander strategies, skills-building activities, and promotion of respectful behaviours. It also works alongside young people to develop their own community education campaign that is connected to national education campaigns including White Ribbon. The programme is primarily delivered in schools as evidence suggests that school-based strategies can lessen relationship violence (Flood et al. 2009). Schools are viewed as a positive site from which to run prevention education as the material can be reinforced by integration within aspects of the curriculum and the systems of the school. School welfare departments can also provide holistic support to young people where needed (WHO 2009b).

Over the past 3 years under the auspices of the National Association for the Prevention of Child Abuse and Neglect (NAPCAN), and with the assistance of International and State government funding, the Love Bites programme has grown comprehensively. It has been implemented in over 80 communities across Australia and has been delivered to over 70,000 young people by trained and supported facilitators.

The training package includes sessions on gender, sexual harassment, ethical bystander behaviour, consenting sexual relationships and what young people want in their emerging relationships. This programme aims to:

- Increase student learning in identifying safe and unsafe feelings
- Encourage the belief that every child has the right to feel safe

- Identify the difference between safe and abusive behaviours in relationships and the features of both
- Talk with a safe and trusted person if they feel unsafe or have experienced abusive behaviours
- Develop skills in managing feelings in safe and respectful ways
- Develop conflict resolution and problem solving skills
- Talk about gender roles and how gender influences relationships
- Develop an ethical framework for their developing relationships

The Love Bites training model provides professional development workshops in local communities for community service providers who work in the area of relationship violence and to school teaching staff. The partnership between service providers and teaching staff implement and deliver the Love Bites sessions in schools. This model has proven to be particularly relevant for rural and remote communities that have high staff turnover in that it ensures a level of sustainability. This model also strives to train male and female facilitators to ensure that male and female role models lead discussions around preventing violence against women with young people (Flood 2008). Online and phone support is available to teachers, community service providers and communities before and after training to provide guidance on troubleshooting if issues arise and also assist with the development of activities for specific issues that communities may be experiencing. NAPCAN works alongside communities so that programming and practices are relevant and culturally inclusive. Reflective practice is also encouraged to ensure high-quality programme facilitation and programme improvement.

Love Bites facilitator-training workshops also include ways to relate to student groups. The NSW Commission for Children and Young People (2003) identified facilitator skills such as active listening, problem solving and good communication. Personal qualities include a sense of humour, energy, enthusiasm and an understanding of the needs of young people. Facilitators are required to:

- Model respectful relationships – speaking to young people as we would like them to speak to each other; having an awareness of the messages communicated by words, tone, body language and attitude
- Be open, calm, receptive and enthusiastic
- Use respectful conflict resolution processes
- Promote open discussion stimulated by actively listening to young people and genuinely respecting their opinions
- Maintain curiosity and wonder about young people's comments allowing critical discussions to flow, not being defensive
- Make young men participating in the sessions feel comfortable and not blamed: giving young men the space to deconstruct societal norms and attitudes empowers them to challenge violence against women, and develop respectful relationships of their own

A strength of Love Bites is child and youth inclusive practice. Programmes are targeted at appropriate developmental stages, and all classroom activities and resources aim to encourage the active participation and voice of each young person. In the creative sessions participants can write, perform and record a hip-hop song, radio advertisement or drama piece, as well as develop art works for posters. These creative works are then used to develop local campaigns, led and delivered by young people, to challenge relationship violence in their communities. Young people contribute to the further development of Love Bites activities and resources through focus groups, ensuring that materials remain relevant and engaging.

As it evolves, Love Bites is moving towards a whole of school and community approach to respectful relationship education. This process includes auditing school readiness for such programmes, participation of all teaching staff in professional development, a comprehensive framework on relationships education, the development of complimentary teaching resources to enhance the existing curriculum and the establishment of support systems for young people who may disclose through the educative process. There is also a connection to parents through school newsletters and events at school assemblies and connection with the local community through respectful relationships community campaigns, led by the young people themselves (White Ribbon Canada 2004). An example of this is in the Northern Territory where the NT Government is funding a Territory-wide youth-led Love Bites poster and radio advertisement campaign.

The Love Bites programme was evaluated independently in 2007. A cross section of students was surveyed across years 10 and 11: a total of 72 responses were recorded. Interviews 6 months after attending the Love Bites programme yielded the following data:

- 93% responded that the programme had improved their knowledge of sexual assault and domestic violence.
- 88.5% indicated that Love Bites had a positive impact on young people's behaviour.
- 76% indicated that since attending the programme, they had seen a positive change in the attitudes and behaviour amongst young people.
- 50% indicated that their friends are more supportive of their relationships.
- 43% indicated that Love Bites had given them more confidence in setting boundaries in their relationships.
- 75% indicated that they would speak up if a friend was in an unhealthy relationship.
- 32% indicated that there was a positive change in relationships since attending the programme.
- 83% indicated they knew of services they could contact and how to contact these services.
- 52.5% had heard of these services from Love Bites.
- 70% indicated that Love Bites is a good way to get the message about healthy relationships across to young people (Spannari-Oxley 2007).

NAPCAN is now developing a more comprehensive behaviour change evaluation framework that will provide data on programme effectiveness and the extent to which attitudes and behaviours in relation to violence against women are changing. This information will further develop programmes and practice.

3.4.4 For the Future

We are experiencing an exciting time in the field of violence prevention/respectful relationships education. Young people, teaching staff and community services are driving change in their communities. The levels of motivation and enthusiasm for change are high, and the belief that we can eliminate violence against women and children is real and growing. With continued leadership from governments and international agencies and sustained financial investment in prevention and evaluation of strategies, there is hope for an end to intergenerational violence against women and children.

3.5 Conclusion

There are those who throw up their hands in horror at the extent of violence in our society and others who say 'what can you do, this is only human behaviour'. This chapter demonstrates that human change is possible given the right conditions and the will to take preventative measures seriously. It is more difficult to measure prevention – to see that when you do something, something else does *not* happen. It may take years to see outcomes in communities whereas grant bodies and politicians often want to see quick results. Despite media coverage that gives the impression that there is more violence in our society than ever before, the opposite is probably true. There is more awareness and more concern about this, especially when it is rife within communities. We now have a better understanding of the factors that promote harmonious and respectful interactions between people. Rather than deal with the aftermath, it is more efficacious to build the knowledge, skills and motivations to establish and maintain positive relationships. In doing this, we must understand the need to promote equality. Healthy relationships need to be embedded in a social milieu where value is accorded to all citizens, not just those with the most power to wield.

References

Amnesty International Australia. (2008). *Setting the standard: International good practice to inform and Australian National Plan to Eliminate Violence Against Women and Children.* Brisbane: QUT.

Australian Bureau of Statistics. (2006). *Personal safety survey.* Canberra: ABS.

Australian Government's National Council to Reduce Violence against Women and Children. (2009a). *The cost of violence against women and their children.* Canberra: Commonwealth of Australia.

Australian Government's National Council to Reduce Violence against Women and Children. (2009b). *Time for action: The National Council's Plan for Australia to reduce violence against women and their children, 2009–2021.* Canberra: Commonwealth of Australia.

Bandura, A. (1986). *Social foundations of thought and action: A social cognitive theory.* Englewood Cliffs: Prentice-Hall.

Benard, B. (2004). *Resiliency: What have we learned?* San Franscisco: WestED.

Blatchford, P. (1998). *Social life in school: Pupils experience of life in school.* London: The Falmer Press.

Blum, R. (2000). *Healthy youth development: Resiliency paradigm for adolescent health development.* Paper presented at the 3rd Pacific Rim Conference of the International Association for Adolescent Health, Lincoln University, Christchurch.

Cam, P. (2006). *Twenty thinking tools.* Melbourne: Australian Council for Educational Research.

Carmody, M., Evans, S., Krogh, C., Flood, M., Hennan, M., & Ovenden, G. (2009). *Framing best practice: The national standards for the primary prevention of sexual assault though education.* Sydney: National Sexual Assault Prevention Education Project for NASASV, University of Western Sydney.

Donnellan, A. M., LaVigna, G. W., Negri-Shoultz, N., & Fassbender, L. L. (1988). *Progress without punishment: Effective approaches for learners with behaviour problems.* New York: Teachers College Press.

Dorling, D. (2005). Prime suspect: Murder in Britain. In P. Hillyard, C. Pantazis, S. Tombs, D. Gordon, & D. Dorling (Eds.), *Criminal obsessions: Why harm matters more than crime.* London: Crime and Society Foundation.

Farmer, T. W., Farmer, E. M., Estell, D. B., & Hutchins, B. C. (2007). The developmental dynamics of aggression and the prevention of school violence. *Journal of Emotional and Behavioral Disorders, 15*(4), 197–208.

Flood, M. (2007, August 13–19). Why violence against women and girls happens, and how to prevent it: A Framework and some key strategies. *Redress.*

Flood, M. (2008, September 10–12). *Involving men in efforts to end violence against women.* Presentation at from Margins to Mainstream: 5th World Conference on the Promotion of Mental Health and the Prevention of Mental and Behaviours Disorders, Melbourne.

Flood, M., & Fergus, L. (2008). *An assault on our future: The impact of violence on young people and their relationships. A White Ribbon Foundation Report.* Sydney: White Ribbon Foundation.

Flood, M., Fergus, L., & Heenan, M. (2009). *Respectful relationships education – Violence prevention and respectful relationships education in Victorian schools.* Melbourne: Victorian Department of Education and Early Childhood Development.

Foshee, V.A., Bauman, K.E., Ennett, S.T., Linder G.F., Benefield, T., & Suchindran, C. (2004). Assessing the long-term effects of the Safe Dates Program and a booster in preventing and reducing adolescent dating violence. *American Journal of Public Health, 94*(4), 619–924.

Frey, K. S., Hirschstein, M. K., & Guzzo, B. A. (2000). Second step: Preventing aggression by promoting social competence. *Journal of Emotional and Behavioral Disorders, 8*(2), 102–112.

Fullan, M. (2003). *The moral imperative of school leaders.* Thousand Oaks: Corwin Press.

Gardner, H., Csikszentmihalyi, M., & Damon, W. (2001). *Good work: When excellence and ethos meet.* New York: Basic Books.

Goldstein, A. P., Glick, B., & Gibbs, J. C. (1998). *Aggression replacement training: A comprehensive intervention for aggressive youth* (Revised ed.). Champaign: Research Press.

Goleman, D. (1996). *Emotional intelligence: Why it can matter more than IQ.* London: Bloomsbury Publishing.

Goleman, D. (2000). Leadership that gets results. *Harvard Business Review, 3*, 78–90.

Grose, M. (2004). *Young leaders program: A leadership programmes for students from Year 5 to Year 8.* Accessed August, 10, 2010 from http://www.parentingideas.com.au/Teachers/Student-Leadership

Hassall, I., & Hanna, K. (2007). *School based prevention programmes: A literature review.* Wellington: Accident Compensation Corporation.

Hromek, R. P. (2004). *Planting the peace virus: Early intervention to prevent violence in schools.* Bristol: Lucky Duck.

Hromek, R. P. (2005). *Game time: Games to promote social and emotional resilience for children age 4–14.* London: Paul Chapman.

Hromek, R. P. (2007). *Emotional coaching: A practical program to support young people.* London: Paul Chapman.

Hromek, R. P., & Roffey, S. (2009). Promoting social and emotional learning with games: "It's fun and we learn things". *Simulation and Gaming, 40*(1), 626–644.

Jennings, P. A., & Greenberg, M. T. (2009). The prosocial classroom: Teacher social and emotional competence in relation to student and classroom outcomes. *Review of Educational Research, 79*(1), 491–525.

Johnson, H., Ollus, N., & Nevala, S. (2008). *Violence against women. An international perspective. HEUNI.* New York: Springer.

Karoly, L. A., Greenwood, P. W., Everingham, S. S., Hoube, J., Kilburn, M. R., Rydell, C. P., & Chiesa, J. (1998). *Investing in our children: What we know and don't know about the costs and benefits of early childhood interventions.* Santa Monica: RAND.

Katz, J. (2006). *The Macho Paradox, why some men hurt women and how all men can help.* Naperville: Sourcebooks Inc.

Leadbeater, B. J., Schellenbach, C. J., Maton, K. I., & Dodgen, D. W. (2004). Research and policy for building strengths: Processes and contexts of individual, family, and community development. In K. I. Maton, C. J. Schellenbach, B. J. Leadbeater, & A. L. Solarz (Eds.), *Investing in children, youth, families, and communities: Strengths-based research and policy* (pp. 13–30). Washington, DC: American Psychological Association.

Maeroff, G. I. (1993). *Team building for school change: Equipping teachers for new roles.* New York: Teachers College Press.

Mayer, G. R., & Sulzer-Azaroff, B. (1990). Interventions for vandalism. In G. Stoner, M. R. Shinn, & H. M. Walker (Eds.), *Interventions for achievement and behaviour problems, monograph* (pp. 559–580). Washington, DC: National Association of School Psychologists.

McCold, P. (2002). *Evaluation of a restorative milieu: CSF Buxmont School/Day Treatment programs 1999–2001 evaluation outcome technical report.* Paper presented at the American Society of Criminology Annual Meeting, Chicago. Accessed February 14, 2006, from http://www.realjustice.org/library/erm.html

McGrath, H., & Noble, T. (2003). *Bounce back! A classroom resiliency program.* Melbourne: Pearson Education Australia.

Mulroney, J. (2003). *Australian prevention programmes for young people.* Sydney: Australian Domestic and Family Violence Clearing House, UNSW.

Noble, T., McGrath, H., Roffey, S., & Rowling, L. (2008). *A scoping study on student wellbeing.* Canberra: Department of Education, Employment and Workplace Relations (DEEWR).

NSW Commission for children and young people. (2003). *Participation: Sharing the stage a practical guide to helping children and young people take part in decision making.* Sydney: NSW Government.

O'Connell, T., & McCold, P. (2004, December 2–5). *Beyond the journey, not much else matters: Avoiding the expert model with explicit restorative practice.* Paper presented at New Frontiers in Restorative Justice: Advancing Theory and Practice, Centre for Justice and Peace Development, Massey University at Albany.

Partnerships against Domestic Violence. (2000). *Strategies and resources for working with young people.* Canberra: Commonwealth of Australia, Strategic Partners Pty, Pirie Printers.

Perry, B. (1996). *The mismatch between opportunity and investment.* Chicago: CIVATAS Initiative.

Post, S., & Neimark, J. (2007). *Why good things happen to good people: How to live a longer healthier happier life by the simple act of giving.* New York: Broadway Books.

Roffey, S. (2002). *School behaviour and families: Frameworks for working together.* London: David Fulton.

Roffey, S. (2006). *Circle time for emotional literacy.* London: Sage.

Ruben, B. D. (1999). Simulation, games, and experience-based learning: The quest for a new paradigm for teaching and learning. *Simulation and Gaming, 30*(4), 498–505.

Scottish Executive. (2003). *Preventing domestic abuse: A national strategy.* Edinburgh: Astron.

Skiba, R., Reynolds, C.R., Graham, S., Sheras. P., Close Conely, J., & Garcia-Vasquez, E. (2006). *Are zero tolerance policies effective in the schools? An evidentiary review and recommendations.* Zero Tolerance Task Force Report for the American Psychological Association.

Spannari-Oxley, M. (2007). *LOVE BiTES evaluation*. Port Macquarie: TAFE.
Surgeon General. (2001). *Youth violence: A report of the Surgeon General, Chapter 5 Prevention and intervention*. US Department of Human Services. Accessed July 20, 2010. http://www.ncbi.nim.nih.gov/bookshelf/br.fegi?book=youth
Ungar, M. (2008). Resilience across cultures. *British Journal of Social Work, 38*, 218–235.
Victorian Health Promotion Foundation (VicHealth). (2008). *Preventing violence before it occurs: A framework and background paper to guide the primary prevention of violence against women in Victoria*. http://www.vichealth.vic.gov.au
Vygotsky, L. S. (1986). *Thought and language*. Cambridge: MIT Press (Original work published 1934).
Walker, H. M., Horner, R. H., Sugai, G., Bullis, M., Sprague, J. R., Bricker, D., & Kaufman, M. J. (1996). Integrated approaches to preventing antisocial behaviour patterns among school aged children. *Journal of Emotional and Behaviour Disorders, 4*(4), 194–211.
White Ribbon Canada. (2004). *White ribbon campaign in a box: Promoting healthy equal relationships*. Ontario: Government of Ontario.
Wilkinson, R., & Pickett, K. (2010). *The spirit level: Why equality is better for everyone*. London: Penguin.
Wolfe, D. A., Wekerle, C., & Scott, K. (1999). *Alternatives to violence: Empowering youth to develop healthy relationships*. Thousand Oaks: Sage Publications.
Wood, M., & Long, N. (1991). *Life space intervention*. Austin: PEO-ED.
World Health Organisation. (2002). *World report on violence and health*. Geneva: WHO.
World Health Organisation. (2005). *Multi countries study on women's health and domestic violence against women: Summary report of initial results on prevalence, health outcomes and women's response*. Geneva: WHO.
World Health Organisation. (2009a). *Violence prevention: The evidence: Promoting gender equality to prevent violence against women*. Geneva: WHO.
World Health Organisation. (2009b). *What is a health promoting school?*. http://www.who.int/school_youth_health/gshi/hps/en/index.html
Zins, J. E., Weissberg, R. P., Wang, M. C., & Walberg, H. J. (2004). *Building academic success on social and emotional learning: What does the research say?* New York: Teachers College Press.

Robyn Hromek is an Honorary Associate of the University of Sydney and an educational psychologist working in Sydney schools. She is also an author, game designer and on the advisory board of the Wellbeing Australia network.
Contact: Robyn.Hromek@det.nsw.edu.au

Angela Walsh has been developing and delivering training in sexual assault and family violence prevention programmes across Australia for 10 years for the National Association for Prevention of Child Abuse and Neglect, and Women's Health (North Coast Area Health Service), NSW. She has also worked as a child protection counsellor and support worker for women escaping family violence.
Contact: angelalovebites@gmail.com

Chapter 4
Learning About Relationships

Gretchen Brion-Meisels and Stephanie M. Jones

4.1 Introduction

In her synthesis of five decades of research on resilience in development, Suniya Luthar (2006) concluded, 'Resilience rests, fundamentally, on relationships' (p. 780). In fact, every major theory of human development identifies relationships as central. In their seminal work, Bronfenbrenner and Morris (1998) encouraged psychologists to consider the reciprocal nature of social, emotional and cognitive growth, describing a nested system of contexts and relationships in which human beings were situated and within which they interacted over the lifespan. Researchers since have expanded upon his framework by: studying the cumulative role of risk factors (Sameroff and Gutman 2004), exploring how protective and promotive systems contribute to resilience (Masten and Wright 2009), articulating the ways in which systems and settings effect development (Tseng and Seidman 2007) and conceptualizing models that integrate the effects of nature and nurture on development over time (Sameroff 2010). Today, across disciplinary fields, practitioners seek to foster healthy relationships in the lives of children.

This chapter provides a discussion of how adults can support children in developing the skills and understandings that enable them to engage in positive relationships. Because adult caretakers shape the relationships of young children (Sameroff 2010), we necessarily highlight the role that adults play in supporting healthy relationships. However, we also speak to the ways that children can learn to play a reciprocal, developmentally appropriate role in their own relationships. We begin by synthesizing traditional research on the stage-salient developmental relationship tasks of early and middle childhood. Next, we highlight dimensions of positive relationships that children must learn from and with adults in order to foster healthy interactions with others. We go on to identify strategies that promote positive

G. Brion-Meisels • S.M. Jones (✉)
Harvard Graduate School of Education, Cambridge, MA, USA
e-mail: gretchen_brion-meisels@gse.harvard.edu; stephanie_m_jones@gse.harvard.edu

S. Roffey (ed.), *Positive Relationships: Evidence Based Practice across the World*,
DOI 10.1007/978-94-007-2147-0_4, © Springer Science+Business Media B.V. 2012

relationships during early and middle childhood and provide examples of programmes that are attempting to improve the quality of children's relationships. Finally, we suggest the need for a shift in how researchers conceptualize the role of early relationships in children's development.

4.2   A Brief Summary of the Stage-Salient Developmental Relationship Tasks of Infancy Through Late Childhood

As human beings transition from the generally helpless state of infancy to the more fully realized autonomy of adulthood, they proceed through a series of interrelated tasks, such as the development of trust, self-regulation and language (Sroufe 1979). This learning is shaped, in part, through the proximal processes of children's primary relationships (Thompson 2006). Although human development is typically seen as continuous and nonlinear, developmental tasks are defined as stage-salient because they become centrally important for the first time during different stages of the lifespan (Aber and Jones 1997). Mastering these tasks is critically important for future development (Masten and Cicchetti 2010). By considering human development in stage-salient terms – and studying contexts, inputs and outputs in these same terms – researchers and practitioners gain an increased ability to think about development from a strengths-based stance (Aber and Jones 1997).

Understanding the developmental tasks necessary for nurturing positive relationships is critical for anyone who hopes to intervene to promote healthy interactions. Because relationships are integral to processes of social, emotional and cognitive development – and may, in fact, be a key mechanism through which these domains of development are linked (Thompson 2006) – research must consider how children's biological and environmental contexts interact to shape these tasks (Table 4.1). We begin by providing a brief overview of the relationship tasks of infancy and childhood (see Sroufe 1979 for a more complete explanation).

4.2.1   Early Relationships and Attachment

During infancy and early childhood, children must develop reliable, reciprocal relationships with their primary caregivers. Commonly referred to as attachment, the development of high-quality primary relationships provides infants with a sense of trust and a foundation from which they can safely explore the world (Bowlby 1969). Research informed by attachment theory has found considerable support for the impact of early primary relationships on the development of children's relational skills. Scholars describe attachment as an emotional bond or tie, characterized by a host of behaviours, including proximity seeking and contact maintenance under stress (Ainsworth et al. 1978). Through early primary relationships, children learn a

Table 4.1 Brief description of the stage-salient relationship tasks of infancy and childhood (Adapted from Aber and Jones 1997)

Transition between stages	Age range	Developmental relationship tasks
Infancy/toddlerhood	0–3	Develop trusting relationship with primary caregivers
		Gain a sense of security from relationship with caregivers
		Begin to self-regulate physiological states
		Practise social referencing
		Develop sense of self as distinct from other
Toddlerhood/preschool	2–5	Balance curiosity and active exploration of the world with sense of security
		Transfer knowledge and relationships from primary caregivers to secondary caregivers
		Develop sensitivity to the needs and expectations of others
		Learn to use others as resources
		Develop increasing sense of autonomy
Preschool/early school age	4–7	Actively engage with surrounds through relationships
		Develop the flexibility to adjust to the demands of different settings
		Manage impulses, especially in the context of peer relationships
		Engage in collective monologues with others
		Learn to follow externally the imposed rules/expectations
		Learn to express empathy and feelings with language
		Begin to categorize self as same as others
Early school-age/middle childhood	6–9	Develop the ability to self-regulate thoughts, behaviours and emotions to flexibly adjust to the demands and opportunities of multiple settings
		Begin to recognize that other peoples' feelings result from their own experiences
		Begin to empathize with groups of people or on the basis of more abstract conditions (e.g. poverty)
		Begin to categorize self as same or different from others
Middle childhood/late childhood	8–11	Develop skills to negotiate conflict and solve interpersonal problems non-aggressively
		Develop an understanding of autonomous morality
		Begin to internalize social/cultural norms
		Become more aware of other peoples' emotions and better able to read a situation
		Begin to consolidate one's self of self as competent and able to handle social and academic spheres of life
		Begin to define one's own identity

strategy of affect regulation that structures their behaviour when confronted with stress. When caregivers are sensitive and responsive in a manner complementary to their infant/toddler's bids for comfort and attention, relationships are thought to be developmentally supportive (Belsky et al. 1984; Egeland and Sroufe 1981). Since children's individual needs differ, early relationships are not characterized by a set of universally 'positive' qualities; rather, they are positive because they are sensitive to the unique individual and contextual needs of infants and children – they exhibit a 'goodness of fit'.[1] When caregivers are inaccessible and unresponsive, infants may learn to regulate their affect by avoiding interactions with their caregivers or come to view the world with anger, mistrust and hostility (Crittenden and Ainsworth 1989; Isabella and Belsky 1991). Without healthy early relationships, children may fail to develop appropriate attention to interpersonal interaction and thereby miss key social cues or become hyper-vigilant to hostile cues in later relationships (Dodge et al. 1990; Shaw and Bell 1993). These processes may also shape neural development in the prefrontal cortex, which has been linked to emotional and cognitive self-regulation later in life (Boyd et al. 2005).

Children and their primary caregivers negotiate strategic interactive patterns over the course of multiple experiences with each other. These interactional patterns become internal working models (cognitions and emotions) that each partner forms of the relationship (Bowlby 1982; Sroufe 1990). These models, which form in a complementary fashion unique to the individual pair, structure and affectively influence social interactions throughout development (Bowlby 1982). For children, they function as a guiding framework for further interaction, becoming a key mechanism through which they learn to be in relationships with others (Shaw and Bell 1993). Early relationships are internalized and affect subsequent social and emotional competence (Lyons-Ruth and Zeanah 1993; Thompson 2006). Characteristics of early relationships often manifest themselves anew over the course of development with new individuals and in new contexts.

4.2.2 Developing Emotional Competence

As children transition into toddlerhood, they must learn to regulate and understand their own emotions with less support from caregivers. For young children, emotional development plays a central role in the growth of social competence (Aber and Jones 1997; Weare and Gray 2003), equal to that of health, formal cognitive ability and achievement (Zigler and Trickett 1978). Emotional competence is generally viewed as encompassing four broad constructs: emotional regulation, emotion

---

[1] In their longitudinal studies of a cohort of infants in New York City, Thomas and Chess (1986) found that 'no one single pattern of person–environment interaction could be applied as a general rule for predicting the developmental course', but rather that healthy development was the result of 'the properties of the environment and its expectations and demands and the subjects temperament and other characteristics' (p. 49). They referred to this as 'goodness of fit'.

recognition and appraisal, emotional expression and empathy/perspective taking (Harris and Saarni 1989; Mayer and Salovey 1997; Saarni 1990). Children who are emotionally competent can identify and understand their own feelings, read and understand emotional states in others, manage strong emotions constructively, regulate their own behaviours and develop empathy for others in the context of relationships (DfES 2005a, DfES 2005b; Hallam 2009). These skills guide children in developing social relationships and managing interactions with others (DfES 2005a, DfES 2005b; Weare and Gray 2003).

To support the development of emotional competence, adults must help children learn to recognize, name and cope with their emotions. Adults also need to model and support the development of empathy for others. Children learn from watching adults; they benefit when adults spend time modelling successful communication and peaceful problem-solving (DfES 2005a, DfES 2005b). Children benefit when parents are responsive to their needs, express interest in their opinions, support their development of communication skills (including the verbal identification of emotional states), celebrate their accomplishments and support them in problem-solving (Boyd et al. 2005). Although preschool-age children are beginning to form relationships outside of the home, primary caregivers often facilitate their relational tasks through direct interaction and modelling and by controlling the settings in which they interact.

Much like parents, early relationships with educational caregivers contribute to children's working models of positive relationships. Teachers must have the time and space to develop one-on-one relationships with young children. As children transition into preschool, they must learn to transfer their knowledge and understanding of relationships from primary caregivers (typically family) to secondary caregivers and eventually peers. For some, this transition includes a shift in contextual or cultural expectations, presenting an additional challenge (Pianta and Cox 1999). Educational caregivers can support this transition by modelling explicit pro-social skills, providing opportunities to practise self-regulation and providing consistent feedback (Weare and Gray 2003). It is important for educational caregivers to value the cultures of their students' families, to partner with parents, to think constructively about issues of language and to collaborate with other professionals in support of children's developmental needs (Clifford 1999; Weare and Gray 2003).

4.2.3 Negotiating Relationships and the Role of Play in Development

During the preschool and early school years, children continue to practise their emotional competencies while adjusting to the demands and opportunities of varied contexts (Aber and Jones 1997). Many children begin to understand that their caregivers' goals may be separate from their own, and that they must negotiate to satisfy both sets of needs (Ainsworth et al. 1978). Increased social interactions require that children negotiate the needs of peers as well, some of whom may struggle with their own emotional competence. Given this, the development of empathy becomes increasingly important. Over time, notions of empathy become more abstract for children, allowing them to empathize with both individuals and groups of people. These expanded feelings of empathy, coupled with increased language agility, often help children to develop contextually appropriate conflict negotiation skills (e.g. avoiding physical aggression in school contexts).

Parents and educators can support children's abilities to build relationships by providing opportunities to: practise self-regulation, identify emotions and develop an understanding of the motivation, needs and skills of others (e.g. DfES 2005a; DfES 2005b). Children can be taught various coping mechanisms for dealing with stress including self-talk, which supports self-regulation (Vygotsky 1978). Since the development of language is critical in allowing children to express empathy and emotions with words (Hoffman 1975), school-based social-emotional learning programmes should provide opportunities to practise verbally communicating one's needs. Similarly, children can benefit from programmes that support their ability to take the perspective of others (Selman et al. 2004).

In addition to modelling and teaching children specific relational skills, a growing body of research documents the foundational role of play in early development (Elkind 2008; NIfP 2009). There is evidence that children learn fundamental self-regulation and pro-social skills through play as this provides an opportunity to: monitor their own and others' performance, reflect on what is happening socially and practise developing skills, maintain rules or instructions that promote executive functioning and use language to structure their own behaviour and influence others (Bodrova and Leong 2007). Research has explored three dimensions of social play – belonging play, rough-and-tumble play, and celebratory play – each of which supports a distinct relational skill-set (NIfP 2009). For example, rough-and-tumble play (e.g. running or wrestling) is thought to support the development of social awareness, cooperation, fairness and altruism (Pelligrini 1988). Panskepp (2008) and others have also connected early play to the epigenetic construction of social brain functions, suggesting that natural play supports critical neurological development. Neurological development is prominent in early childhood, and studies suggest a physiological basis for the development of self-regulation and empathy (Blair 2002). While processes in the prefrontal cortex affect children's self-regulation skills, these skills (in turn) affect their relationships with others (Jones and Zigler 2002).

4.2.4 *Looking Towards Adolescence*

During late childhood, children must learn to balance the contextual and cultural norms of their environment with their growing sense of self. This is often a period of development when adults play less of a mediatory role in relationships. As a result, older children must develop an ability to 'read' situations and predict appropriate and effective emotional and behavioural reactions for specific contexts. As children gain more control over the settings and people with whom they interact, their primary relationships begin to shift towards peers. School and community-based settings can provide important opportunities for older children to practise positive relational skills with the support of adult caregivers. This is also a period when children begin to integrate understandings of self with understandings of their social and academic lives, cultural contexts and relationships.

Having reviewed some of the stage-salient relational tasks of development, we turn our attention now towards the dimensions of positive relationships, more broadly. What types of processes and environments support positive relationships?

4.3 Qualities of Positive Relationships Within and Across Contexts in Early and Middle Childhood

Although the specific qualities of positive relationships vary across ecological and developmental contexts, there are several dimensions of relationships that universally support children's development: relationships work best when they are *developmentally and contextually appropriate, reciprocal, reliable* and *flexible* (Jones and Zigler 2002). Here, we explore these dimensions generally rather than attempting to highlight characteristics of positive relationships in specific contexts, because we believe that they can be actualized differently, dependent upon contextual needs. In describing these dimensions of positive relationships, we draw on the stage-salient developmental tasks summarized above.

One of the most important qualities of positive relationships is that they are *developmentally appropriate*. As evidenced above, children's relational needs change dramatically between birth and adolescence. While toddlers require a secure base from which to explore the world, school-age children benefit from increased autonomy and support in negotiating new relationships. Positive relationships adjust to these varying tasks, are sensitive to children's individual needs and help children prepare for the next steps in their development. For example, while caregivers may support a toddler's development of relational skills by modelling the use of language to identify emotional states, adults are more likely to support adolescents' relationships by encouraging the use of conflict resolution strategies. Similarly, social emotional interventions must provide children with developmentally appropriate skills.

Just as relationships must be developmentally appropriate, so too must they be *contextually or culturally relevant*. The power of thoughts, emotions and behaviours lies in the way people make meaning of them. For example, in their study of differences in early childrearing practices of Japanese and American children, Rothbaum et al. (2000) found that parents chose different ways of exercising control, with American parents being more likely to directly confront their children and Japanese parents being more likely to model deference. Both of these parenting styles are effective in their cultural context (Lewis 2000); but, one can imagine the difficulties a child might face if placed in a classroom with a teacher who employed a form of management different from that used at home. Because primary caregivers typically transmit cultural norms to very young children through everyday interactions, these early relationships are (by nature) contextually appropriate. However, as children get older, they begin to interact with secondary caregivers and peers and are required to adjust to varying expectations around communication and behaviour. Research on the transition into kindergarten, for example, suggests that children who experience incongruence between the settings of home and school are often seen as less successful than those whose family cultures mirror those of their school (Christenson 1999). Because children must learn to transfer knowledge of relationships from primary to secondary caregivers, it is easy to imagine the challenges that students face when school settings are not sensitive to home cultures.

Relationships are interactional by nature, but positive relationships are *explicitly reciprocal*; they provide opportunities for each party to influence and learn from the other. In his chapter on early social and personality development, Thompson (2006) suggests that positive relational experiences are 'generative of new understanding, whether of emotions, self, morality or people's beliefs' (p. 25). Relationships are most generative when they foster learning for *all* of those involved. Even very young children influence the ways that adults respond to their needs; for example, parents' perceptions of their children's temperaments can affect their choice of parenting styles (Rubin et al. 1999). Positive relationships acknowledge and build on their own interactional nature in developmentally appropriate ways. This type of reciprocity is difficult for many secondary caregivers to provide, as they must balance the relational needs of multiple children. At the same time, it may be critical to learning: research suggests that effective teachers are sensitive and responsive to their students' needs (Pianta and Allen 2008).

Finally, positive relationships are *reliable*: as children adapt to changes in their environments over time, sustained relationships can provide critical developmental supports (Benard 1991). For example, in their study of the effects of mentoring relationships on a national sample of adolescents, DuBois and Silverthorn (2005) found that teenagers who reported being in mentoring relationships characterized by consistent, positive interaction were more likely to report positive outcomes in terms of education, work or psychological wellbeing, and less likely to report problem behaviours. Other studies have noted that the longevity and intensity of mentoring relationships can vastly impact their effect on adolescents (Rhodes and DuBois 2008):

> "Close and enduring ties appear to be fostered when mentors adopt a flexible, youth centered style in which the young person's interests and preferences are emphasized, rather than when they focus predominantly on their own agendas or expectations for the relationship" (p. 255)

Similar benefits emerge from sustained positive relationships with parents and teachers. In fact, research suggests that the effects of mentoring relationships may be mediated by children's perceptions of their relationships with parents, peers and school-based adults (Rhodes and DuBois 2008). The importance of reliable relationships has implications for policies that aim to help children: it suggests the need for policies that provide economic and social stability for families and encourages us to align relationship structures across contexts and developmental periods.

In sum, positive relationships take into account children's ecologies by providing *developmentally and culturally relevant, reciprocal* and *reliable support* across the lifespan. As a result, children learn to recreate these dimensions of positive relationships in their future interactions.

4.4 A Closer Look at the Context of School: Positive Relationships in Educational Settings

School is a critical setting for relational learning, but it is also a setting deeply influenced by relationships. Children learn many of their social and emotional skills in school contexts by watching adults and peers or through direct instruction. In addition, relationships between parents and teachers play a significant role in shaping students' outcomes (Henderson and Mapp 2002).[2] As many educators find it difficult to build *developmentally and culturally relevant, reciprocal and reliable relationships,* in part because the needs of individual children are so varied, this section considers several factors that can support this endeavour.

First, schools need to build trust amongst individuals to support the emergence of *reciprocity* and the maintenance of *reliable* relationships. Trusting relationships have critical effects on cognitive, social and emotional development (Thompson 2006). At the same time, trust between children shapes their interactions with each other (Goddard 2003; Kahn and Turiel 1988) as well as the interactions of adults around them (Dunsmuir et al. 2004; Goddard 2003). Classrooms nurture pro-social skills and positive peer relationships when children engage in structured activities that help them to develop trust and connectedness (Jones et al. 2008). Teachers can build trust in their classrooms through scaffolding pro-social behaviours (e.g. group work), building a sense of collective responsibility for success, providing psychological safety (often, through consistency) and modelling language that supports nonviolent communication; in turn, positive relationships with teachers support student learning (Pianta and Allen 2008; Weare and Gray 2003). Students who report their school environment to be 'supportive and caring' are less likely to engage in violence and substance abuse, more likely to develop positive attitudes towards self and others and more likely to engage in school (Schaps 2005). Often, this distinction is given to schools where students have strong relationships with at least one adult, feel psychologically safe, are given structured opportunities to connect with peers and feel as though their needs are met. In addition, evidence suggests that trust amongst parents and teachers increases positive outcomes for children (Dunsmuir et al. 2004; Weare and Gray 2003) and is an important prerequisite for collaboration (Voltz 1994).

Critical to the development of trust is the development of *cross-cultural understanding,* a concept that overlaps with the notion of *culturally relevant relationships.* Research suggests that schools are structured in ways that value certain types of social and cultural capital over others (Bourdieu 1984). Children who arrive at school

---

[2]For example, when parents are involved in school, students show improvement in grades and test scores, increased motivation and self esteem, higher attendance rates and lower dropout rates (Christenson 1999).

with different types of social and cultural capital often experience schooling as a series of micro-aggressions (Delgado-Bernal 2002; Solorzano 1997). For example, a child used to looking down when he addresses adults and speaking softly to show respect may be told to 'Look up!' and 'Speak up!' by teachers in his elementary classroom. There is a vast body of research on culturally relevant pedagogy, which provides examples of ways in which teachers can nurture and value the multiplicity of cultures represented by students in their classrooms (e.g. Gay 2000; Maina 1997; Winch-Dummett 2006). Positive relationships are nurtured when: teachers work to understand children in the context of the norms and communities where they have been raised; children have opportunities to *both* teach and learn from their classmates, recognizing the value of different contributions to a classroom community; high expectations are held for all children; classroom norms draw from relational patterns in children's home cultures; content reflects students' cultural histories; and instruction provides an opportunity to understand the world from multiple perspectives (Education Alliance 2006). Schools that foster a sense of cross-cultural understanding amongst adults are best able to support the development of healthy relationships for children; for example, children benefit when teachers take the time to understand parents' hopes and concerns about their child's development (Education Alliance 2006). When the cultures of families are not respected and valued, schools and children suffer.

Finally, critical to the development of trust is the existence of *democratic, collaborative school structures*; these structures help to ensure that classrooms and schools are *developmentally appropriate* and *flexible* to the needs of students. A growing body of research suggests that children's participation in school and community-based organizations can positively affect communities (Ginwright and James 2002), organizations/schools (Mitra 2008) and the healthy development of children themselves (O'Donoghue et al. 2003). Children benefit from the opportunity to voice their opinions, contribute to the good of the community, collaborate with adults on projects and gain an understanding of ways to create change in their own lives. These activities help improve communication skills and build feelings of connectedness. Research on families and schools also suggests that moving towards a 'partnership approach' (Christenson 1999) enhances relationships between parents and teachers, improving student-level outcomes (Henderson and Mapp 2002). Here, parents and teachers 'model collaboration by: listening to each other's perspective and viewing differences as strengths; sharing information to co-construct the "bigger picture" about children's performance; respecting the skills and knowledge of each other; and planning and making decisions cooperatively' (Christenson 1999: 148). Schools can improve relationships by building structures that allow parents and children to authentically participate in educational processes.

Of note, the field of positive youth development has identified qualities of schools and community organizations that promote positive relationships. For example, the *Developmental Assets* (Scales and Leffert 2004), used regularly in the United States and Canada, highlights external and internal factors that support children's development. Many of these speak to the question of positive relationships. This work echoes our calls for *developmentally and culturally appropriate* relationships that are *reciprocal, reliable* and *flexible* in nature.

4.5   Programmes That Help Children Learn to Be in Positive Relationships

There is a growing body of evidence suggesting that early intervention and prevention programmes can enhance children's relationships (Diekstra 2008; Durlak et al. 2011; Elias 2003; Ferrer-Wreder et al. 2004). In Great Britain, for example, the Social and Emotional Aspects of Learning programme has reduced emotional and behavioural difficulties for students needing extra support (Humphrey et al. 2010) and has increased staff understanding of the social and emotional aspects of learning, which has changed their behaviour with students (Hallam 2009). In many countries, similar programmes have been implemented to improve children's relational skills; unfortunately, there are limited evaluations of these programmes. In this section, we provide a brief overview of three school-based interventions that have been shown to improve children's outcomes through the nurturing of positive relationships: *Responsive Classroom, the 4Rs Program* and Colombia's *National Program of Citizenship Competencies*. These programmes are distinct in that Responsive Classroom targets positive relationships through classroom processes, 4Rs targets positive relationships through teachers' competencies and instruction and the National Program of Citizenship Competencies targets positive relationships through national standards.

4.5.1   Responsive Classroom

Started in 1981, Responsive Classroom is an approach to teaching that integrates social and emotional learning throughout the school day in developmentally and contextually appropriate ways. The programme builds relationships amongst students, between teachers and students and between parents and teachers, by creating space for children to practise social interaction. Teachers dedicate time to building community and setting up classroom rituals; students participate in creating classroom rules; and all consequences are 'logical' to 'allow children to fix and learn from their mistakes while preserving their dignity' (Responsive Classroom 2010). In addition, teachers hold Morning Meetings daily, where students engage in structured activities that help support their academic and pro-social skills. During the remainder of the day, teachers present students with developmentally appropriate learning activities that provide opportunities for social interaction. Students are given academic choices to encourage independence and responsibility and support their individual learning styles and interests. The physical layout of responsive classrooms supports these pedagogical priorities. Evaluations demonstrate programmatic gains in students' social, emotional and cognitive development (Rimm-Kaufman 2006).

Responsive Classroom is designed to create organizational change in elementary schools: all grade-levels participate, and school-wide community-building activities support cross-grade and home-school collaboration. Rituals and daily activities are designed to be developmentally appropriate and to support students in transitioning between their home and school cultures. Although these activities may not be culturally relevant for all students, they become a means of fostering a classroom culture in which all students are included. In addition, curricular flexibility allows students to choose activities that match their learning styles and interests, promoting responsibility and autonomy. Across grades, a similar set of classroom practices support peer relationships that are reliable over time. Responsive Classroom practices give students a chance to learn from peers who have different relational needs. By valuing each student and family, the Responsive Classroom approach highlights the benefit of reciprocity in relationships. In this way, the school community comes to prioritize relationship-building.

4.5.2 The 4Rs Program

Like Responsive Classroom, the 4Rs Program (Reading, Writing, Respect and Resolution) integrates a social-emotional curriculum with traditional academic learning. The programme trains teachers to implement a curriculum that supports the development of pro-social skills, including social competence and peer cooperation. For example, teachers are taught to model good listening skills (direct eye contact, paraphrasing, acknowledging comprehension) through their interactions with other adults and students and to explicitly teach these skills using real-life examples in their classrooms. During teacher training, teachers reflect on their own social and emotional experiences, attitudes and competencies, while learning explicit strategies for improving classroom social-emotional learning (Jones et al. 2008). In class, high-quality children's stories and other literacy-based activities are used to teach and model relational skills. By changing teachers' relationships and their curricular content, the programme targets classroom pedagogies and the transactional social processes in the setting overall.[3] Initial findings from a school-randomized evaluation suggest that the programme results in increases in both individual- and classroom-level positive outcomes (Jones et al. 2011).

The 4Rs Program aims to support teachers and students in developing relationships that are developmentally and culturally appropriate, reliable and flexible; by targeting all classrooms, it creates organizational-level change in a school community. The programme supports reciprocal relationships by teaching pro-social skills to both children and staff, asking teachers to reflect on their own relationships, as well as to support their students' developing relationships. In addition, its literacy-based curriculum increases teachers' capacities to support students' relationships across domains. Finally, the programme serves as a reliable source of social-emotional support for students since it spans multiple grade levels within a school.

---

[3] One example of this type of effect is that children who have positive relationships with their teachers tend to be more accepted by their peers (Ladd et al. 1999) and to be well-liked and considered socially competent by other students in the classroom (Hughes et al. 2001).

4.5.3   The National Program of Citizenship Competencies

Our last highlighted social-emotional intervention emerges from a different cultural context, Colombia, and operates at a different ecological level (the macro-system). Responding to the effects of more than four decades of violent political conflict in Colombia, in 2004, the Colombian Ministry of Education developed a National Program of Citizenship Competencies (Ministerio de Educación de Nacional 2004; Patti and Espinosa 2007). The competencies outline a set of standards organized by developmental stage (3rd–11th grade), which include cognitive, emotional, communicative and integrative competencies.[4] The competencies span developmental domains, touching upon the themes of peace and peaceful interactions, democratic participation and diversity (Chaux 2009; Ministerio de Educación Nacional 2004). By focusing on the development of standards rather than the transmission of values, the Ministry of Education holds that students can 'develop their competencies by practising them in simulated or real-life situations', an assertion that differs from many past efforts to promote citizenship (Chaux 2009: 88; Patti and Espinosa 2007). The government does not dictate the pedagogical approach of specific school communities, although it is supporting the evaluation and expansion of specific programmes (Chaux 2009) and the development of local curricula.

The National Program of Citizenship Competencies supports the development of positive relationships amongst children, as well as between children and adults. In fact, the competencies speak to the elements of positive relationships highlighted above: they are developmentally and culturally appropriate, reliable and flexible. The standards differ across developmental periods; for example, while a 4th grader is expected to learn to address daily conflict in school and family using peaceful strategies, a 10th grader is called upon to 'explicitly reject all forms of discrimination of social exclusion' (Patti and Espinosa 2007: 113); by spanning grade-levels, the competencies are structured to be reliable supports. Also, the competencies are broad enough to allow communities to determine their own pedagogical approaches (Patti and Espinosa 2007). Finally, the competencies are explicitly reciprocal in that they aim to empower students and recognize the role that children can play in shaping their relationships.

4.6   (Re)conceptualizing Positive Relationships: A Shifting Focus on Supporting Development

The research presented in this chapter suggests that positive relationships are critical for children's healthy development *and* that healthy development is critical for children's positive relationships. As cascade theories suggest (Masten and Cicchetti 2010),

---

[4]Here, cognitive competencies develop skills and understandings that support active participation in civic life; emotional competencies develop skills and understandings that support one's ability to respond to his/her own emotions as well as others' emotions; communicative competencies develop the capacity to have productive dialogues; and integrative competencies develop skills that require social, emotional and cognitive competencies (e.g. brainstorming compromises to a conflict).

positive relationships yield positive relationships. Because relationships serve as a primary proximal process for all domains of development, nurturing positive relationships is one of the most powerful means of supporting children.

In 2006, Ross Thompson suggested the need for 'a developmental relational science' (2006: 25), which would integrate important parts of 'attachment theory, neo-Vygotskian thinking, sociolinguistic approaches to cognitive growth, and other perspectives into a thoughtful understanding of how early relational experience contributes to fundamental competencies and the emergence of individual differences in thinking, sociability, and personality development' (p. 25). By studying relationships, Thompson argued, we might better understand the interrelated pathways of development. Recently, Sameroff (2010) articulated a theory of development that begins to pull together these empirical understandings of personal change, ecological context, self-regulation and representation, highlighting the role of relationships in them.[5] Whether in the largely dependent state of infancy or the largely autonomous state of adulthood, relationships remain central to human's social, emotional and cognitive growth. Sameroff suggests the need for future research to integrate additional perspectives of human development from sociology and anthropology[6]; these perspectives can help us to understand how relationships between and amongst individuals shape the social, emotional and cognitive development of children. In this sense, Sameroff's (2010) conclusion echoes Thompson's (2006) call for a 'developmental relational science' (p. 25). By carefully articulating pathways to relationships that are developmentally and culturally relevant, reciprocal, reliable and flexible, researchers and practitioners can more fully support the healthy development of children across the world.

References

Aber, J. L., & Jones, S. M. (1997). Indicators of positive development in early childhood: Improving concepts and measures. In R. M. Hauser, B. V. Brown, & W. R. Prosser (Eds.), *Indicators of children's well-being* (pp. 395–408). New York: Russell Sage.

Ainsworth, M. D. S., Blehar, M. C., Waters, E., & Wall, S. (1978). *Patterns of attachment: A psychological study of the strange situation*. Hillsdale: Erlbaum.

Belsky, J., Taylor, D., & Rovine, M. (1984). The Pennsylvania infant and family development project, III: The origins of individual differences in infant-mother attachment: Maternal and infant contributions. *Child Development, 55*, 718–728.

---

[5] According to Sameroff (2010), self-regulation occurs in the context of 'other regulation' as children rely on adults, peers and teachers to learn about the 'range and limits of their behaviour' (p. 15).

[6] Specifically, Sameroff discusses the 'opportunity structure' construct from sociology and the 'meaning making' construct from anthropology. These constructs centre relationships in the process of development by reinforcing the mediating role that relationships have on individual growth. Sociology, Sameroff (2010) writes, can teach us that 'individuals are embedded in networks of relationships that constrain or encourage different aspects of individual behaviour'; anthropology can help us explore the differences in meaning systems across groups of people, or "how different cultures think about their practices" (p. 20).

Benard, B. (1991). *Fostering resiliency in kids: Protective factors in the family, school and community*. Portland: Northwest Educational Research Laboratory.

Blair, C. (2002). School readiness: Integrating cognition and emotion in a neurobiological conceptualization of children's functioning at school entry. *American Psychologist, 57*(2), 111–127.

Bodrova, E., & Leong, D. J. (2007). *Tools of the mind: The Vygotskian approach to early childhood education* (2nd ed.). New Jersey: Prentice Hall.

Bourdieu, P. (1984). *Distinction: A social critique of the judgment of taste*. Cambridge: Harvard University Press.

Bowlby, J. (1969/1982). *Attachment and loss: Vol. 1. Attachment; Vol. 2. Separation; Vol. 3 Loss*. New York: Basic Books.

Boyd, J., Barnett, W. S., Bodrova, E., Leong, D. J., & Gomby, D. (2005, March). *Promoting children's social and emotional development though preschool education. Preschool policy brief*. New Brunswick: National Institution for Early Education Research.

Bronfenbrenner, U., & Morris, P. (1998). The ecology of developmental process. *The Handbook of Child Psychology, 1*, 993–1029.

Chaux, E. (2009). Citizenship competencies in the midst of a violent political conflict: The Colombian educational response. *Harvard Educational Review, 79*(1), 84–93.

Christenson, S. L. (1999). Families and schools: Rights, responsibilities, resources and relationships. In R. C. Pianta & M. J. Cox (Eds.), *The transition to kindergarten* (pp. 143–178). Baltimore: Paul H. Brookes Publishing Co.

Clifford, R. M. (1999). Personal preparation and the transition to kindergarten. In R. C. Pianta & M. J. Cox (Eds.), *The transition to kindergarten* (pp. 317–324). Baltimore: Paul H. Brookes Publishing.

Crittenden, P. M., & Ainsworth, M. D. S. (1989). Child maltreatment and attachment theory. In D. Cicchetti & V. Carlson (Eds.), *Handbook of child maltreatment* (pp. 432–463). New York: Cambridge University Press.

Delgado-Bernal, D. (2002). Critical race theory, Latino critical theory, and critical raced-gendered epistemologies: Recognizing students of color as holders and creators of knowledge. *Qualitative inquiry, 8*(1), 105–126.

Department for Education and Skills (DfES). (2005a). *Excellence and enjoyment: Social and emotional aspects of learning: Relationships theme overview*. Nottingham: DfES Publications.

Department for Education and Skills (DfES). (2005b). *Excellence and enjoyment in social and emotional aspects of learning: Guidance*. Nottingham: DfES Publications.

Diekstra, R. F. W. (2008). *Social and emotional education: An international analysis*. Retrieved on December 10, 2010, from http://educacion.fundacionmbotin.org/index.php?a=educacion_responsable_evaluacionandl=EN

Dodge, K. A., Bates, G. S., & Pettit, G. S. (1990). Mechanisms in the cycle of violence. *Science, 250*, 1678–1683.

DuBois, D. L., & Silverthorn, N. (2005). Natural mentoring relationships and adolescent health: Evidence form a national study. *American Journal of Public Health, 95*(3), 518–524.

Dunsmuir, S., Frederickson, N., & Lang, J. (2004). Building home-school trust. *Educational and Child Psychology, 21*(4), 109–128.

Durlak, J. A., Weissberg, R. P., Dymnicki, A. B., Taylor, R. D., & Schellinger, K. B. (2011), The impact of enhancing students' social and emotional learning: A meta-analysis of school-based universal interventions. *Child Development, 82*(1), 405–432.

Education Alliance. (2006). *Principles for culturally responsive teaching*. Retrieved October 11, 2010, from http://www.alliance.brown.edu/tdl/tl-strategies/crt-principles.shtml#expectations

Egeland, B., & Sroufe, L. A. (1981). Attachment and early maltreatment. *Child Development., 52*(1), 44–52.

Elias, M. J. (2003). *Academic and social-emotional learning*. Brussels: International Academy of Education.

Elkind, D. (2008). The power of play: Learning what comes naturally. *American Journal of Play, 1*(1), 1–7.

Ferrer-Wreder, L., Stattin, H., Lorente, C. C., Tubman, J. G., & Adamson, L. (2004). *Successful prevention and youth development programs across borders.* New York: Kluwer Academic/ Plenum Publishers.

Gay, G. (2000). *Culturally responsive teaching: Theory, research and practice.* New York: Teachers College Press.

Ginwright, S., & James, T. (2002). From assets to agents of change: Social justice, organizing and youth development. In B. Kirshner, J. F. O'Donoghue, & M. McLaughlin (Eds.), *Youth participation: Improving institutions and communities* (pp. 27–46). Danvers: Wiley Periodicals.

Goddard, R. D. (2003). Relational networks, social trust, and norms: A social capital perspective on students' chances of academic success. *Educational Evaluation and Policy Analysis, 25*(1), 59–74.

Hallam, S. (2009). An evaluation of the Social and Emotional Aspects of Learning (SEAL) programme: Promoting positive behaviour, effective learning and well-being in primary school children. *Oxford Review of Education, 35*(3), 313–330.

Harris, P. L., & Saarni, C. (1989). Children's understanding of emotion: An introduction. In C. Saarni & P. L. Harris (Eds.), *Children's understanding of emotion* (pp. 3–24). Cambridge: Cambridge University Press.

Henderson, A. T., & Mapp, K. L. (2002). *A new wave of evidence: The impact of school, family and community connections on student achievement.* Austin: National Center for Family and Community Connections with Schools.

Hoffman, M. L. (1975). Altruistic behaviour and the parent-child relationship. *Journal of Personality and Social Psychology, 31*, 937–943.

Hughes, J. N., Cavell, T. A., & Wilson, V. (2001). The developmental significance of the quality of teacher–student relationships. *Journal of School Psychology, 39*, 281–301.

Humphrey, N., Kalambouka, A., Wigelsworth, M., & Lendrum, A. (2010). Going for goals: An evaluation of a story, social-emotional intervention for primary school children. *School Psychology International, 31*(3), 250–270.

Isabella, R. A., & Belsky, J. (1991). Interactional synchrony and the origins of infant-mother attachment: A replication study. *Child Development, 62*, 373–384.

Jones, S. M., & Zigler, E. (2002). The Mozart effect: Not learning from history. *Journal of Applied Developmental Psychology, 23*, 355–372.

Jones, S. M., Brown, J. L., & Aber, J. L. (2008). Classroom settings as targets of intervention and research. In H. Yoshikawa & M. Shinn (Eds.), *Toward positive youth development: Transforming schools and community programs* (pp. 58–77). New York: Oxford University Press.

Jones, S. M., Brown J. L., & Aber, J. L. (2011). Two year impacts of a universal school-based social-emotional and literacy intervention: An experiment in translational developmental research. Child *Development, 82*, 533–554.

Kahn, P. H., & Turiel, E. (1988). Children's conceptions of trust in the context of social expectations. *Merrill-Palmer Quarterly, 34*(4), 403–419.

Ladd, G. W., Birch, S. H., & Buhs, E. S. (1999). Children's social and scholastic lives in kindergarten: Related spheres of influence? *Child Development, 70*(6), 1373–1400.

Lewis, C. S. (2000). Human development in the United States and Japan: New ways to think about continuity across the lifespan. *Child Development, 71*(5), 1152–1154.

Luthar, S. S. (2006). Resilience in development: A synthesis of research across five decades. In D. Cicchetti & D. J. Cohen (Eds.), *Developmental psychopathology: Risk, disorder, and adaptation* (2nd ed., pp. 739–795). New York: Wiley.

Lyons-Ruth, K., & Zeanah, C. H. (1993). The family context of infant mental health: Affective development in the primary caregiving relationship. In C. H. Zeanah (Ed.), *Handbook of infant mental health* (pp. 14–37). New York: The Guilford Press.

Maina, F. (1997). Culturally relevant pedagogy: First nations education in Canada. *The Canadian Journal of Native Studies, XVII*(2), 293–314.

Masten, A. S., & Cicchetti, D. (2010). Developmental cascades. *Development and Psychopathology, 22*, 491–495.

Masten, A. S., & Wright, M. O'. D. (2009). Resilience over the lifespan: Developmental perspectives on resistance, recovery, and transformation. In J. W. Reich, A. J. Zautra, & J. S. Hall (Eds.), *Handbook of adult resilience* (pp. 213–237). New York: Guilford Press.

Mayer, J. D., & Salovey, P. (1997). What is emotional intelligence? In P. Salovey & D. J. Sluyter (Eds.), *Emotional development and emotional intelligence: Educational implications* (pp. 3–34). New York: Basic Books.

Ministerio de Educación Nacional. (2004). *Estándares Básicos de Competencias Ciudadanas. Formar para la Ciudadanía…; Sí es Posible. Lo que Necesitamos Saber y Saber Hacer* [Basic standards in citizenship competencies. Education for citizenship is possible: What we need to know and know how to do]. Colombia: Espantapájaros Taller, 2003. Colombia: Ministerio de Educación Nacional.

Mitra, D. L. (2008). *Student voice in school reform: Building youth-adult partnerships that strengthen schools and empower youth.* Albany: State University of New York Press.

National Institute for Play (NIfP). (2009). *Social play. Play science – The patterns of play.* Retrieved December 9, 2010, from http://www.nifplay.org/states_play.html#_4

O'Donoghue, J. F., Kirshner, B., & McLaughlin, M. (2003). Introduction: Moving youth participation forward. In B. Kirshner, J. F. O'Donoghue, & M. McLaughlin (Eds.), *Youth participation: Improving institutions and communities* (pp. 15–25). Danvers: Wiley Periodicals, Inc.

Panskepp, J. (2008). Play, ADHD, and the construction of the social brain. *American Journal of Play, 1*(1), 57–81.

Patti, J., & Espinosa, A. C. (2007). Citizenship competencies in Colombia: Learning from policy and practice. *Conflict Resolution Quarterly, 25*(1), 109–125.

Pelligrini, A. D. (1988). Rough-and-Tumble play from childhood through adolescence. In D. Fromberg & D. Bergen (Eds.), *Play from birth to twelve and beyond: Contexts, perspectives, and meanings* (pp. 401–408). Garland: New York.

Pianta, R. C., & Allen, J. P. (2008). Building capacity for positive youth development in secondary school classrooms: Changing teachers' interactions with students. In H. Yoshikawa & M. Shinn (Eds.), *Toward positive youth development: Transforming schools and community programs* (pp. 21–39). New York: Oxford University Press.

Pianta, R. C., & Cox, M. J. (Eds.). (1999). *The transition to kindergarten.* Baltimore: Paul H. Brookes Publishing.

Responsive Classroom. (2010). *Guiding principles.* Retrieved on October 11, 2010, from http://www.responsiveclassroom.org/about/aboutrc.html

Rhodes, J. E., & DuBois, D. L. (2008). Mentoring relationships and programs for youth. *Association for Psychological Sciences, 17*(4), 254–258.

Rimm-Kaufman, S. E. (2006). *Social and academic learning study on the contribution of the responsive classroom approach.* Turners Falls: Northeast Foundation for Children.

Rothbaum, F., Pott, M., Azuma, H., Miyake, K., & Weisz, J. (2000). The development of close relationships in Japan and the US: Pathways of symbiotic harmony and generative tension. *Child Development, 71*, 1121–1142.

Rubin, K. H., Nelson, L. J., Hastings, P., & Asendorpf, J. (1999). The transaction between parents' perceptions of their children's shyness and their parenting styles. *International Journal of Behavioural Development, 23*(4), 937–957.

Saarni, C. (1990). Emotional competence: How emotions and relationships become integrated. In R. A. Thompson (Ed.), *Socio-emotional development: Nebraska symposium on motivation, 1988* (pp. 115–182). Lincoln: University of Nebraska Press.

Sameroff, A. (2010). A unified theory of development: A dialectic integration of nature and nurture. *Child Development, 81*(1), 6–22.

Sameroff, A. J., & Gutman, L. M. (2004). Contributions of risk research to the design of successful interventions. In P. Allen-Meares & M. W. Fraser (Eds.), *Intervention with children and adolescents: An interdisciplinary approach* (pp. 9–26). Boston: Pearson.

Scales, P. C., & Leffert, N. (2004). *Developmental assets: A synthesis of the scientific research on adolescent development.* Minneapolis: Search Institute.

Schaps, E. (2005). Chapter 3: The role of supportive school environments in promoting academic success. In *Getting results: Developing safe and healthy kids, update 5* (pp. 37–56). Sacramento: California Department of Education.

Selman, R. L., Watts, C. L., & Schultz, L. H. (2004). *Fostering friendship: Pair therapy for treatment and prevention*. New Brunswick: Transaction Publishers.

Shaw, D. S., & Bell, R. Q. (1993). Developmental theories of parental contributors to antisocial behaviour. *Journal of Abnormal Child Psychology, 21*(5), 493–518.

Solorzano, D. G. (1997). Images and words that wound: Critical race theory, racial stereotyping and teacher education. *Teacher Education Quarterly, 24*(3), 5–19.

Sroufe, L. A. (1979). The coherence of individual development. *American Psychologist, 34*(10), 834–841.

Sroufe, L. A. (1990). An organizational perspective on the self. In D. Cicchetti & M. Beeghly (Eds.), *The self in transition: Infancy to childhood* (pp. 281–308). Chicago: University of Chicago Press.

Thomas, A., & Chess, S. (1986). The New York longitudinal study: From infancy to early adult life. In R. Plomin & J. Dunn (Eds.), *The study of temperament: Changes, continuities and challenges* (pp. 39–53). Hillsdale: Lawrence Erlbaum.

Thompson, R. A. (2006). The development of the person: Social understanding, relationships, self, conscience. In W. Damon & R. M. Lerner (Eds.), & N. Eisenberg (Vol. Ed.) *Handbook of child psychology: Vol. 3. Social, emotional, and personality development* (6th ed., pp. 24–98). New York: Wiley.

Tseng, V., & Seidman, E. (2007). A systems framework for understanding social settings. *American Journal of Community Psychology, 39*, 217–228.

Voltz, D. L. (1994). Developing collaborative parent-teacher relationships with culturally diverse parents. *Intervention in School and Clinic, 29*(5), 288–291.

Vygotsky, L. S. (1978). *Mind in society: The development of higher psychological processes*. Cambridge: Harvard University Press.

Weare, K., & Gray, G. (2003). *What works in developing children's emotional and social competence and wellbeing?* Southampton: DfES Publications.

Winch-Dummett, C. (2006). Successful pedagogies for an Australian multicultural classroom. *International Education Journal, 7*(5), 778–789.

Zigler, E., & Trickett, P. K. (1978). IQ, social competence, and evaluation of early childhood intervention programs. *American Psychologist, 33*, 789–798.

Gretchen Brion-Meisels is a doctoral student at the Harvard Graduate School of Education. Her research seeks to explore holistic student support processes that build on the knowledge of students and communities. She is a former editor of the *Harvard Educational Review* and helped edit a volume entitled, *Humanizing Education: Critical Alternatives to Reform* (2010).
Contact: gretchen_brion-meisels@gse.harvard.edu

Stephanie M. Jones is an assistant professor of Education at the Harvard Graduate School of Education. Jones' research focuses on the developmental impact of educational interventions targeting children's social-emotional and academic skills. She is involved as Principal Investigator or Co-Investigator in a number of evaluation studies of preschool and school-based programmes in social-emotional learning and literacy.
Contact: stephanie_m_jones@gse.harvard.edu

Chapter 5
Positive Couple Relationships: The Evidence for Long-Lasting Relationship Satisfaction and Happiness

Vagdevi Meunier and Wayne Baker

5.1 Introduction

The field of positive psychology is painting a new picture of what it takes to create lasting, stable and, more importantly, enjoyable relationships (Gable and Haidt 2005). To create happiness with an intimate partner, it is not enough to simply learn how to get rid of negative behaviours (Gottman 1995; Gottman and Silver 2000). There is a critical need to build a positive psychology of relationships, one that details the behaviours happy couples engage in that accentuate the positive and ignore or reduce the impact of the negative.

5.2 A Positive Psychology of Relationships

Psychology has long been a science of healing and has tried to follow in the footsteps of medical science. The literature and research has focused almost entirely on the cause and elimination of suffering. There has been little focus on the 'fulfilled individual and thriving community' (Seligman and Csikszentmihalyi 2000). This has been particularly true in the field of relationship science, where concerns about violence, depression, divorce, betrayals and other negative human experiences have held centre stage for many decades (Gable and Haidt 2005). We know more about couples in distress, who come to marital therapy because they could not handle what life had to offer, than we do about the couples who are quietly managing all the same

V. Meunier (✉)
St. Edwards University, Austin, TX, USA
e-mail: vagdevim@gmail.com

W. Baker
Austin, TX, USA
e-mail: wayne@waynebakerlpc.com

S. Roffey (ed.), *Positive Relationships: Evidence Based Practice across the World*,
DOI 10.1007/978-94-007-2147-0_5, © Springer Science+Business Media B.V. 2012

challenges and transitions of life and maintaining their relationships over a long time. We know little about couples who are managing to thrive and grow despite setbacks, and who are finding ways to enjoy, support and nurture each other as well as their children (Tucker and Crouter 2008), even under circumstances one would not expect to offer contentment such as slum dwellers in Calcutta (Gable and Haidt 2005).

Divorce rates have risen at an alarming rate in the past century in most industrialized countries, and have caused great concern for the impact not only on individual stress and mental health but also on relationships, families and social communities as a whole (Kaslow 2001; Coontz 2006). In recent decades, non-industrialized countries have also begun to see rising divorce rates. For example, India, which had the lowest divorce rates in the world for many decades, has begun to see a sharp rise in divorces in urban cities (Shetty 2009). Similarly in Japan and China, the rate of relationship breakup has gone up enough to cause concern about the social impact of this phenomenon on childbirth, children's mental health, the stability of extended family structures, and even productivity in the workplace (Kaslow 2001).

The rising concern about relationship breakup hides an important finding. The majority of couples in committed, intimate relationships are doing well. Research from eight different countries (US, Canada, Germany, Sweden, the Netherlands, Israel, South Africa and Chile) found the divorce rate to be between 20% and 50% (Sharlin et al. 2000). What is exceptional about these findings is that, in most parts of the world, 50–80% of couples are in lasting relationships that they find quite satisfying. That is a fact worth celebrating but it is often ignored or lost in the mountains of writing about divorce and distress in relationships.

We are now beginning to see a growing body of sociological as well as psychological research that speaks to the value of being in long-term committed relationships both for men and women (Waite and Gallagher 2001; O'Connell 2008). We are learning that social support from close positive relationships has positive impact on longevity, wellbeing, productivity and immune function (Kantrowitz and Wingert 1999). Once we know that committed relationships are beneficial and that happy committed relationships 'make life worth living' (Waite and Gallagher 2001; Seligman and Csikszentmihalyi 2000), the next step is understanding what it takes to create that happiness, positivity and stability in committed relationships.

There are a few researchers who have made it their career goal to study and understand positive intimate relationships. One of them is Dr. John Gottman, who has spent more than three decades studying over 3,000 married couples using multi-method and multi-dimensional research methods and built a solid scientific model of healthy relationships that he calls the Sound Relationship House (Gottman 1995, 1999, 2007) (see Fig. 5.1). The Sound Relationship House model is a template for healthy, satisfying and lasting relationships.

Gottman is able to predict with over 94% accuracy which relationships are likely to remain intact and those that will not. He also replicated his findings in six separate studies (2007). Gottman discovered early in his research that helping couples have positive relationships is not just about preventing or eliminating negative behaviours. He found a group of couples he called Masters of Relationship who were engaging in specific behaviours that were enhancing or maintaining the positivity of the relationship.

Fig. 5.1 The Sound
Relationship House
(Reprinted with permission
from The Gottman
Relationship Institute: www.
gottman.com. Copyright
© 2008 by Dr. John M.
Gottman and Dr. Julie
Schwartz Gottman)

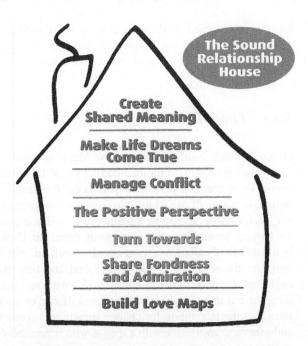

Barbara Fredrickson's research confirms that when flourishing relationships go above
a tipping point of 3:1 positive to negative experiences they are a qualitatively different
experience (2009). Similarly, Amy Strachman and Shelly Gable (2006), who have
been studying positive behaviours in a variety of relationships, have found that happy
couples tend to demonstrate specific behaviours that go beyond avoiding behaviours
that might cause pain and suffering to each other. Based on the work of these major
researchers as well as other emerging research on positivity in relationships, the following sections offer an overview of the factors and behaviours that can be found in
positive couple relationships.

5.3   Qualities of Positive Couple Relationships: The Friendship Dimension

Most committed, intimate and romantic relationships begin with a foundation of
friendship. Even in cultures where marriages are arranged, the couple that builds a
strong friendship in the early years of marriage will be more likely to weather the
challenges of the later years (Sharlin et al. 2000; Sandhya 2009). Unfortunately,
many couples believe that finding one's soul mate is the goal, and that once they
have found the perfect mate, the love between the two of them will take care of
any challenges that arise. Empirical research on relationships shows that love has
to be nurtured and savoured and preserved through regular actions that build the
foundation of friendship (Gottman 1999, 2007). Gottman's research found that there

are three components to the marital friendship that form the foundation of the sound relationship house: Love Maps, Fondness and Admiration and Turning Towards (the latter also known as the emotional bank account).

5.3.1   Love Maps

Gottman (1995) coined the term 'Love Maps' to denote the cognitive space that one partner has in their mind for their partner's world. In other words, how well does one spouse know the other person's experiences, likes and dislikes and personality quirks or unique talents. 'Love Maps' also refers to the awareness and sensitivity one partner has for his or her partner's inner world – what is making them happy, what they are looking forward to, what is stressing them, etc. During the courtship period and in the throes of early love, most couples work on love maps quite easily and regularly. As the relationship gets established and time passes, these love maps are neglected. Couples forget to update their love maps, and believe they know everything there is to know about their partners. However, people grow and change all the time, and the inspiration for change sometimes comes from having an energizing, enthusiastic conversation with a spouse who is genuinely interested in one's story, as much as it comes from intrinsic motivations. Gottman found that master couples maintained this regular interest in their partner's lives and built rituals of connection that kept their love maps updated (1999).

Other researchers have substantiated the importance of these love maps, albeit in different terms. Diener and Seligman (2002) found that the 10% of students with the highest levels of happiness and fewest symptoms of depression had strong ties to family and friends and made a commitment to sharing time with them. Australian researchers Halford et al. (2007) confirmed that newly married couples who worked on their relationship were more successful in maintaining satisfaction despite stressful life events over a 5-year period.

5.3.2   Fondness and Admiration

The second component of the friendship dimension is maintaining fondness and admiration. This is a simple concept to understand but challenging to maintain over the long term. Maintaining admiration is critical to preventing the loss of respect or empathy towards one another. Research has shown that emotional expressiveness is positively correlated with marital satisfaction, and that the sense of stability that comes from regular experience of feeling loved (and admired) in a relationship is the best predictor of long-term commitment (Sharlin et al. 2000). People are usually drawn into relationships because of feelings of fondness and admiration. However, over time, partners begin to notice and react to small irritations and disappointments more than positive behaviours. As the number of negative experiences are noted and added to, fondness and admiration can be eroded. Scanning the environment for what is not going well enhances negative thinking and feeds negative emotional states, which can become quite absorbing. In fact, negative emotional states are more intense and likely to dampen any positive emotions that may also be present (Gottman 1995; Johnson 2008; Hanson and Mendius 2009). In order to overcome this negative bias, it is important to maintain generous praise and appreciation for each other.

Maintaining admiration also has the added benefit that spouses who admire each other are more likely to accept and even celebrate their differences and enjoy the diverse interests and opinions they offer each other (Gottman 2007). Spouses who feel fondness and admiration and make an effort to express these positive feelings are also likely to see the positivity add up over time leading to a longevity bonus of about 10 years (Fredrickson 2009). A key ingredient in maintaining positivity is to express positive feelings either verbally or in some other form, and to make an effort to express specific, recent and timely praise rather than global or general admiration. Lyubomirsky (2007) found that deliberately counting one's blessings on a regular basis, for example in a gratitude diary, once a week, increased participants' feelings of satisfaction about their life. In order to express positive thoughts and feelings in a relationship, it is important to cultivate and maintain internal positive thoughts and perceptions. Research shows that positivity engenders success and more positivity in a nurturing feedback loop (Fredrickson 2009; Lyubomirsky et al. 2005). Rehman and Holtzworth-Munroe (2007), in a cross-cultural study of American and Pakistani couples, found a strong association between positive marital communication and satisfaction indices. In a relationship, positive expression leads to gratitude and appreciation from the spouse, which then enhances self-esteem in both partners and leads to increased positive thinking and perceptions.

Robinson and Price (1980) showed that couples who had high adjustment (or satisfaction in the marriage) where the fondness and admiration was intact, had the same count of both positive and negative interactions in the relationship as independent observers. Distressed couples underestimated the positive interactions by up to 50%. Spouses in positive relationships accentuate the positive, maintain positive illusions and admiration for their partners, and this helps them have a more realistic or balanced view of experiences in the relationship. They find the good in whatever has happened to them: researchers call this 'benefit finding'.

Research shows that there are some specific positive behaviours that are more impactful. For example, expressing gratitude appears to be more important than seeking happiness (Algoe and Haidt 2009). Individuals who encourage feelings of gratitude towards another person tend to experience more closeness, more affection and tend to have positive thoughts and feelings about the other's motives or personality. Individuals who focus on happiness tend to be more self-centred – concerned about what they are getting in a relationship (Algoe et al. 2008; Katzir et al. 2010).

Positivity doesn't just reflect success and happiness in life, it produces success and happiness too. A meta-analysis of positivity research confirmed this finding (Lyubomirsky et al. 2005). Positivity does not only reflect a current state, it draws in and produces that state. Barbara Fredrickson has created the Broaden and Build theory of positivity based on two decades of empirical research. Maintaining positive emotions (internally) and expressing positivity (towards others) help to broaden one's perspective, see the big picture, think more creatively and find solutions and new ideas more easily. Broadening then leads to building more positivity, creating new pathways towards happiness, serenity, joy, etc. As the positivity ratio approaches the tipping point, which is 3:1 positive to negative thoughts or moments, it creates flourishing individuals as well as relationships (Fredrickson 2009; Cohn et al. 2009).

5.3.3   The Emotional Bank Account

Researchers have believed for a long time that the fundamental unit of intimacy is verbal and reciprocal self-disclosure (Jourard 1959). Driver and Gottman (2004) showed, through research on couples' mundane interactions throughout the day, that the fundamental unit of intimacy is actually the Bid and the Turn. This is a concept they developed to explain the simple, often subtle, interactions that happen between two people who are sharing time and space together. Couples who are in the same room together, even if they are engaged in individual pursuits such as reading or watching television, will be making small gestures to each other, both verbal and nonverbal that function as invitations to connect. For example, one spouse who is reading the newspaper starts to chuckle and the other spouse who is reading something else says, 'What?' The first spouse shares the article in the newspaper that caused the chuckle and both of them have a moment of shared laughter before going back to their individual reading. The first spouse made a bid and the partner turned towards their spouse rather than turning away (ignoring the chuckle) or turning against (hushing their partner). Driver and Gottman found that happy couples respond to their partner's bid for attention about 85% of the time with a positive response. The frequency of bids and turns can be 20 times greater in happy couples, which creates an upward spiral of bids and turns, often up to 77 times in 10 min contrasted with 10–20 bids in 10 min for distressed couples (Driver et al. 2003). This high level of positive reciprocity leads to deposits in the 'emotional bank account' in the relationship. If the emotional bank account is filled to the brim, conflict, stress and other misfortunes of life tend to have a lower impact. If the emotional bank account is running on empty, every argument has the potential to derail the relationship.

The hallmark of positive relationships is that partners not only notice these small invitations but turn towards each other enthusiastically. They show willingness and delight in being invited to share in a personal experience with their spouse and have no hesitation in laughing loudly, complimenting their spouse or showing a high level of interest and engagement in the interaction. High level bids and enthusiastic 'turning towards' behaviour lead to relationships that become rich environments of intimacy, lightheartedness and enjoyment.

Strachman and Gable (2006) found a similar distinction in their research on couples that they labelled approach- or avoidance-oriented behaviour. A person is using approach skills when he or she is demonstrating motivations that are connected to rewards or positive outcomes, which, in turn, was related to greater happiness in the relationship. For example, I call my husband to find out how his day is going, to let him know I am thinking of him fondly or to share something interesting or exciting from my day. The motivation here is to seek out connection or share my experience. On the other hand, avoidance-oriented skills are those that help us avoid pain or suffering, or, to prevent something bad from happening. If I call my husband but my motivation is to check upon him because I worry that he is engaging in an affair, I am likely to communicate a different message. The behaviours might be the same – I called my husband – but the motivations and intentions are quite different. One will enhance the positivity in the relationship and the other might result in conflict (because of the fearful motivation) or maintain the relationship at a price. Strachman and Gable found that some people had high approach-oriented skills, which increased the likelihood of their receiving support, positive feedback and enjoyment from relationships. Capitalization, which is the retelling of a positive event to your spouse, is likely to generate more positive affect that is over and above the initial positive affect of the event itself (Fredrickson and Joiner 2002; Gable et al. 2004). The partner's supportive response must be seen as supportive of the event and of the relationship. There is a basking effect of the positive emotions for both partners.

5.3.4 Play, Fun and Humour

Positive relationships are often characterized by play and humour because both individuals in the relationship are prone to scanning their environment for success and opportunities for gratitude rather than the reverse (Gottman 2007). Positivity research confirms that injecting humour into a conflictual or distressing situation has multiple benefits for both partners (Fredrickson 2009, Lyubomirsky 2007) including increased immune function, lowered cortisol, reduced risk of depression or stress-related illness and increased likelihood of relationship satisfaction. In fact, Gottman (1999) found that the first 3 minutes of a conflict conversation can be used to predict the trajectory of the conversation as well as the relationship itself because the lack of humour, a harsh opening or start-up to the discussion and the use of negative conflict strategies are powerful determinants of relationship pathways and health.

Playfulness and humour in relationships have other significant consequences. They are often present when partners are enthusiastically turning towards each other, which then leads to a greater sense of intimacy and closeness (Gottman and Silver 2000). These behaviours are also likely to be associated with more sexual desire, affectionate touch and greater sexual satisfaction (McCarthy and McCarthy 2009). A study of older Israeli couples in enduring marriages found that sexual pleasure as well as affection, trust, openness and consideration were important factors in marital satisfaction throughout the lifespan and not just in earlier stages of relationship (Cohen et al. 2009).

5.4   The Conflict Dimension

Healthy relationships are not 100% positive or full of playfulness and humour at the expense of other emotions (Wallerstein and Blakeslee 1995). Researchers have found that in general there is a positivity offset of about 2:1, suggesting that on average most people experience about two positive events for each negative event (Fredrickson 2009). Flourishing relationships exceed the tipping point of three positives to every negative. However, even in flourishing relationships, the negative side of the ratio is never zero. Positive relationships are healthy because both partners in the relationship have the capacity to recognize, honour and work with the negative moments or emotions that come up in life. As Fredrickson (2009) found, individuals in healthy relationships are characterized by less reactivity to negative circumstances, an ability to see positive alternatives or return to positive perceptions of the relationship quickly and an emotional agility that allows them to spend less time worrying about the past or the future and being able to count their blessings in the present.

In Gottman's (1999) sound relationship model, the middle two levels represent the conflict dimension and include skills such as learning how to manage conflict that is unsolvable, effectively repairing negative interactions and avoiding relationship-damaging behaviours during conflict. Gottman found that couples who thrive have a softer, gentler approach to conflict, inject humour, diffuse tensions at low levels of negativity and avoid the four horsemen of the apocalypse. The four horsemen – criticism, defensiveness, contempt and stonewalling – are the four behaviours that predict the deterioration of a relationship. A detailed description of the four horsemen can be found in Gottman's book, *Why Marriages Succeed or Fail* (1995). Conflict in itself is not a sign of deterioration because conflict often allows partners to air grievances that may be building in the background (Kesner 2008).

Building a lasting vision of the relationship and putting conflict into perspective are important tasks in healthy relationships (Fincham et al. 2004). When we open ourselves to knowing and being known deeply by our partner, we are likely to encounter differences in opinion, values or emotional and relational templates (Banse 2004). Expressing the different facets of our personality can be risky if differences are seen as threatening (Johnson 2008). Conflict then becomes a vehicle for real and enduring growth if the partners can use their differences as opportunities to build a stronger base for their intimacy and admiration for each other.

5.4.1   Positive Sentiment Override

Gottman (1999) found that marriages exist in two kinds of steady states or set points he called Positive Sentiment Override (PSO) and Negative Sentiment Override (NSO). These states are called sentiment overrides because the prevailing sentiment, whether positive or negative, tends to override the momentary experiences, colours the neutral moments or helps filter the incoming communication from the partner. Flourishing relationships that exist in a state of PSO are often characterized by 1.93

positive interactions or gestures per minute (about 115 per hour) which is significantly higher than distressed relationships (Gottman et al. 1998). In other words, these relationships offer rich environments of affection, positivity, humour and appreciation that override the more mundane challenges in life. The PSO becomes a sort of filter that allows partners to see even negative communications in a positive light because each negative experience is seen within the context of a rich database of positive experiences. PSO can alter the way in which a couple remembers past events or can create a positive container that can weather challenging interactions (Gottman 2007). A positive sentiment override is not something a couple can consciously create in a relationship because it is the indirect outcome of many positive elements in the relationship. In other words, PSO is like the weather of a relationship that requires many conditions coming together at the right time and in the right mixture to form the clouds of happiness. A strong friendship system characterized by updated love maps and regular expressions of fondness and appreciation are critical to creating the positive weather in the relationship. For PSO to exist there must also be an absence of serious unresolved or gridlocked conflict as a result of well-established and regular conflict management strategies (Gottman 2007).

5.4.2 Softened Start-Up

Softened start-up is the term coined by Gottman (1999) to denote a gentle opening in the first 3 minutes of a conflict discussion. This is the critical period during conflict when exercising tact in opening a conversation, maintaining a calm, open mental state and managing one's emotional reactivity has significant pay-off. A necessary skill in starting and managing conflict discussions well is being able to manage one's physiological reactivity. In one study, Gottman and associates (1995) found that listener positivity and neutrality during conflict discussions were more prevalent in happy marriages. Gottman (1999) and other researchers (Atkinson 2005) have shown that conflict discussions in committed relationships can have the same physiological signature as combat stress, which includes symptoms such as elevated heart rate (typically over 95 beats per minute), agitation, misperceptions of incoming information and flight or fight thinking.

Any understanding of safety in relationships has to take into account some of our evolutionary legacies. Our brains are wired to keep us safe (Hanson and Mendius 2009). The entire limbic system functions on the basis of the danger signals that are picked up by the amygdala and then transmitted across the brain, shutting down thinking centres and heightening the survival mechanisms of flight, fight, or freeze. Couples who know how to argue productively seem to understand this intuitively and develop strategies to diffuse tensions at low levels of negativity, have low thresholds for hurtful communication, take breaks in conversations when the conflict seems gridlocked and balance their complaints with statements of love or appreciation and humour. Gottman and Krokoff (1989) found that in satisfied relationships, men defuse negativity in low-conflict situations while women de-escalate negativity in high-conflict contexts.

5.4.3   Unsolvable Problems

Gottman (1999, 2007) found that about two-thirds of all conflicts across both happy as well as distressed couples are not resolvable. In other words, the topics that cause conflict in the relationship are likely to endure for many years, and there may be no good solutions to be found. Couples who understand this learn to manage conflicts the same way they manage chronic illnesses, by learning strategies to keep the conflict at bay, reducing the impact of the conflict on other aspects of their relationship and learning ways to negotiate compromises in place of trying to solve unsolvable problems.

Experimental studies have repeatedly shown that individual positive moods or internal positivity has a large impact on conflict management and negotiation. In fact Gottman et al. (1998) found that amongst newlyweds positive affect, when used as a contingent emotion to diffuse negativity or soothe a partner, was the only predictor of both marital stability and satisfaction 6 years later. Positivity on an individual or relationship level reduces aggressive tactics, increases cooperation, curiosity and willingness to look at new solutions, decreases use of avoidance or manipulation strategies and increases the desire to help others. This effect is so prevalent it has been dubbed the 'feel good, do good' phenomenon (Lyubomirsky et al. 2005). Since a person's positive mood or state increases the ability to negotiate conflict more productively, it also enhances feelings of gratitude and appreciation in the partner (Fredrickson 2009; Cohn et al. 2009) and the likelihood that each partner considers the other's point of view and 'accepts influence'. Accepting influence or being willing to take a partner's suggestion and be influenced by their perceptions were predictive of long-term relationship satisfaction for men (Gottman and Silver 2000).

5.4.4   Repair

Relationship repair is a critical aspect of healthy conflict management (Gottman 1999). In Gottman's research, the master couples were repairing and de-escalating the conflict during the argument as well as making effective repairs after a negative interaction. Repair attempts during the conflict include efforts to interject humour, conceding a point, or apologizing for hurting the partner's feelings. There is typically one effort to repair about every 3 minutes for most couples (Gottman 2007). Repair attempts can also include bids for connection through a joke, a quick peck on the cheek or a smile that is received and returned.

Conflict in long-term committed relationships is unavoidable, at least in most healthy relationships. This is because life itself brings ups and downs in addition to differences in individuals within a relationship who bring diverse points of view, differences in upbringing and social and moral values, and predictable mishaps in attunement or communications. A German study found that distressed and non-distressed couples have many similarities in their conflict management strategies: the important difference was that non-distressed couples had more predictability and trust that a positive gesture will be reciprocated by the spouse (Hahlweg et al. 1984).

The key to successful conflict management is not avoiding conflict but maintaining reciprocal, fair and respectful conflict management methods that avoid the four horsemen of the apocalypse (Gottman 1995). One is likely to find criticism (treating a relationship problem like it is a defect in the partner), defensiveness (not taking responsibility for even a small part of the problem) or stonewalling (shutting down during a conversation) in happy and unhappy couples. Gottman et al. (1998) found that a softened start-up in a woman's approach to conflict and a man's ability to accept influence from his partner were positive predictors of a lasting relationship.

What one is not likely to find in happy satisfied relationships is contempt. Contempt is any behaviour, gesture or non-verbal signal that communicates that one partner is on a superior plane compared to the other partner. Contempt is the most corrosive of conflict strategies used during arguments because it erodes the respect, the equality and the sense of safety in a relationship (Gottman 1999; Johnson 2008). Couples in positive relationships rarely feel contempt towards their partners both because of their own internal positivity but also because they make efforts to maintain admiration, affection and respect in the relationship even when they are fighting. They also recognize the harm caused by contemptuous behaviour and either avoid it altogether during conflict or recognize when they have crossed the line and quickly retract or repair the hurt. In fact, the absence of contempt can be seen as a positive prognostic indicator of health in a relationship.

5.4.5   Forgive and Give Thanks

Any discussion of conflict management in committed relationships has to pay special attention to the concepts of forgiveness and expressions of gratitude. These two behaviours or attitudes are absolutely essential for the success of long-term relationships and also mark the major challenges of maintaining positivity in a relationship over time (Algoe et al. 2010; Luskin 2003; Kornfield 2008). Everyone at some point feels hurt, let down, betrayed, disappointed or wronged by his or her partner. Spouses report that the capacity to seek and offer forgiveness is one of the most important factors contributing to marital longevity and marital satisfaction (Fincham et al. 2004). Research consistently shows that forgiving the spouse enhances relationship intimacy and commitment, promotes better conflict resolution and has a positive influence on marital quality over the long haul (Fincham and Beach 2007; Fincham et al. 2004). Closely related to forgiveness is gratitude, the virtue of learning to give thanks. As a positive emotion, gratitude helps to create an upward spiral of relational wellbeing (Fredrickson et al. 2008; Fredrickson and Joiner 2002).

Injury in an intimate relationship engenders strong negative emotions. Sometimes, forgiveness or gratitude cannot be achieved immediately because the wounding or injury is of great significance to the person who is wounded (Johnson 2008). While any long-term relationship has to weather periodic disappointments, mishaps or mistakes, there are some moments that cause more emotional injury than others such as affairs, abandonment or abuse. Johnson describes these as attachment injuries because the negative interaction ruptures the attachment bond between the two partners in the relationship (Johnson 2008). In such circumstances, the wounded partner may justifiably react with anger or resentment, emotions Johnson refers to as secondary emotions that protect and hide the primary, more vulnerable emotions such as sadness, helplessness or hurt. Couples in healthy relationships recognize that replacing anger and resentment with grief or sadness ultimately allows movement towards a radical acceptance and healing (O'Connell 2008).

5.4.6 Empathic Attunement

Another key element of successful conflict management is empathic attunement (Gottman 2007). Attunement to each other's emotional experience, being able to imagine what the other person is thinking and feeling and being able to respond to the emotional needs of the partner rather than get caught up in defensiveness and blame can build relationship safety, regulate negative emotions in both self and others through positive limbic resonance (Hanson and Mendius 2009) and even heal attachment injuries (Johnson 2008). Empathic attunement also conveys the idea that one partner may not be able to prevent wounds or disappointments from happening, but will be emotionally present and willing to participate in the healing process. When one person hurts another in a committed relationship, no one else can offer the kind of healing the wounded partner needs more than the one attachment figure who caused the injury. This is the primary gift offered by empathic attunement, which is why couples that offer this are more likely to overcome negative experiences successfully.

Individual positivity and emotion regulation help each partner see the conflict in a balanced manner, reduce overreaction, recover quickly from negative events, repair successfully and maintain closeness even through difficult events (Fredrickson 2009). Fincham and Beach (2010) note that flourishing relationships are ones where each partner takes the responsibility and puts forth the effort to keep the relationship high in health and low in distress. When the two, individual skills and relational skills, are present in each partner, the relationship becomes resilient, which leads to flourishing, when conflict can be transformed into opportunities for greater intimacy and understanding (Fredrickson 2009; Gottman 2007), which in turn makes each person feel like they are part of a relational experience that has greater meaning, a life purpose or a spiritual bond.

5.5 Shared Meaning Dimension

Shared meaning is the aspect of a committed relationship that creates meaning and purpose to an intimate partnership. In the Sound Relationship House model, shared meaning has two levels or components. The first one is supporting and making each other's dreams come true. The second component is creating a shared culture, which is often done through the roles, rituals and traditions that are honoured within the family life of the partnership.

5.5.1 Making Dreams Come True

In order to support each other's dreams, each partner in the relationship has to maintain an active engagement and commitment to the relationship. Through that active commitment, and the safety and trust that are built in the relationship, each partner then has the opportunity to articulate their life dreams and try to be all that they can be. Research done in several cultures (Sharlin et al. 2000) found that couples in almost every culture spoke of being supportive of each other's wishes, careers and dreams as a key component of relationship satisfaction. Research shows that positivity within oneself breeds compassion and kindness which engenders gratitude with one's partner and pride in oneself for acting from a place of integrity or wholeness (Lyubomirsky 2007). The pride in one's actions then inspires visions of greater action, lofty dreams of action within the world and self-confidence and efficacy in carrying out these dreams. Again, one sees the positive feedback loop that helps individuals grow in themselves and in relationship through the practice of internal and external positive thoughts and actions. As Fredrickson (2009) found in her research, since positivity at the individual and relationship level broadens and builds physical, intellectual, psychological and social resources, couples in positive relationships develop the ability to be more flexible, creative, adaptive, receptive and far thinking, all of which has a direct correlation with success in life. This finding was confirmed through a meta-analysis of both experimental and correlational research that showed that happy people have greater levels of satisfaction with all spheres of experience including family, love, social support system, education and work, leisure activities and even housing and transportation (Lyubomirsky et al. 2005).

5.5.2 Building Shared Meaning

Individual dreams or successes are just one of the aspects of shared meaning in a committed relationship. When two adults join together to build a family bond with each other, the more their life together is characterized by symbolic actions and demonstrations of that family bond, the more meaningful the relationship feels to each partner (Gottman 2007). Seligman et al. (2005) found three main components to happiness: pleasure, engagement (or depth of involvement in family, work, hobbies, etc.) and meaning. Engagement and meaning were more important in the pursuit of happiness than pleasure (Wallis 2004). Shared meaning in a couple is created through mutual engagement in meaningful activities.

Bill Doherty (1997) wrote a book called *The Intentional Family*, where he affirms this notion that two people in a marriage are creating a new culture between them.

When this relational culture is characterized by roles, rituals, traditions or regular patterns of symbolic behaviour that has meaning, purpose or cultural context for each of them, the emotional bond between the partners feels stronger and more resilient. Roles represent the kind of explicit and implicit arrangements between partners for tasks and responsibilities within the relationship. If these roles capitalize on each person's strengths or interests and create a harmonious working arrangement, each partner's sense of stability and accountability within the relationship is enhanced. The roles do not need to follow a prescribed set of cultural values. The roles have to suit the two individuals in the relationship and honour each partner's upbringing, values, interests and strengths. As Wallerstein and Blakeslee (1995) found in their qualitative research, 'Every good marriage must adapt to the developmental changes in each partner, bending and yielding to the redefinitions that all men and women go through'. In a similar fashion, rituals are regular patterns of action that each person can count on as a symbol of what is important, meaningful and purposeful in their lives. Rituals can be formal and significant such as religious participation, holiday rituals, family events and other developmental moments or informal such as mundane or simple repeated acts that carry symbolic meaning such as waking up together, having meals together, parting and reunion rituals, shared chores or family play time. The richness of a family life can be measured by the quantity and quality of these moments of shared meaning that all members of the couple or family participate in and enjoy.

Shared meaning in flourishing relationships can also be about activities or rituals that occur outside the context of the couple relationship. As Fincham and Beach (2010) point out, in flourishing relationships the partners reward themselves with the kinds of friendships and activities that make them whole and more interesting. Partners do not depend only on each other to fulfil all of their needs. We become interesting to others when we thrive and grow by having outside interests and relationships that meet our needs in a healthy manner and help us feel alive, vital and productive. In that context, each partner brings something fresh and rich to the primary relationship from their other activities and network of relationships that feeds the primary relationship. It also means that each partner in the relationship asks for what they need and want from their partners but can tolerate disappointment or temporary unavailability by their partner because they have multiple avenues for meeting their needs. Honesty, transparency, trust and fidelity would, of course, be important elements that allow each person to trust that they can have many pathways to happiness and fulfilment that include the spouse or partner as a primary but not exclusive figure. Flourishing relationships are born out of flourishing human beings. Fincham and Beach (2010) suggest that a dynamic balance between one's focus on spousal relationship, family subsystems, other relational networks and community are aspects of healthy individual functioning. Individuals who feel part of a broad and complex relationship container are able to be productive citizens of their communities and societies and bring value to the world and not just their immediate circle of influence. Fincham and Beach also suggest that if we promote the 'mini-memes' of commitment, forgiveness, gratitude and sacrifice, then we have the ability to create a forward momentum in society that is based on positivity. If we could all live our lives as ambassadors of positivity, we stand a good chance of creating a huge impact in the world.

5.6   Summary

Love encompasses all other positive emotions such as awe, inspiration, pride, joy, hope, gratitude, serenity, interest and inspiration (Fredrickson 2009). The context in which these positive emotions are experienced, i.e. in an attachment bond, transforms them into love. Because of this multifaceted nature of love, it is more accurate to think of love as a journey through the many faces of positive emotions, some of them intense and dramatic such as joy or pride or awe and others more calming and soothing such as contentment, serenity and gratitude. Flourishing relationships are created through the positive emotional experiences and energy created both within a person and between two people. Relationships that thrive offer friendship, intimacy, affection, passion and hope. Individuals in thriving relationships don't just survive; they overcome and conquer the challenges of life and relationships. They feel like 'champions of love' (Fredrickson 2009) and they bring this pride, self-confidence and resilience to all aspects of their lives. Two adults choosing a filial relationship with each other in an equal, romantic and primary attachment bond form the kernel of society. From this adult attachment relationship arise the dreams, visions and actions that create family, community, society and the world culture. When we are able to teach adults to have positive thriving relationships, we are changing the world one couple at a time.

References

Algoe, S. B., & Haidt, J. (2009). Witnessing excellence in action: The 'other-praising' emotions of elevation, gratitude, and admiration. *The Journal of Positive Psychology, 4*(2), 105–127.

Algoe, S. B., Haidt, J., & Gable, S. L. (2008). Beyond reciprocity: Gratitude and relationships in everyday life. *Emotion, 8*(3), 425–429. doi:10.1037/1528-3542.8.3.425.

Algoe, S. B., Gable, S. L., & Maisel, N. (2010). It's the little things: Everyday gratitude as a booster shot for romantic relationships. *Personal Relationships, 17*(2), 217–233.

Atkinson, B. J. (2005). *Emotional intelligence in couples therapy: Advances in neurobiology and the science of intimate relationships.* New York: W.W. Norton and Company.

Banse, R. (2004). Adult attachment and marital satisfaction: Evidence for dyadic configuration effects. *Journal of Social and Personal Relationships, 21,* 273–282.

Cohen, O., Geron, Y., & Farchi, A. (2009). Marital quality and global well-being among older adult Israeli couples in enduring marriages. *American Journal of Family Therapy, 37,* 299–317.

Cohn, M. A., Fredrickson, B. L., Brown, S. L., Mikels, J. A., & Conway, A. M. (2009). Happiness unpacked: Positive emotions increase life satisfaction by building resilience. *Emotion, 9*(3), 361–368.

Coontz, S. (2006). The origins of modern divorce. *Family Process, 46*(1), 7–16.

Diener, E., & Seligman, M. E. P. (2002). Very happy people. *Psychological Science, 13*(1), 81–84.

Doherty, W. (1997). *The intentional family: How to build family ties in our modern world.* New York: Perseus Books.

Driver, J. L., & Gottman, J. M. (2004). Daily marital interactions and positive affect during marital conflict among newlywed couples. *Family Process, 43*(3), 301–314.

Driver, J., Tabares, A., Shapiro, A., Nahm, E. Y., & Gottman, J. M. (2003). Interactional patterns in marital success and failure: Gottman laboratory studies. In F. Walsh (Ed.), *Normal family processes: Growing diversity and complexity* (3rd ed., pp. 493–513). New York: Guilford Press.

Fincham, F. D., & Beach, S. R. H. (2007). Forgiveness and marital quality: Precursor or consequence in well-established relationships? *The Journal of Positive Psychology, 2*(4), 260–268.

Fincham, F. D., & Beach, S. R. H. (2010). Of memes and marriage: Towards a positive relationship science. *Journal of Family Theory and Review, 2*, 4–24.

Fincham, F. D., Beach, S. R. H., & Davila, J. (2004). Forgiveness and conflict resolution in marriage. *Journal of Family Psychology, 18*(1), 72–81.

Fredrickson, B. (2009). *Positivity: Groundbreaking research reveals how to embrace the hidden strength of positive emotions, overcome negativity, and thrive.* New York: Crown Publishing.

Fredrickson, B., & Joiner, T. (2002). Positive emotions trigger upward spirals towards emotional wellbeing. *Psychological Science, 13*(2), 172–175.

Fredrickson, B. L., Cohn, M. A., Coffey, K. A., Pek, J., & Finkel, S. M. (2008). Open hearts build lives: Positive emotions, induced through loving-kindness meditation, build consequential personal resources. *Journal of Personality and Social Psychology, 9*(5), 1045–1062.

Gable, S. L., & Haidt, J. (2005). What (and why) is positive psychology? *Review of General Psychology, 9*(2), 103–110. doi:10.1037/1089-2680.9.2.103.

Gable, S. L., Reis, H. T., Impett, E., & Asher, E. R. (2004). What do you do when things go right? The intrapersonal and interpersonal benefits of sharing positive events. *Journal of Personality and Social Psychology, 87*(2), 228–245.

Gottman, J. M. (1995). *Why marriages succeed or fail: And how you can make yours last.* New York: Simon and Schuster.

Gottman, J. M. (1999). *The marriage clinic: A scientifically based marital therapy.* New York: Norton.

Gottman, J. M. (2007). *Marital therapy: A research-based approach. Training manual for the level I professional workshop for clinicians.* Seattle: The Gottman Institute.

Gottman, J. M., & Krokoff, L. J. (1989). Marital interaction and satisfaction: A longitudinal view. *Journal of Consulting and Clinical Psychology, 57*(1), 47–52.

Gottman, J. M., & Silver, N. (2000). *The seven principles for making marriage work: A practical guide from the country's foremost relationship expert.* New York: Three Rivers Press.

Gottman, J. M., Coan, J., Swanson, C., & Carrere, S. (1998). Predicting marital happiness and stability from newlywed interactions. *Journal of Marriage and the Family, 60*, 5–22.

Hahlweg, K., Revenstorf, D., & Schindler, L. (1984). Effects of behavioural marital therapy on couples' communication and problem-solving skills. *Journal of Consulting and Clinical Psychology, 52*(4), 553–566.

Halford, K. W., Lizzio, A., Wilson, K. L., & Occhipinti, S. (2007). Does working at your marriage help? Couple relationship self-regulation and satisfaction in the first 4 years of marriage. *Journal of Family Psychology, 21*(2), 185–194.

Hanson, R., & Mendius, R. (2009). *The Buddha's brain: The practical neuroscience of happiness, love, and wisdom.* Oakland: New Harbinger Publications.

Johnson, S. (2008). *Hold me tight: Seven conversations for a lifetime of love.* New York: Little Brown and Company.

Jourard, S. (1959). Self-disclosure and other-cathexis. *Journal of Consulting and Clinical Psychology*, February 1980, *48*(1), 117–118.

Kantrowitz, B., & Wingert, P. (1999, April 19). The science of a good marriage. *Newsweek, 133*(16), 52–58.

Kaslow, F. (2001). Families and family psychology: Intersecting crossroads. *American Psychologist, 56*(1), 37–46.

Katzir, M., Eyal, T., Meiran, N., & Kessler, Y. (2010). Imagined positive emotions and inhibitory control: The differentiated effect of pride versus happiness. *Journal of Experimental Psychology. Learning, Memory, and Cognition, 36*(5), 1314–1320.

Kesner, J. (2008). Why happy couples fight. *Prevention, 60*(9), 144.

Kornfield, J. (2008). *The art of forgiveness, loving kindness, and peace.* New York: Bantam.

Luskin, F. (2003). *Forgive for good.* New York: HarperOne.

Lyubomirsky, S. (2007). *The how of happiness: The scientific approach to getting the life you want.* New York: The Penguin Press.

Lyubomirsky, S., King, L., & Diener, E. (2005). The benefits of frequent positive affect: Does happiness lead to success? *Psychological Bulletin, 131*(6), 803–855.

McCarthy, B. W., & McCarthy, E. (2009). *Discovering your couple sexual style: Sharing desire, pleasure, and satisfaction.* New York: Routledge.

O'Connell, M. (2008). *The marriage benefit: The surprising rewards of staying together.* New York: Springboard Press.

Rehman, U. S., & Holtzworth-Munroe, A. (2007). A cross-cultural examination of the relation of marital communication behaviour to marital satisfaction. *Journal of Family Psychology, 21*(4), 759–763.

Robinson, E. A., & Price, M. G. (1980). Pleasurable behaviour in marital interaction: An observational study. *Journal of Consulting and Clinical Psychology, 48*(1), 117–118.

Sandhya, S. (2009). The social context of marital happiness in urban Indian couples: Interplay of intimacy and conflict. *Journal of Marital and Family Therapy, 35*(1), 74–96.

Seligman, M. E. P., & Csikszentmihalyi, M. (2000). Positive psychology: An introduction. *American Psychologist, 55*(1), 5–14. doi:10.1037//0003-066X.55.1.5.

Seligman, M. E. P., Steen, T. A., Park, N., & Peterson, C. (2005). Positive psychology progress: Empirical validation of interventions. *American Psychologist, 60*(5), 410–421. doi:10.1037/0003-066X.60.5.410.

Sharlin, S. A., Kaslow, F. W., & Hammerschmidt, H. (2000). *Together through thick and thin: A multinational study of long-term marriages.* Binghamton: Haworth Clinical Practice Press.

Shetty, P. (2009). India learns the meaning of divorce. *The Guardian.* guardian.co.uk, Wednesday February 25, 2009, 13.00 GMT.

Strachman, A., & Gable, S. L. (2006). Approach and avoidance relationship commitment. *Motivation and Emotion, 30*(2), 117–126. doi:10.1007/s11031-006-9026-9.

Tucker, M. B., & Crouter, A. C. (2008, April). Enduring couples in varying sociocultural contexts. *Family Relations, 57,* 113–116.

Waite, L. J., & Gallagher, M. (2001). *The case for marriage: Why married people are happier, healthier, and better off financially.* New York: Broadway.

Wallerstein, J. S., & Blakeslee, S. (1995). *The good marriage: How and why love lasts.* New York: Houghton Mifflin.

Wallis, C. (2004). The science of happiness. *Time Magazine,* January 17, 2005.

Vagdevi Meunier is a clinical psychologist and Associate Professor at St. Edwards University in Austin, Texas. She has a private clinical and consulting practice in Austin where she specializes in couples and family therapy, couples workshops, training and supervision, and organisational consultation. She is a consultant and trainer with the Gottman Institute.
Contact: vagdevim@gmail.com

Wayne Baker is a professional counsellor and in private practice in Austin, Texas. He specializes in working with couples surviving the damage of infidelity and adult trauma survivors. He leads groups for men and couples.
Contact: wayne@waynebakerlpc.com

Chapter 6
Positive Parent–Child Relationships

Kimberley O'Brien and Jane Mosco

6.1 Parenting in the Twenty-First Century

Family relationships in the Western world have been affected by rapid social and technological changes. Parents are pressured to work longer hours while young children spend more time with alternative carers both within and outside the home. While there is ongoing political pressure in several Western countries to improve maternity and paternity leave and provide subsidised childcare, the majority of families make do with minimal economic and practical assistance when raising infants and toddlers.

Parents usually want the best for their children whatever they conceive this to be. Unlike previous generations, today's parents are faced with an information industry offering suggestions on every angle of the parenting process. Parenting 'gurus' proliferate, sometimes giving different advice or emphasising different aspects of the role. Although the word 'parents' is commonly used, there is still an expectation that it is women who take on this primary responsibility with men being the main breadwinners. This division of labour is less and less the norm, although there are clear indications that even where women are working full time outside the home, they still do most of the work within it and take on the primary responsibility for many of the tasks inherent in parenting (Crompton 2006).

More children than ever spend time being cared for outside the family, and there are a plethora of recommendations concerning the quality of that care. Other specific issues that impact the modern parent–child relationship include work demands, greater mobility, the scattering of the extended family, family breakdown and single parenthood. There is regular media coverage on family life; from the general problems of parenting and growing up in today's world to the need to protect children

K. O'Brien (✉)
Quirky Kid Clinic, P.O. Box 598, Woollahra, NSW 2025
e-mail: kimberley@quirkykid.com.au

J. Mosco
Bishop Druitt College, P.O. Box 8004, 111 North Boambee Rd, Coffs Harbour, NSW 2450
e-mail: jmosco@bdc.nsw.edu.au

S. Roffey (ed.), *Positive Relationships: Evidence Based Practice across the World*,
DOI 10.1007/978-94-007-2147-0_6, © Springer Science+Business Media B.V. 2012

from abuse and neglect. This chapter explores the evidence, rather than any current zeitgeist on factors and approaches that enable parents to be the best they can be – in order to facilitate the authentic wellbeing of their children (Suldo 2009).

6.2 Parenting Styles

Parental responsibility for children and their development varies in emphasis across time and culture. It includes foci on physical health, spiritual development, cultural transmission, socialisation, emotional health and cognitive development. Here we explore what is of benefit to children in all domains of their development – enhancing their ability to flourish and achieve authentic wellbeing.

Parents' relationships with their children are strongly linked with outcomes (Amato 2000; Demo and Cox 2000). The most harmonious and positive parent–child relationships share similar qualities from birth to adolescence although specific practices change as children grow. Baumrind's (1967) classic research identified four styles of parenting in preschool-age families. These are:

- The neglectful *uninvolved* parent
- The controlling and detached *authoritarian* parent
- The warm *permissive* parent with low expectations for their children and weak boundaries for behaviour
- The warm, responsive and encouraging *authoritative* parent with high age-appropriate expectations and limits for their children and the provision of support to meet these (DeHart et al. 2000)

Baumrind found that preschool children in *authoritarian* households were more hostile and less independent, while *permissive* parents were more likely to raise children who were less achievement-oriented and did not develop appropriate independence or resilience. The most self-reliant, content, adaptable and cooperative children were raised by *authoritative* parents. This theory has now extended to children of all ages (Baumrind 1989; Maccoby and Martin 1983) confirming that authoritative parenting predicts healthy child adjustment (Amato 2000; Demo and Cox 2000).

Numerous 'parenting experts' have since explored positive strategies to complement this parenting style, with 'step-by-step suggestions' for raising happy kids (Hartley-Brewer 2004) and creating a 'phenomenal family' (McGraw 2004). These approaches regularly refer to positive strategies such as giving praise and devoting time, enhancing motivation and self-confidence, building respect, trust and security and encouraging independence and self-reliance. Popular catch phrases are littered within parenting literature, such as purposeful parenting: 'the modelling of good emotional and mental stability in order to be the role model your children will remember' (McGraw 2004); proactive parenting: 'we don't wait for things to go wrong before we reflect on our parenting strategies' (Walker 2010); unconditional parenting: 'children shouldn't have to earn a parents approval and they should always feel loved' (Kohn 2005) and positive parenting: 'parents who do not overplay their role of police for civilization, lest they invite avoidable resentment, resistance and hostility' (Ginott and Goddard 2003). A warm, responsive, supportive parenting style with high expectations is also referred to as 'facilitative' in some of the literature (Bryant 2001; Roffey 2011).

6.3   Learning Parenting Styles

Parenting styles develop from a combination of the parents' own experiences as children and the society in which they live, including the books they read, the friends they keep and their exposure to different expectations within the community (Buss 2005). Although these influences are usually found locally, ideas about parenting may accumulate through exchanges with other cultures or through extended family, such as grandparents of migrants who remain in the country of origin. This may cause conflict for parents who may need to reflect on what is the best interests of the child in the setting in which they are being raised. Parenting styles are often not questioned until something goes awry. A parent may seek help to change their child in some way and discover they need to change how they are parenting.

6.4   Core Principles Underpinning Positive Parent–Child Relationships

Understanding: All human relationships are perpetually changing. Maintaining a healthy and enduring relationship requires the ability to empathise with someone, understand their needs and appreciate their alternative perspectives. Effective parenting includes an understanding of how children develop and learn, and what motivates them. Children are also individuals – tuning into their specific likes, dislikes, sensitivities and strengths builds the ability to respond well to their needs as they grow. We must also understand ourselves – what we can expect of ourselves as parents and what support we will require along the parenting pathway (Walker 2010).

Mutual respect: This is vital in any healthy relationship. Parents who try to impose their own will on a child are likely to be met with resentment or a simmering sense of frustration (Kohn 2005). Respect means being willing to listen to children and look at situations from their perspective. Even if a parent has the final say in making decisions in the best interest of the child, showing that views of the child are taken into consideration reduces potential power struggles. Self-determination theory (Ryan and Deci 2000) indicates that young people need to feel autonomous, experience choice and feel listened to. Conversely, where parents use a controlling parenting style, children may learn to try to control others through bullying behaviours (Assor et al. 2002). By acknowledging children's feelings, desires and questions, parents model ways that promote both prosocial behaviour and authentic independence. Positive parents are flexible, able to compromise and work towards mutual goals. For example, if there is a need to reorganise bedroom allocations, the whole family can discuss alternative solutions together. Although parents might make the final decision, this is likely to be more acceptable to the children when authentic consultation has taken place. With an authoritarian parent, the decision may be made without reference to anyone else in the family, who are then expected to comply, often with resentment.

Open communication: The quality of communication between parent and child is an indicator of the mutual respect and dignity existing within the parent–child relationship. Adults with the skills to enter the world of children in a compassionate and caring way are helping children to trust their inner reality and develop self-confidence (Ginott 1965). Parents who reflect on themselves and the relationships they share with their children are less likely to be rigid, impatient or negative. This may involve admitting they made a wrong decision or apologising for an unthoughtful comment. These interactions help children learn richer and more developed interpersonal and intrapersonal skills. A parent who listens well and is open to questions teaches the child to articulate emotions safely.

Time: Setting aside time to nurture the parent–child relationship is another key to continuing good communication as children mature into young adults (Sanders 2008). Simply spending time with a parent makes children feel valued and worthy of attention particularly where parents follow the young person's lead and participate in an activity the child has chosen. For those who have to compete for their parent's attention this is especially valuable (McNeely and Barber 2010). Giving children attention in the absence of distractions, such as television or competing siblings, provides opportunities for developing new mutual interests, resolving any conflict, maintaining trust, accessing emotional availability and providing close proximity for physical affection. Children also like to be included in adult activities, such as building projects and cooking. Being given responsibilities in such joint endeavours promotes a sense of connection essential for wellbeing and resilience and can foster a sense of independence and confidence – especially if the child is allowed to make and learn from mistakes.

6.5   Family Resilience

The literature on family resilience indicates common factors across diverse cultural and ethnic groups that are globally recognisable (Patterson 2002).

Family resilience factors are described as:

- *Having a positive outlook*: such as looking for the best in a situation, acting as though you imagine that things will turn out well.

- *Having consistency of family member accord*: working consciously to reduce stress in the household and use positive conflict resolution techniques.
- *Engaging in flexibility*: being open to spontaneous plans, or changing your mind when it seems appropriate.
- *Using positive family communication*: noticing and acknowledging when children are behaving well, using positive and reinforcing language. Having many more positive than negative statements in daily interactions.
- *Practising sound financial management*: use budgets and forward planning to ensure you can meet your financial commitments.
- *Participation in shared recreation*: going fishing, swimming or baking a cake together.
- *Following regular routines and rituals*: these may include having a regular bedtime routine (game, bath, book, bed) special dinners or celebrations.
- *Being engaged in spirituality*: this may involve saying blessings before meals, engaging in regular meditation or discussing mindfulness around the dinner table.
- *Belonging to wider support networks*, such as a local soccer club, faith-based community or community garden. (Black and Lobo 2008).

These qualities of family resilience are essential tools for leading a meaningful life as well as benefiting the positive development of our children. Although the family unit has gone through many developments and changes, the depth of special meaning it has for people hasn't changed. Family life is reported to be responsible for many significant aspects of our lives, and for many people, positive family experiences are focused around love and security (DCSF 2010).

6.6   Parenting Style and Prosocial Behaviour

The relationship between parenting style and a child's prosocial behaviour-behaviour has been studied extensively (e.g. Eisenberg and Fabes 1998; Bierhoff 2002; Grusec et al. 2002). Parental warmth, use of reasoning and autonomy support enhance a child's ability to empathise and adopt prosocial behaviour (Clark and Ladd 2000; Krevans and Gibbs 1996) where a power-assertive behaviour management approach is much less effective – especially over time. Where parents provide children with a caring model this increases both the child's willingness to attend to parental messages and their accuracy in detecting these messages (Knafo and Schwartz 2003; Smetana et al. 2009; Staub 1979). In one example, children observed to have a warm relationship with their parents were rated by their teachers as more prosocial in that their considerate behaviour was intended to benefit others (Clark and Ladd 2000). Parents who express negative feelings toward their children are more likely to raise children with less prosocial behaviour (Deater-Deckard et al. 2001). Authoritative parents also set clear limits and standards of behaviour and utilise an approach that aims to explain and teach the preferred behaviour. This encourages learning and forgiving, allowing children to engage in problem solving and increase their independence.

6.7   A Focus on Fathers

Although fathers are less often the focus of parenting research, studies confirm the value of active and authoritative parenting styles for both parents.

When fathers are more involved in children's lives, children experience better friendships and more empathy, have increased educational achievement and a positive sense of self (Flouri 2005). Today's fathers are being more involved in children's lives (Gray 2006) and research suggests that engaging fathers throughout pregnancy and the birth of babies, is more likely to lead to fathers remaining actively involved in bringing up their children (May 1978). There are indications (Craig 2006; Tan 1997) that the higher a father's educational qualification, the more time he will spend with his children. The quality of that relationship remains crucial. Data from an urban Southern Visayan region supported Filipino fathers' involvement in parenting with regards to positive outcomes for school age and adolescent children. This was particularly so for boys when fathers utilised an authoritative style (Harper 2010). Although the best outcome for adolescents results from having two authoritative parents, Simons and Conger (2007) found that having just one could generally protect young people from the more negative impacts of other less preferable styles of parenting.

6.8   Ecological Factors That Contribute to Positive Parent–Child Relationships

To better understand how broader social systems contribute to child development, Urie Bronfenbrenner (1979) developed *The Ecology of Human Development* theory. He identified four levels within nested systems. The *microsystem* (such as the family or classroom); the *mesosystem* (which is the interaction between those at the microsystem, such as a teacher and parent); the *exosystem* (external environments which indirectly influence development, e.g. parental workplace); and the *macrosystem* (the larger sociocultural context). Bronfrenbrenner later added a fifth system, called the *chronosystem* (the evolution of the external systems over time).

Each system contains roles, norms and rules that can powerfully shape development. Although the biggest impact on children is centred around what happens in the home, parents also make important decisions external to family interactions for their children, including which educational philosophy, sport or political party to embrace.

Empirical research suggests that strong and stable relationships in the family home have the greatest impact on a child's happiness and healthy development (DCSF 2009). As 'the conductor of the family orchestra' (Harold 2001), positive adult relationships set the tone of children's family experiences as does the level of marital accord (Walsh 1998, 2002).

Parents who are happier in their relationships participate in more positive relationships with their young children (Simons et al. 1993), so it is not surprising that there is a strong association between the quality of the partners' relationship and better child outcomes (Coleman and Glenn 2009). Children report that the experience of parental conflict is stressful for them, and as a result children can withdraw, become anxious or aggressive (DCSF 2009).

Even in families where parents have separated, when the adults involved manage to work co-operatively, children cope better (Rodgers and Pryor 1998). It is the quality of the relationship with the non-resident parent rather than the frequency of the contact that is important (Gilmore 2006). Positive and consistent parenting with regards to behaviour, support and involvement, is linked with increased academic and behavioural outcomes (London Economics 2007).

Children's happiness also depends on the relationships they witness between other adults residing in their home environment, such as grandparents or alternative carers (DCSF 2010), and the relationships these adults have with them. It is the quality of the relationships not the form of family unit itself that is important.

Children and adolescents are particularly vulnerable to the impact of tension between adults and to the reactions or mood swings of carers experiencing stress or tiredness. Parents exhibiting erratic or extreme responses to their child's behaviour are likely to trigger fear, confusion or mistrust within the parent–child relationship. Children's wellbeing depends on the adults in their life being reliable and predictable, providing guidance, meeting both emotional and material needs as well as setting reasonable limits on behaviour. Finkenauer and colleagues (2004) reported that when children from Holland shared sensitive and personal information with a parent, they reported increased family contentment.

As internal family dynamics are impacted by external factors including alternative care arrangements and extended working hours for parents, we need to consider the impact of factors beyond the immediate care-giving environment.

6.9 Parent Support

The more supported parents are, the better placed they are to support children and to parent more positively (DCSF 2010).

There are key developmental periods and pressure points where additional education and support are most beneficial. These include the steep learning curve of becoming a new parent, of managing the toddler years, starting school and during the transition at adolescence from child to adulthood. Educational programmes on positive parenting skills can be successful in supporting parents at these times (Moran et al. 2004; de Graaf et al. 2008)

When parents are able to access practical support such as flexible work practices, assistance with caring for children during holidays, times of ill health, or attending school occasions, children benefit. This relieves stress and enables parents to be more involved in their children's lives.

6.10 Developmental Aspects of Positive Parent–Child Relationships

6.10.1 Bonding and Attachment – The First 9 Months

Parents begin their journey before their child is born, with quality health care for mind and body during pregnancy and birth. Stress reduction and extra support at this stage can make a difference to how a mother feels about her role and this in turn may impact on how she responds to her baby.

Securing a healthy and enduring attachment with a child occurs between birth and 9 months (Ainsworth and Bowlby 1991). These early months and the baby's first experiences of the world are crucial. Babies respond to the levels of responsiveness of their carers. Between 6 and 10 weeks there is engagement with the social smile (Sroufe and Waters 1976), by 3 months babies are smiling when they are socialising and interacting with other people (Ellsworth et al. 1993). When parents are playful with their child they can influence a baby's reactions (Repacholi 1998).

According to Bowlby's Attachment Theory, infants require a close and continuous care-giving relationship with a supportive and stable parental figure in order to thrive both physically and emotionally (Bowlby 1973; Ainsworth et al. 1978). In some cases, the bonding process between mother and baby is disrupted through separation, deprivation, depression or bereavement. For infants living in alternative care, primary attachment figures are still essential in the development of security, trust and self-worth (Cassidy 1999; Verschueren and Marcoen 1999). It does not have to be the biological mother.

Gerhardt (2004) highlighted the importance of 'love' in healthy infant brain development. By this she means the extent to which a baby needs are met and ways in which these are met. Emotional nurturing and responsiveness to an infant's attempt to make connections is fundamental and when these needs are unmet there is a rise in stress and levels of cortisol, which has implications for future development. Gerhardt explored how a baby's earliest relationships shape their nervous system and how the development of the brain can affect future emotional wellbeing with particular reference to the way children (and adults) later respond to stress.

Summarising the empirical research on secure and insecure attachments, Sroufe and colleagues (2005) conclude that the beneficial effects of secure attachments are observed in harmonious parent–child relationships and in satisfying, close friendships at later stages of development. A parent's ability to assess a situation from the child's perspective enhances attachment and a positive parent–child relationship (Velderman et al. 2006). A mother's ability to respond promptly to signs of fear, stress, tiredness and hunger for example are fundamental to secure attachment. Research suggests more empathic parents are better able to form close, mutually responsive relationships with their young children (Kochanska 1997).

6.10.2   Toddlers in Today's World

Toddlers are busy people, responding to physical play, seeking out parental affection, and learning new skills. Parenting that results in shared positive affect – when both parent and child experience positive emotions – has broad adaptive consequences for development, including children's security, early morality and eagerness to imitate parents (Kochanska and Aksan 1995; Aksan and Kochanska 2004). Proactive and responsive parenting, which 'tracks' the child during the day, allows adults to anticipate child needs, notice subtle cues such as tiredness and ensure safety, including encounters with peers. This helps toddlers cope with distress before it becomes intense.

Mothers' internal knowledge of attachment seems important. Vaughn et al. (2007) found that in three sociocultural groups, the mother's ability to create stories rich in attachment themes about everyday events predicted children's ability to use their mother as a secure base when at home, coming to her when they were distressed or needed support. Maternal responsiveness to distress is linked positively with the development of empathic abilities and prosocial behaviours in young children (Davidov and Grusec 2006). For young children in care, quality care can be determined in part by the carer's ability to be responsive to the child's needs.

Early childhood is a time to experience autonomy and become more independent. Some children do this with passion. 'No, me do it' every other minute can be frustrating for busy parents. Children are also naturally curious and want to explore in areas that parents may see as risky. This boundary pushing can involve seemingly challenging behaviours. The key is to recognise this developmental stage and not misinterpret the behaviours as 'naughty', disobedient or disrespectful. Having a clear and structured response to issues of challenging behaviour supports parents to maintain positive parent–child relationships.

Understanding their child's temperament can help parents have realistic expectations. Fearfulness in shyer infants can be reduced by warm, supportive parenting that lowers cortisol (Gunnar et al. 1997). Other strategies include using regular routines and rhythms and responding to needs of the child as they arise. As well as setting age appropriate guidelines, distraction, imitation and modelling reinforces desired behaviour as does noticing when the sought after behaviour is practised.

Parenting can at times hamper healthy development even though intentions are caring. The phenomenon of anxious parents hovering over their own children is sometimes known as 'helicopter parenting' resulting in 'bubble-wrapped kids'. Risk-taking is inhibited and children lack opportunities to explore their own capacities, particularly in terms of physical play. Occupational therapists (Jackson-King 2010) have identified delays in developmental milestones, such as walking, running and climbing due to these inhibitions. Gill (2007) also gives evidence that children's restricted experiences of childhood are hampering their natural development as parents are fearful of the potential risks involved in explortion and experimentation. Children need encouragement to test out their growing capacities. Too much restriction not only impairs physical wellbeing but also ultimately children's social and psychological wellbeing including their relationship with their parents (Nelson 2010).

6.10.3 Positive Parenting in Middle Childhood

As children develop to school age and beyond, the same key concepts of warmth, support, high expectations, boundary setting and responsiveness remain critical to effective relationships. When family life has supported children positively in early childhood, this stage of middle childhood (6–11 years) can focus on mastery of skills and increased peer interactions both in school and home, as physical, social and cognitive abilities increase. Across cultures, children this age take on greater responsibilities in the family. In Malawi, when Ngoni children lose their first teeth around 6 years, this indicates their new role. Boys move away from family groupings, independence is encouraged and children are now held accountable for their behaviour (Read 1968; Rogoff 1996)

Parents assist children in developing both independence and competence by teaching skills around the house and monitoring schoolwork. Parents who are firm but have reasonable expectations of behaviour and standards and support children in meeting these, this helps children feel good about their developing skills (Dekovic and Meeus 1997; Feiring and Taska 1996). A controlling style reinforces children's non-competence, either through having things done for them by adults or by belittling their efforts, whilst a permissive style encourages a false sense of self, leading the child to doubt themselves as they get older (Damon 1995). Positive communication is important. Letting children know that it is ok to make mistakes strengthens children's ability to bounce back and try again.

Although parents remain highly influential at this time, peers are also increasing in focus as a key area of feedback for children. Many spend more time with their siblings than with their parents (McHale and Crouter 1996). While most parents strive to maintain a positive relationship with their children, there is greater variability in the degree brothers and sisters get along. Evidence suggests that problematic parent–child relationships go hand in hand with more hostile sibling relationships (Brody et al. 1994; Easterbrooks and Emde 1988), whereas the most positive sibling relationships typically evolve in households with positive parent–child relationships. There is a bidirectional influence between positive relationships within the family and prosocial behaviour outside the family. Parents who encourage and foster cooperative and pretend play between siblings are more likely to raise children with greater social understanding and enhanced social skills in peer group situations (Downey and Condron 2004). Positive dynamics between all family members is not only dependent on the parent–child relationship, but also related to how much parent's foster positive relations between siblings in early/middle childhood.

6.10.4   Journeying Towards Adolescence and Beyond

Adolescent development involves complex changes in many areas. Young people are not only maturing physically and biologically, they are increasingly using abstract thinking to explore their understanding of the world and their own identity. The transition from child to adult involves freedoms and responsibilities associated with this bumpy terrain and the parent–child relationship often needs to change in response. These changes are often linked with the cultural milieu. For example Hispanic adolescent boys' relationships with parents were found to improve, as this reflects the cultural traditional status of male roles in the society (Molina and Chassin 1996).

Fuller (2008) points out that the frontal lobes are the last part of the brain to fully mature. This leaves adolescents primed for emotions, romance and running away but not so much for planning, being in control of impulsive reactions and thinking ahead (Dahl 2004; Geidd 2004). Parents can assist their offspring create cognitive pathways that support positive, helpful thinking and learning habits. One way of doing this is to develop co-regulation, in which young people are increasingly encouraged to make their own decisions about things that affect them (Masten 2004). This needs to start in middle childhood and gradually increase as they grow towards adulthood. Rather than tell their teenager what to do, parents ask questions about the things that need to be taken into account, consequences of different decisions and how these help to meet long term goals, not just short term outcomes. This encourages thinking rather than impulsivity and helps the young person feel parents are listening to them. Although teenagers may still make what adults consider to be 'bad' decisions at times this approach leaves the door open for continuing conversation.

Not surprisingly this period of time can be confusing for everyone. It is helpful for parents to be aware of teenage development so interactions are based on realistic expectations. Studies identify adolescents asserting their independence as one of the greatest sources of conflict within the family unit and the greatest threat to an otherwise positive parent–child relationship. In a large cross-sectional study that spanned ages 6 through 18 years, Loeber et al. (2000) found that positive aspects of parenting decreased markedly through middle adolescence.

The life tasks of adolescents are to explore, take risks, become more autonomous and develop their own unique identity. The task of parents is to keep their child safe, on the pathway to healthy wellbeing and coach them well for adulthood. Conflict is therefore often part of the journey. The research also points out, however, that positive relationships with parents can act as a mediator for outcomes of wellbeing (Hayes et al. 2004). Even in this heavily influenced peer environment parenting practices and family belonging do still have a significant effect on wellbeing outcomes for young people (Csikszentmihalyi and Schneider 2001) during this intense developmental stage.

Promoting resilience strategies enables young people to maintain a sense of belonging to the family and reassured that their views matter and are taken into account. This can include having meals together and celebrating birthday and family customs. Spending time with teenagers on their own (Ashbourne and Daly 2010), engaging positively with their friends and encouraging them to actively engage with a variety of people and other organisations are all effective strategies. Adolescents also learn about themselves and relationships from parents who attend to their own wellbeing and social life, including caring for their adult marital relationship.

The parent–child relationship continues to change as adolescents mature. For young adults who chose to leave home and become more independent, there is another shift as both parties explore new roles, such as friend or mentor (Peel 2003). Dornbusch et al. (1987) suggest that authoritative parenting maintains its effectiveness across the developmental journey and is particularly valuable during the adolescent stage in its more democratic nature.

6.11   Cultural Influences on Parenting

Although some literature discusses differences in parenting practices across cultures, ethnic and religious groups, research also indicates some similarities. One such area is that of parental support. Adolescents across diverse groups showed that different parental support can elicit the same meaning in young people from other cultural backgrounds, indicating that instrumental support and emotional support are connected. For example in countries where money or education may be rare and valued, this is seen as an example of parental support by adolescents, whilst in another country, quality time with one another may be rare and valued, and this is seen as parental support (McNeely and Barber 2010).

Just as every parent–child relationship is different, parents from different racial and ethnic communities may attach different priorities to different aspects of parenting. For example, according to Spicer (2010), African–American parents are less likely than Hispanic and white parents to see routines and discussions of feelings as centrally important in the earliest years, whereas white parents are more likely than African–American and Hispanic parents to see setting and enforcing rules, comforting an upset child, and encouraging a child to persist in difficult tasks as important. In all cases, the majority of parents in any population endorse the importance of supportive parenting behaviours, but these subtle differences may indicate potential targets for increased dialogue and understanding on how parents can shape early social and emotional development.

In a literature review of intercultural marriages, Crippen and Brew (2007) found that cultural differences can become amplified when parenting children, each developmental stage potentially triggering new conflicts. Addressing these cultural differences ensures that children have a way to express their feelings and assist with identity formation. When culturally assertive behaviours are expressed in a helpful and respectful way, the parenting process itself can be the medium for passing on the cultural values and practices between parents and children (Keller et al. 2004). Other benefits of intercultural parenting (Vivero and Jenkins 1999) are promoting 'broader, stronger, social and cognitive skill sets, greater interpersonal flexibility and less ethnocentric attitude'. Johnson (1995) noted that these challenges and diversity led to family resilience in the areas of creative problem solving and drawing on strengths to overcome difficulties. Again, the conscious choice of parenting style can focus on the positive things that unite us, resulting in a healthier and stronger family.

6.12   Conclusion

A wealth of evidence points to a positive, balanced and facilitative approach to parenting as fostering a constructive and effective relationship between parent and child, leading to the best outcomes for children and young people. This warm and caring approach accompanied by high expectations and clear boundaries, supports the journey of development from the key attachment period in infancy, to the school-age years and into adolescence. Positive parenting encompasses the flexibility to respond to each unique stage with mutual respect and open communication. Throughout different cultures and ethnic groups, taking the essence of this facilitative approach provides a compass for navigating the way to wellbeing for parents, carers and children alike.

References

Ainsworth, M. D. S., & Bowlby, J. (1991). An ethological approach to personality development. *American Psychologist, 46*, 331–341.

Ainsworth, M. D. S., Blehar, M. C., Waters, E., & Wall, S. (1978). *Patterns of attachment: Psychological study of the strange situation*. Hillsdale: Erlbaum.

Aksan, N., & Kochanska, G. (2004). Heterogeneity of joy in infancy. *Infancy, 6*(1), 79–94.

Amato, P. R. (2000). The consequences of divorce for adults and children. *Journal of Marriage and Family, 62*, 1269–1287.

Ashbourne, L. M., & Daly, K. (2010). Parents and adolescents making time choices: "Choosing a relationship". *Journal of Family Issues, 31*(11), 1419–41.

Assor, A., Kaplan, H., & Roth, G. (2002). Choice is good but relevance is excellent: Autonomy effecting teacher behaviours that predict students' engagement in learning. *British Journal of Educational Psychology, 72*, 261–278.

Baumrind, D. (1967). Child care practices anteceding three patterns of preschool behaviour. *Genetic Psychology Monographs, 75*, 43–88.

Baumrind, D. (1989). Rearing competent children. In M. Damon (Ed.), *Child development today and tomorrow* (pp. 349–378). San Francisco: Jossey-Bass.

Bierhoff, H. W. (2002). *Prosocial behaviour*. Hove: Psychology Press.

Black, K., & Lobo, M. (2008). A conceptual review of family resilience factors. *Journal of Family Nursing, 14*, 33.

Bowlby, J. (1973). *Attachment and loss: Vol 2. Separation: Anxiety and anger*. New York: Basic Books.

Brody, G. H., Stoneman, Z., & McCoy, J. K. (1994). Forecasting sibling relationships in early adolescence from child temperaments and family processes in middle childhood. *Child Development, 65*, 771–784.

Bronfenbrenner, U. (1979). *The ecology of human development*. Cambridge: Harvard University Press.

Bryant, K. E. (2001). *Parenting styles and spiritual maturity*. Ph.D. Thesis, University of Texas, Austin.

Buss, D. M. (Ed.). (2005). *The handbook of evolutionary psychology*. Hoboken: Wiley.

Cassidy, J. (1999). The nature of the child's ties. In J. Cassidy & P. R. Shaver (Eds.), *Handbook of attachment: Theory, research and clinical applications* (pp. 3–20). New York: Guilford Press.

Clark, K. E., & Ladd, G. W. (2000). Connectedness and autonomy support in parent-child relationships: Links to children's socio-emotional orientation and peer relationships. *Developmental Psychology, 36*, 485–498.

Coleman, L., & Glenn, G. (2009). *When couples part: Understanding the consequences for adults and children*. London: One Plus One.

Craig, L. (2006). Parental education, time in paid work and time with children: An Australian time-diary analysis. *The British Journal of Sociology, 57*(4), 553–575.

Crippen, C., & Brew, L. (2007). Intercultural parenting and the trans-cultural family: A literature review. *The Family Journal, 15*(107).

Crompton, R. (2006). *Employment and the family: The re-configuration of work and family life in contemporary societies*. Cambridge: Cambridge University Press.

Csikszentmihalyi, M., & Schneider, B. (2001). Conditions for optimal development in adolescence: An experimental approach. *Applied Developmental Science, 5*(3).

Dahl, R. E. (2004). Adolescent brain development: A period of vulnerabilities and opportunities. *Annals of the New York Academy of Science, 1021*, 1–22.

Damon, W. (1995). *Greater expectations: Overcoming the culture of indulgence in America's homes and schools*. New York: Free Press.

Davidov, M., & Grusec, J. (2006). Untangling the links of parental responsiveness to distress and warmth to child outcomes. *Child Development, 77*, 44–58.

DCSF. (2009). *Impact of family breakdown on children's wellbeing evidence review* (Researcher report DCSF-RR113). London: Department for Children, Schools and Families.

DCSF. (2010). *UK families and relationships green paper*. London: Department for Children, Schools and Families.

de Graaf, I., Speetjens, P., Smit, F., de Wolff, M., & Tavecchio, L. (2008). Effectiveness of the Triple P Positive Parenting Program on Behavioural Problems in children: A meta anaylsis. *Behaviour Modification, 32*(5).

Deater-Deckard, K., Dunn, J., O'Connor, T. G., Davies, L., & Golding, J. (2001). Using the stepfamily genetic design to examine gene-environment processes in child and family functioning. *Marriage and Family Review, 33*, 131–156.

DeHart, G., Sroufe, L., & Cooper, T. (2000). *Child development: It's nature and course* (4th ed.). Boston: McGraw Hill.

Dekovic, M., & Meeus, W. (1997). Peer relations in adolescence: Effects of parenting and adolescents' self-concept. *Journal of Adolescence, 20*, 163–176.

Demo, D. H., & Cox, M. (2000). Families with young children: A review of research in the 1990s. *Journal of Marriage and the Family, 62*, 876–895.

Dornbusch, S. M., Ritter, P., Leiderman, P. H., Roberts, D. F., & Fraleigh, M. J. (1987). The relation of parenting style to adolescent school performance. *Child Development, 58*, 1244–57.

Downey, D. B., & Condron, D. J. (2004). Playing well with others in kindergarten: The benefit of siblings at home. *Journal of Marriage and Family, 6*, 333–350.

Easterbrooks, M. A., & Emde, R. N. (1988). Marital and parent-child relationships: The role of affect in the family system. In R. Hinde & J. Stevenson-Hinde (Eds.), *Relationships within families: Mutual influences* (pp. 83–102). Oxford: Oxford University Press.

Economics, L. (2007). *Cost benefit analysis of interventions with parents*. London: Department for Children, Schools and Families.

Eisenberg, N., & Fabes, R. A. (1998). Pro-social development. In N. Eisenberg & W. Damon (Eds.), *Handbook of child development* (Vol. 4: Social, emotional and personality development 5th ed., pp. 707–778). New York: Wiley.

Ellsworth, C. P., Muir, D. W., & Haynes, S. M. J. (1993). Social competence and person-object differentiation: An analysis of the still face effect. *Developmental Psychology, 29*, 63–73.

Feiring, C., & Taska, L. S. (1996). Family self-concept: Ideas on its meaning. In B. Bracken (Ed.), *Handbook of self-concept* (pp. 317–373). New York: Wiley.

Finkenauer, C., Engels, C. R. M. R., Branje, S. J. T., & Neeus, W. (2004). Disclosure and relationship satisfaction in families. *Journal of Marriage and Family, 66*(1), 195–209.

Flouri, E. (2005). *Fathering and child outcomes.* Chichester: Wiley.

Fuller, A. (2008) Into the mystery of the adolescent mind. In T. Hanson (Ed.), *The bereavement buddy issue 2.* Dubbo: NALAG Centre for Loss and Grief, National Association for Loss and Grief (NSW) Inc.

Geidd, J. (2004). Structural magnetic resonance imaging of the adolescent brain. *Annals of the New York Academy of Sciences, 1021*, 77–85.

Gerhardt, S. (2004). *Why love matters: How affection shapes a baby's brain.* London: Routledge.

Gill, T. (2007). *No fear: Growing up in a Risk Averse Society.* Calouste Gulbenkian Foundation, p. 81. http://www.gulbenkian.org.uk/media/item/1266/223/No-fear-19.12.07.pdf

Gilmore, S. (2006). Contact/shared residence and child well being: Research evidence and its implications for legal decision-making. *International Journal of Law, Policy and the Family, 20*, 344–365.

Ginott, A. (1965). Between parent and child. In A. Ginott & H. W. Goddard (Eds.), *Between parent and child: Updated and revised (2003).* New York: Three Rivers Press.

Ginott, A., & Goddard, H. W. (Eds.). (2003). *Between parent and child: Updated and revised.* New York: Three Rivers Press.

Gray, A. (2006). The time economy of parenting. *Sociological Research, 11*(3).

Grusec, J. E., Davidov, M., & Lundell, L. (2002). Prosocial and helping behaviour. In P. K. Smith & C. H. Craig (Eds.), *Blackwell handbook of childhood social development* (pp. 457–474). Malden: Blackwell.

Gunnar, M., Tout, K., De Haan, M., Peirece, S., & Stanbury, K. (1997). Temperament, social competence and adrenocortical activity in preschoolers. *Developmental Psychobiology, 31*(1), 65–85.

Harold, G. (2001). What matters about conflict? In J. Reynolds (Ed.), *Not in front of the children? How conflict between parents affects children.* London: One Plus One.

Harper, S. E. (2010). Exploring the role of Filipino fathers: Paternal behaviours and child outcomes. *Journal of Family Issues, 31*(1), 66–89.

Hartley-Brewer, E. (2004). *Raising happy kids: Over 100 tips for parents and teachers.* New York: Da Capo Press.

Hayes, L., Smart, D., Toumbourou, J. W., & Sanson, A. (2004). *Parenting influence on adolescent alcohol use* (Australian Institute of Family Studies Report 10). Melbourne: Australian Institute of Family Studies.

Jackson-King, J. (2010). *Raising the best possible child: How to parent happy and successful kids.* Sydney: ABC Books.

Johnson, A. C. (1995). Resiliency mechanisms in culturally diverse families. *The Family Journal: Counselling and Therapy for Couples and Families, 3*(4), 316–324.

Keller, H., Lamm, B., Abels, M., Yovsi, R., Borke, J., Jensen, H., Papaligoura, Z., Holub, C., Lo, W., Tomiyama, A. J., Su, Y., Wang, Y., & Chaudhary, N. (2004). The bio-culture of parenting: Evidence from 5 cultural communities. *Parenting: Science and Practice, 4*(1), 25–50.

Knafo, A., & Schwartz, S. H. (2003). Parenting and accuracy of perception of parental values by adolescents. *Child Development, 73*, 595–611.

Kochanska, G. (1997). Mutually responsive orientation between mothers and their young children: Implications for early socialisation. *Child Development, 68*(1), 94–112.

Kochanska, G., & Aksan, N. (1995). Mother –child mutually positive affect, the quality of child compliance to requests and prohibitions and maternal control as correlates of early internalisation. *Child Development, 66*(1), 236–54.

Kohn, A. (2005). *Unconditional parenting: A provocative challenge to the conventional wisdom about discipline.* New York: Atria Press.

Krevans, J., & Gibbs, J. C. (1996). Parents' use of inductive discipline: Relations to children's empathy and prosocial behaviour. *Child Development, 67,* 3263–3277.

Loeber, R., Drinkwater, M., Yin, Y., Anderson, S. J., Schmidt, L. C., & Crawford, A. (2000). Stability of family interaction from ages 6 to 18. *Journal of Abnormal Child Psychology, 28,* 353–369.

Maccoby, E. E., & Martin, J. A. (1983). Socialization in the context of the family: Parent–child interaction. In P. Mussen & E. M. Hetherington (Eds.), *Handbook of child psychology* (Vol IV: Socialization, personality, and social development, pp. 1–101). New York: Wiley.

Masten, A. S. (2004). Regulatory processes, risk and resilience in adolescent development. *Annals of the New York Academy of Sciences, 1021,* 310–319.

May, K. A. (1978). Active involvement of expectant fathers in pregnancy: Some further considerations. *Journal of Obstetric, Gynecologic, and Neonatal Nursing, 7*(2), 7–12.

McGraw, P. C. (2004). *Family first: Your step-by-step plan for creating a phenomenal family.* New York: Free Press.

McHale, S. M., & Crouter, A. C. (1996). The family contexts of children's sibling relationships. In G. H. Brody (Ed.), *Sibling relationships: Their causes and consequences* (pp. 173–196). Norwood: Ablex.

McNeely, C. A., & Barber, B. K. (2010). How do parents make adolescents feel loved? Perspectives on supportive parenting from adolescents in 12 cultures. *Journal of Adolescent Research, 25,* 601.

Molina, B. S. G., & Chassin, L. (1996). The parent-adolescent relationship at puberty: Hispanic ethnicity and parent alcoholism as moderators. *Developmental Psychology, 32,* 675–686.

Moran, P., Ghate, D., & van de Merwe, A. (2004). *What works in parenting support? A review of the international evidence* (Research report RR574). London: DES Policy Research Bureau.

Nelson, N. K. (2010). *Parenting out of control: Anxious parents in uncertain times.* New York/London: New York University Press.

Patterson, J. M. (2002). Integrating family resilience and family stress theory. *Journal of Marriage and Family, 64*(2), 349–360.

Peel, K. (2003). *Family for life: How to have happy, healthy relationships with your adult children.* New York: McGraw-Hill.

Read, M. (1968). *Children of their fathers: Growing up among the Ngoni of Malawi.* New York: Holt, Rinehart and Winston.

Repacholi, B. M. (1998). Infants use of attentional cues to identify the referent of another person's emotional expression. *Developmental Psychology, 34,* 1017–1025.

Rodgers, B., & Pryor, J. (1998). *Divorce and separation: the outcomes for children.* York: Joseph Rowntree Foundation.

Roffey, S. (2011). *The new teachers' survival guide to behaviour* (2nd ed.). London: Sage Publications.

Rogoff, B. (1996). Developmental transitions in children's participation in sociocultural activities. In A. J. Sameroff & M. M. Haith (Eds.), *The five to seven year shift. The age of reason and responsibility* (pp. 273–294). Chicago: University of Chicago Press.

Ryan, R. M., & Deci, E. L. (2000). Self determination theory and the facilitation of intrinsic motivation, social development, and well-being. *American Psychologist, 55,* 68–78.

Sanders, M. (2008). Triple P-Positive Parenting Program as a public health approach to strengthening parenting. *Journal of Family Psychology, 22*(3), 506–517.

Simons, L. G., & Conger, R. D. (2007). Linking mother-father differences in parenting to a typology of family parenting styles and adolescent outcomes. *Journal of Family Issues, 28,* 212.

Simons, R. L., Beaman, J., Conger, R. D., & Chao, W. (1993). Children's experiences, conceptions of parenting and attitudes of spouse as determinants of parental behaviour. *Journal of Marriage and Family, 55*(1), 9.

Smetana, J. G., Tasopoulos-Chan, M., Gettman, D. C., Villalobos, M., Campione-Barr, N., & Metzger, A. (2009). Adolescents' and parents' evaluations of helping versus fulfilling personal desires in family situations. *Child Development, 80,* 280–294. doi:10.1111/j.1467-8624.2008.01259.x.

Spicer, P. (2010). *Cultural influences on parenting. Zero to three.* Norman: University of Oklahoma Press.

Sroufe, L. A., & Waters, E. (1976). The ontogenesis of smiling and laughter: A perspective on the organization of development in infancy. *Psychological Review, 83*, 173–189.

Sroufe, L. A., Egeland, B., Carlson, E., & Collins, W. A. (2005). *The development of the person: The minnesota study of risk and adaptation from birth to adulthood*. New York: Guilford Press.

Staub, E. (1979). *Positive social behavior and morality: Vol. 2* (Socialization and development). New York: Academic.

Suldo, S. M. (2009). Parent-child relationships. In R. Gilman, E. S. Huebner, & M. J. Furlong (Eds.), *Handbook of positive psychology in schools*. New York: Routledge.

Tan, E. A. (1997). Economic development and well-being of women. In *Philippines human development report*. Peru: Human Development Network and United Nations Development Program.

Vaughn, B. E., Coppola, G., Verissimo, M., Monteirio, L., Jose Santos, A., Posada, G., Carbell, O. A., Plata, S. J., Waters, H. S., Bost, K. K., McBride, B., Shine, N., & Korth, B. (2007). The quality of maternal secure-base scripts predicts children's secure-base behavior at home in three sociocultural groups. *International Journal of Behavioural Development, 31*(1), 65–76.

Velderman, M. K., Bakermans-Kranenburg, M. J., Juffer, F., & van IJzendoorn, M. H. (2006). Effects of attachment-based interventions on maternal sensitivity and infant attachment: Differential susceptibility of highly reactive infants. *Journal of Family Psychology, 20*(2), 266–274.

Verschueren, K., & Marcoen, M. (1999). Representation of self and socioemotional competence in kindergarteners: Differential and combined effects of attachment to mother and father. *Child Development, 70*, 183–201.

Vivero, V. N., & Jenkins, S. R. (1999). Existential hazards of the multi-cultural individual: Defining and understanding the "cultural homelessness". *Cultural Diversity and Ethnic Minority Psychology, 5*(1), 6–26.

Walker, K. (2010). *Parenting: A practical guide to raising preschool and primary-school children*. Melbourne: Penguin.

Walsh, F. (1998). *Strengthening family resilience*. New York: Guildford.

Walsh, F. (2002). A family resilience framework. Innovative practice applications. *Family Relations, 51*(2), 130–137.

Kimberley O'Brien is a child psychologist and Director of the Quirky Kid Clinic in Sydney. She is currently completing her Ph.D. at Monash University.
Contact: kimberley@quirkykid.com.au.

Jane Mosco is a psychologist and school counsellor working at Bishop Druitt College, Coffs Harbour. She also works in private practice with children and their families in Bellingen.
Contact: jmosco@bdc.nsw.edu.au.

Chapter 7
Promoting Positive Outcomes for Children Experiencing Change in Family Relationships

Emilia Dowling and Diana Elliott

7.1   Introduction

The aim of this chapter is to explore what parents and other family members and professionals can do to ensure that the needs and wellbeing of children are held in mind throughout what can be a lengthy and tortuous process: the separation and divorce of their parents and therefore, the end of the family as children know it.

Whilst discourses in western society emphasise that each and every child matters, in practice, it is often the adult perspective that takes precedence in the decisions that in turn affect children's lives and wellbeing. How can we ensure that the voice of the child is heard and taken into account? How can we best protect the child and their relationships in the future?

Drawing on the international evidence, together with our knowledge and experience through many years of working with families during and in the aftermath of separation and divorce, this chapter will address:

- Separation and divorce as a process rather than an event
- Our conceptual framework: divorce as a transition
- What the international research indicates promotes children's wellbeing in these circumstances
- What helps children during and after separation and divorce
- What practice has taught us
- What parents tell us
- A framework for professionals
- What is needed for children and parents

E. Dowling (✉)
Tavistock Clinic, London, UK
e-mail: emilia@dowling2901.plus.com

D. Elliott
Institute of Family Therapy, London, UK
e-mail: di_elliott23@hotmail.com

S. Roffey (ed.), *Positive Relationships: Evidence Based Practice across the World*,
DOI 10.1007/978-94-007-2147-0_7, © Springer Science+Business Media B.V. 2012

The chapter will conclude with some signposts that hopefully will contribute to enable parents, professionals and children to make sense of the experience and utilise their resources, knowledge and skills to manage these difficult transitions in family relationships.

7.2 Separation and Divorce as a Process

When a family separates, it is a form of bereavement at many levels for individuals in the family. Each family member will also be experiencing this at different times and in different ways. The impact of the separation extends to other family members including grandparents, aunts, uncles, cousins and beyond that to the community, school and workplace. It affects relationships at many levels and in many ways. The process gives rise to strong emotions including despair and anger, distress and sadness and sometimes relief. There is potential for many conflictual situations. The losses are potentially enormous, of partners, children, extended family, friends, home and school.

Often, children are the last to know that their parents are parting, or have not been told, in an effort to avoid the pain. Sometimes, this ending is a surprise to children; sometimes, they have experienced the turbulence preceding it. It takes emotional as well as physical energy to travel through this life experience, and again it can be different for each family member. It is a process over time rather than a one-off event. The experience can be likened to the image of throwing a stone into still water and witnessing the endless rippling effect.

A helpful frame is that of a process of change over time – a separation/divorce cycle that progresses from recognising the breakdown, deciding to separate, planning and preparing for the outcome, the legal process and beyond into the post-divorce family. At each stage, there are emotional and practical tasks to be achieved. It is in recognising this process of change over time that can help parents and practitioners make sense of the complexity of the emotions involved whilst managing some of the tasks to be undertaken by members of the family at each stage of this cycle (Robinson 1991).

It has to be understood that 'few people are able to behave totally rationally and unselfishly at times of crisis, uncertainty and great unhappiness in their life…' (King and Trowell 1992).

Whilst friends and relatives may be highly supportive, the other possibility is that they may line up behind the protagonists and become partisan and adversarial. Practitioners who become involved in the process of separation and divorce and who are not versed in the complexities of family processes and the power of the wider family system may speak of the individuals involved as 'reasonable' or 'unreasonable'. This occurs when they see the situation through the lens of one individual and in this way escalate conflict and become themselves part of the problem rather than a helpful resource.

We know from practice that couples rarely set out together as partners envisaging that the partnership will not endure. When the relationship falters and ends, it is initially a very private, personal matter. Sometimes, it is a mutual decision, often not. Even so, many partners manage to sort out all the necessary arrangements for family and finance without professional help. Some seek professional help, and their personal sadness becomes public and involved in the legal system if they decide to divorce. The journey through divorce, whilst a psychological process, then moves into the legal framework. The legal process seeks to ensure that arrangements are made for children and their support, and that financial matters are also settled by the couple. It can become adversarial, and if so, counterproductive for families in distress. However, many family lawyers are committed to a conciliatory approach, and an increasing number of family lawyers are becoming family mediators too in several countries. The courts encourage mediation, and there is a positive growth of information sessions for parents, often in groups, which empower parents not only with information but also skills to talk to their children and ex-partners.

7.3   Conceptual Framework: Divorce as a Transition

The consequences of divorce and separation are felt by an increasing number of children who are growing up in different family configurations from the traditional nuclear family (Dowling and Gorell Barnes 2000). 'Research in the UK estimated that 19% of children born to married couples will experience parental divorce by the age of ten and 28% by age sixteen. However, these figures may underestimate the rate of family dissolution, since they do not include the separation of cohabiting parents' (Rodgers and Pryor 1998:4).

A recent review of international literature into the consequences of couple relationship breakdown for adults and children by One Plus One, the UK's leading relationships research organisation, concludes that 45% of marriages in the UK will end in divorce (Coleman and Glenn 2009).

No doubt these statistics will continue to increase as the traditional nuclear family is replaced by a variety of family forms, but what is most important is not so much the statistics, but our concern as professionals about the stories that lie behind the research headlines on divorce and remarriage, and in particular the experience of children who go through this transition as they grow up.

The ideas we are sharing in this chapter are based on many years of experience of working with families living through processes of separation and divorce, as well as subsequent family reconstruction. Our practice is informed by many ideas as well as the experience of working with a wide range of families at different stages in the transition. In particular, we have been influenced by the following conceptual frameworks:

7.3.1 Attachment Theory

John Bowlby's ideas have been crucial to the understanding of children's needs at different developmental stages, and we know from research on attachment that children who experience their parents as unresponsive or unavailable will tend to see themselves as unlovable or unworthy. On the other hand, children whose parents are perceived as available and helpful will develop a narrative about themselves as coping but also worthy of help (Bowlby 1977, 1988).

Parents need to understand that children's wish for proximity and responsiveness is a developmental expression of their needs, rather than construe it as 'naughty' or 'attention-seeking' behaviour. They also need to recognise that the commonest source of anger is connected with anxiety and uncertainty about parents' or caregivers' availability (Dowling and Gorell Barnes 2000).

Gill Gorell Barnes (2005) uses the framework of attachment when assessing the possibility of post-divorce contact when a parent is pursuing contact after a long absence of two or more years. In her work as an expert witness advising the courts in the UK as to whether re-establishing contact is in the child's best interest, she pays particular attention to the way the parent seeking contact expresses his/her attachment and whether it is primarily directed to the child or to the ex-partner. When there has been violence, is there acknowledgement of the effect on the child and the other parent's concern about the child's safety?

Gorell Barnes also considers each parent's capacity to, at least minimally, understand the other's point of view in order to serve the child's best interests and the way in which children themselves express their own attachment to the absent parent and their wish to re-establish contact.

7.3.2 Systems Theory

Systems theory has been a crucial influence in the development of family therapy (Rivett and Street 2003). It involves an emphasis on the effect of relationships on relationships and a focus on what takes place between people rather than on the individual's inner world. The importance of the connection between systemic and narrative ideas and their application to practice when working with families has been emphasised by Vetere and Dallos (2003) and Vetere and Dowling (2005).

7.3.3 Social Constructionist Ideas

A basic premise of the social constructionist view is that reality is constructed in interaction through language (Campbell 2000). Therefore, in our clinical work we endeavour to listen to different voices, different views, different realities. This means giving up the notion of one truth.

We pay attention to different narratives: fathers, mothers, children, school. We try to elicit the different discourses paying attention not only to the dominant but also the marginalised voices. One of the main aims of our work with families in transition has been to enable the voice of the child to be heard.

7.3.4 Narrative Theory

The central tenet of narrative theory is that 'the self is constructed, storied through interaction with others and that in this context language produces meaning not just reflects experience' (Burck 1997:64).

These theories suggest that the stories people develop about themselves do not encompass the totality of their experience. Therefore, it is part of our professional task to elicit other stories that may have been submerged, which contribute to a wider and more useful narrative. In post-divorce work, it is often the story of acrimony and resentment that prevails, and it is important, particularly for children, to incorporate positive elements that may have been present in the relationship in order to widen the story and enable children to have a more balanced perspective of the parental relationship.

When using a narrative approach as the focus of our intervention, we must be aware that when we listen to a story, it will be from one person's perspective and that decisions about who is invited to an interview or a meeting determine who we listen to and therefore whose voice might remain unheard. A particular danger might be the temptation to privilege adult over children's voices.

In our work with families during and in the aftermath of separation and divorce, we endeavour to pay attention to the following:

- The importance of working towards a coherent story about the separation for children. This is sometimes difficult to achieve as children find themselves caught up in the middle of oppositional narratives held by each parent.
- The importance of listening to different narratives: fathers, mothers, children, school.
- Different beliefs: the dangers and pitfalls of privileging some narratives over others (negative aspects of a parent, marital dispute over parent–child relationship).
- Dominant and marginalised discourses.
- Power and silencing of voices.
- Giving children a voice.

Blow and Daniel (2005) emphasise the importance of recognising that children have a mind of their own and may have different ideas about what is best for them. In their work, they aim to understand the impact the parental separation has had on children and assess their sense of agency in relation to the future. It is their experience, as is ours, that children caught in the middle of an adversarial process very rarely feel heard. They have found in their work that children's narratives are often constrained by their parents' polarised views, and therefore, they might not feel free to say everything they think either to parents or professionals.

7.4 Post-divorce Narratives

In a previous publication, three main groups of parental relationship narratives were identified (Gorell Barnes and Dowling 1997) that highlighted the dilemmas for children having to reconcile the very entrenched positions that their parents take.

The first group involves competing parental narratives with the children having to sacrifice their own view in order to fit in with and please each parent.

The second group involves the obstinate refusal to provide children with a story about the absent parent. The absence of meaning and the inability to make sense of their experience lead to confusion and lack of concentration in children.

The third group represents those parents who continue to compete with each other as to who is the better parent with the inevitable triangulation of the children, who take on the task of filtering information and adapting their own views and wishes in order to 'keep the peace'.

Sometimes, the children are caught in the middle of conflicting narratives and are left confused and bewildered, even blaming themselves for the changes occurring around them.

The following is an example of conflicting narratives and their effect on the children:

Sam, 8, and his younger brother Ben were very confused about the fact that father was not living at home any longer. On the one hand, the parents had played down the changes – 'dad has moved out because he has a lot of work to do'; on the other hand, the children seemed to be seeing more of him, and at the same time, they were noticing how often mum got upset and they saw her crying. Despite these very evident changes, no adequate explanation was provided for the boys. The school were concerned about Sam's disruptive behaviour and Ben's 'dreamy attitude' and difficulty in concentrating. During the work with the family, it proved very difficult to openly address the changes. Father, whose new partner was expecting a new baby, had not even told the boys he was living with someone else and his way of managing was never to take the children to his new place. Mother found it very difficult to help the children make the connection between her sadness and the end of her marriage; therefore, it had not been possible for them to express their sadness about their parents' separation or even make sense of it.

Research and clinical experience indicate that it is important to listen and keep in focus the child's perspective whilst paying ongoing attention to the differing dilemmas affecting mothers, fathers and stepparents in the evolution of the idea of ongoing 'family life' after divorce.

In relation to practice, this has made us pay attention to the hierarchy of discourses in a family, the way in which certain stories about children's lives and parental functioning dominate over other stories and the effects of such dominance on potential stories, which have become silenced or submerged.

7.5   Multiple Voices, Multiple Perspectives

How can we develop our practice, widening the narratives, bringing forth silent voices and enabling marginalised discourses to emerge?

We have found the following guiding principles to be very useful in our understanding and helping families in transition:

- Maintaining a systemic approach, based on an interactional framework which focuses on the relationships between people and the patterns of interaction that maintain behaviour rather than apportioning blame to an individual
- Viewing separation and divorce as a transition and therefore avoiding pathologising the process and its consequences
- Striving towards a collaborative and respectful practice, paying attention to the different voices and different perspectives
- Giving up the notion of one truth.
- Aiming to reach families outside the consulting room, the general separating population, through parent and children groups, working with schools and in the community.

In our work with families and schools, we find it helpful to invite participants to identify stories which may not have been verbalised before but which will contribute to widen the narrative and introduce new meanings, and therefore opening up possibilities for change.

No narrative should be privileged over any other, and it is important to allow different voices to emerge in order to enrich the story. Young people benefit from this approach as often the adult discourse is privileged over the children's discourse.

We need to be curious about who has been silenced: whose voices have become marginalised? How are we, as professionals, going to empower those voices to emerge and be heard? It may be that discourses of gender, race and difference are being marginalised by the dominant, powerful voices.

7.6   What the Research Shows

There is now an extensive body of research that shows divorce as a risk factor in the psychological wellbeing of children. Studies have shown higher incidence of physical and psychological ill health, lower performance at school, substance abuse and behavioural problems (Rodgers and Pryor 1998; Cockett and Tripp 1994). However, the evidence is complex, and we as professionals need to focus on the protective factors which promote resilience and enable children to adjust to the transition.

Some recent studies have shown interesting findings that throw new and more detailed light on the consequences of divorce for children:

Coleman and Glenn (2009) carried out a comprehensive review of the research evidence on the consequences of divorce for adults and children. They identify parental *conflict* as a crucial issue but, interestingly, conclude that the way conflict is *dealt with* is what matters more than the conflict itself. They also found that *low level of conflict* prior to divorce seemed to be more detrimental to the wellbeing of children than high conflict. This is because the children do not have much time to anticipate the divorce of their parents, and therefore might even blame themselves for it. The authors also identified a useful distinction between *destructive* conflicts, for example when violence is involved, and *constructive* conflicts, when the level of conflict is mild and can be resolved, as this provides the children with a model for resolving disputes effectively.

They highlight the negative effects of prolonged conflict that involves children in the role of messengers or as recipients of negative information. They also conclude that the risks for children increase when the experiences of parental relationship breakdown are repeated.

This review helpfully reminds us that the negative effects of marital breakdown on children are not universal, and many children are able to adjust to the transition. It is important to remember that as the review points out and our clinical experience shows, a crucial moderating factor in terms of outcomes for children is the quality of parent–child relationship. Therefore, good and effective parenting is a powerful and positive way to reduce the negative impact of divorce and separation on children.

McIntosh (2007) reports that in Australia, 25% of children of divorced parents developed mental health difficulties such as emotional and behavioural problems compared with 12% of children in intact families. She describes a 'child-inclusive', evidence-based model of intervention with divorce and separated families and shows positive outcomes for parents and children. Her study of 142 families compared outcomes for two treatment groups of separated parents who attended mediation: child-focused intervention and child-inclusive intervention. The former focuses on the parenting arrangements that best support the children's needs, but the children are not seen. The latter includes a brief assessment of the child's experience of the separation. Follow up data 1 year after the mediation showed reduction in the level of conflict and improved capacity to manage and resolve the initial disputes. Children in both groups perceived a reduction in the intensity and frequency of conflict between their parents, which resulted in a lowering of their own distress about their parents' disagreements.

McIntosh highlights the importance of *parental attunement* or *reflective function*, which refers to a parent's capacity to put themselves in their child's shoes and see things from their point of view, as a crucial factor in promoting children's security. She describes as 'secure base parents' those who are able to regulate emotions for themselves and their children.

7.7 What Helps Children During and After Separation and Divorce

- An age appropriate explanation for the family break-up
- Absence of conflict between parents after divorce
- Good relationships and easy contact with both parents

- Knowledge about the absent parent, even if there is no contact
- How well a parent adjusts has a significant impact on how well children adjust (Dowling and Gorell Barnes 2000: 41)

It is a significant leap from being a couple with children to parenting apart. When working with separating/divorcing families, it is clear that many parents seek to do their best but feel they have no signposts as to what to say and do to help their children, particularly when they are in distress themselves. Sometimes, they think that their children will know about the situation when they have not actually spelt it out to them. As a contrast, others will want to inform children of 'the truth', i.e. detailed accounts about the failure of the parent–adult relationship which, as children tell us, is unwelcome.

In offering group meetings to parents, it is our experience that they welcome informing themselves of the reactions and needs of their children appropriate to age and stage and to hear what helps. Information about research, books, videos, websites and help lines are well received, and parents share their own knowledge with each other in such a setting.

7.7.1   The Voice of the Child

The voice of the child/young person can be heard in different ways. Ideally, the child is included in family discussions so that there are understandings about what is happening, and the child is able to participate and have a voice. This may not be possible initially or in high-conflict situations.

There are different models developing which include the child in mediation. This may be inclusion as a principle (McIntosh 2007) or inclusion by invitation where the child has the right to accept or not. The child thus may be seen directly in the process of mediation or indirectly when the mediator helps parents focus on plans to include the needs of their particular and individual children.

In England, if parents can't agree, the Family Court may appoint a Family Court Advisor to talk with the child and report to the Court. On some occasions, judges also talk with children when deciding on arrangements for future residence and contact.

There are growing resources for parents, practitioners and policy makers ranging from research studies, videos made by young people (e.g. *When Parents Part* by Young Voice), pocket guides, direct lists compiled by young people to help parents and check lists. Below we cite a few examples.

Dr. Joan Kelly, a clinical psychologist, researcher and practitioner based in California, USA, who has worked in the field of separation and divorce and has studied the impact of divorce on children for four decades, offers the following 'Ten top ways to protect your kids from the fallout of a high-conflict break-up' (Kelly 2009): The headings of these helpful tips are: 'Talk to your children about your separation; Be discreet; Act like grown-ups; Keep conflict away from the kids; Dad stay in the picture, Mom deal with anger appropriately; Be a good parent; Manage your own mental health; Keep the people your children care about in their lives; Be thoughtful about your future love life; and Pay your child support'.

In her review of the empirical evidence on the longer term adjustment of children of divorce, Joan Kelly highlights the stressors of the initial separation such as the fact that the majority of children seem to have little emotional preparation for the separation of their parents and often lack essential information regarding the practical changes affecting their lives. A particular stressor is the abrupt departure of one parent, usually the father (Kelly and Emery 2003).

Kelly, like other researchers, emphasises the adverse effect of persistent conflict between the parents following separation and divorce. She points out that the children of divorce face the loss of important relationships with friends and extended family members, and moving away can be a factor. In her research, she found that in Virginia, USA, for example, the average distance between fathers and children, 10 years after divorce, was 400 miles (Hetherington and Kelly 2002). In terms of balance between risk and resilience, Kelly makes a useful distinction between painful memories and longer term pathological effects.

7.7.2 Parenting Coordinator

High-conflict couples tend to use the Court system as a means of continuing their disputes for some years post divorce. This perpetual cycle puts children in the middle of the conflict, and whilst there has been development in alternative dispute resolution such as family mediation and divorce education programmes, there has also been a growing need to address the distress of high-conflict parents. Over the last decade, the role of the Parenting Coordinator has been developing in many states in the USA (Mitcham and Henry 2007). The role is a mix of counselling, family mediation and the Court in dealing with parenting plans and contact issues.

The Parenting Coordinator, mandated by the Court, is often a highly experienced mental health professional. Help is given to parents to put their parenting plans in place by facilitating disputes, making recommendations where there is an impasse and offering education in a collaborative way. Judges, lawyers and mental health professionals are recognising the value of the Parent Coordinator in cases of high-conflict families where they are helped to focus on their children's needs.

7.7.3 A Research Study

A study seeking views on what children thought of post-divorce family life focused on what worked well in addition to what was problematic. A few of the points made by children were that they valued mutual respect between parents and emphasised their wish to participate in family discussions rather than in making choices.

However, some children who felt unheard or frightened did wish to make their own choices. The preference was for conversations to take place within the family, seeing the involvement of outside agencies as a last resort. They valued the quality rather than the quantity of time with parents (Smart and Neale 2000).

7.7.4   A Pocket Guide

A pocket guide for parents, *What Most Children Say*, has been devised by Kent Family Mediation Service, UK. It gives clear and simple messages from children which the Guide links directly with relevant research findings (see website). Some of the messages are:

- Try not to argue in front of us.
- Tell us what is happening.
- Keep talking together about things that affect us.
- We can cope and get on with our lives, as long as you do too; if you don't, we can't.
- We don't want to be involved in what went wrong or whose fault it is (Kent Family Mediation Service (2010).

7.7.5   Messages from a Group of School Children

We worked with a group of school children aged 14–15 who had experience of divorce in the family. They eagerly put together the following list for parents and generously agreed to its wide distribution.

Questions are 'What should young people be told when their parents separate or divorce?' and/or 'What should parents be told to bear in mind about their young people?':

- That they are still loved
- That they don't want to hear one parent 'slagged off' by the other
- How courts work
- That they don't have to pretend that one parent doesn't exist when they are talking with the other parent
- That they are still loved by both parents
- Young people should be told that their parents have grown apart, not that they can't stand being with each other anymore
- The child that stays with the parent should not be expected to take on the responsibility of the parent who has gone, e.g. the eldest son should not have to take the place of the father
- That it is not their fault
- That they will get over it – there is light at the end of the tunnel

- That they should not feel guilty about going out with their friends and leaving Mum or Dad in
- That they don't have to be down and morbid all the time
- That they are not social outcasts, and they need to be able to rely on their friends

7.7.6 An Innovative Initiative

An association of mediation practitioners in the South of England found that they were on occasions working with families with maybe three or four children/young adults, where one or more could not attend by reason of being away at school or college. By agreement, they completed a questionnaire which was to be used in a mediation session for parents to include this in their planning. This device proved fruitful and was pronounced helpful by parents and the rest of the family. This has been developed further and used with children who may decide not to accept an invitation to attend mediation but are willing to include their thoughts by completing the questionnaire. It may also be used when they do attend – an initiative taken up with enthusiasm by children. The practitioners have given permission to reproduce the questions:

1. What is your understanding of the present situation?
2. What hopes do you have about family life in the future?
3. What worries, if any, do you have about family life in the future?
4. What would you like more of or less of, or to be different?
5. If Mum and Dad asked for your advice, what would you say?
6. Is there anything else?

7.8 What Practice Has Taught Us

Over the years, we have seen many families consulting over their children's difficulties or attending mediation either during or after prolonged and painful court cases. There is little doubt that the adversarial context in which the courts usually operate is detrimental to conflict resolution and contributes to reinforce the entrenched positions taken by parents who are in the middle of a process where hurt, rage, resentment and other powerful feelings dominate.

Our clinical experience shows that what is needed is a more collaborative stance by practitioners, where adults are helped to manage their differences and concentrate on the needs of their children who are the most vulnerable party when the family breaks up. Resources need to be available, *early on in the process*, in order to help parents move from a fighting position where the most important factor is to 'win' or to 'be right' to a more cooperative parenting position where they can begin to work together for their children, even if profound differences between them as partners remain.

It is important to stress that parents are also vulnerable at this time, and, although they might feel self-indulgent, they need to take care of themselves physically and mentally so that they can look after their children. Support systems such as family, friends and colleagues can be invaluable.

We know from our work with families that children often find themselves in:

A *loyalty bind*, over what parent to please or what to say in order not to upset the other: this puts an intolerable burden of responsibility for filtering their emotions in order not to upset their parents and keep conflict at bay.

Confusion and anger: children often find themselves confused over the reasons for the separation and lacking a coherent story that helps them to make sense of the crisis in the family. Parents can help children by tolerating and acknowledging their angry feelings and providing a *developmentally appropriate story* of what has happened. This need not involve blame, but it needs to acknowledge that the marital relationship has come to an end. However, it is important to emphasise that the parent–child relationship will continue and that children are never to blame for the divorce or separation of their parents.

Difficulties to concentrate/achieve at school: when children are preoccupied with conflict at home, this has a detrimental effect on their capacity to concentrate and learn, particularly if they feel responsible for the psychological wellbeing of a parent or parents and adopt a care taker role in relation to a parent who might be depressed or anxious.

7.9 What Parents Tell Us

In working with groups of separating and divorcing parents, we have found that their main preoccupation is to do their best for their children. We have worked with groups where participants are at different stages of the divorce process, and they are able to help and learn from each other and generally gain confidence in their own abilities as parents.

They are thirsty for information about loss for family members: age and stage reactions of their children and what they can do to help. A gender mix helps them to look at situations from the other's perspective and therefore contributes to a better and different understanding of what might have been previously perceived as simply an ex-partner's negative behaviour. We are acutely aware that being part of a group enables them to gain a wider lens on male and female responses and to reflect and modify previously fixed views.

As well as gaining information, parents consistently ask for skills and ideas on what to say to children and how to manage communication with an ex-partner. They find it useful to experiment with specific examples of situations and explore together different ways of handling them.

We think it is important to emphasise that it is crucial for those who facilitate these groups to have the necessary skills to manage and contain the very strong emotions and highly charged climate that can develop in the group process.

We seek to set up a nurturing, collaborative experience, acknowledging emotions whilst keeping the focus mainly on what children need from parents. Alongside this, it is essential to acknowledge parents' efforts, skills, commitment and creativity in finding solutions for themselves and their families. We try to maintain a balance between respect for both parents whilst keeping children in mind.

7.10 Post-divorce Re-partnering and Remarriage

It is beyond the scope of this chapter to elaborate in detail on the transition to becoming a 'reconstituted family' with the various permutations and additions to family relationships. However, in the context of the risk factors affecting children, the evidence shows that the post-divorce stage creates the potential for children to experience changes and disruptions in family life when one or both parents introduce new partners, cohabit, remarry or re-divorce. The re-partnering of parents is particularly stressful for children if it occurs soon after divorce (Hetherington and Kelly 2002).

In her research on children's perspectives of family relationships in the UK, Judy Dunn found that it was common for children of single parents to feel displaced when their mothers re-partnered, for children to feel less important than step and half siblings and many children wished more contact with their non-resident parents. However, she found that these concerns decreased over time. Shared family activities as well as communication between children and parents were found to be very important (Dunn 2008).

7.11 Signposts for the Future

7.11.1 For Practitioners

Practitioners need a framework for thinking and reflecting about their work. Ongoing supervision and consultation are essential. In their paper on 'Frozen Narratives', Blow and Daniel (2002) remind us of the emotionally draining nature of this work: 'This is partly because of the enormous distress caused to children in the name of love, and partly because the levels of hostility and mistrust are such that making a therapeutic alliance with one partner is seen as betrayal by the other' (p. 94).

Policy makers, practitioners, lawyers, schools and all those who, as a result of their work, come into contact with families during and in the aftermath of separation and divorce need to understand the psychological processes involved over time for parents and children alike. The assumption that this can be a single event to be dealt with rationally and practically is unhelpful. The level of conflict can vary in each unique situation and Bernard Mayer (2009) encourages practitioners to ask themselves: 'How can we help people to engage with this issue over time?' rather than

'What can we do to resolve or de-escalate this conflict?' (Preface, p. x). 'I focus on conflicts as enduring, ongoing or long term rather than intractable or irresolvable, because I think the latter terms suggest that conflict duration is in itself a problem or that progress is hopeless' (Preface, p. xiv).

7.11.2   For Parents and Children

The process of separation is complex and cannot be addressed with a one-size-fits-all model of mediation or parent/children information programmes. A more thera-peutic model of mediation may take root. This model has been developed by Irving and Benjamin (2002) and is not to be confused with therapy. They propose that they use therapeutic techniques to 'advance the objectives of family media-tion' (p. 10). There is a possibility of pre-mediation, which enables clients to feel heard in a way which is meaningful to them, and to find avenues for managing conflicts in a different way so that mediation itself can become more possible. There is also development of one-stop-shop agencies where there is a menu of services available by entering one door. Indeed, this was proposed by Dr. Janet Walker in her original research in Ogus et al. (1989). One example of this was a government-funded initiative in which one of us was involved (DE) called *Family Focus – One Stop Shop* which was an integral part of a family mediation service. The report at the end of the 3-year project was compiled in 2005. There was a menu of services which were considered at an initial consultation. At that time, a decision was made to engage in one of the following: work with couples, indi-viduals or families – a relationship review which considered whether or not the relationship was over or if it could continue – and the other option offered was for separation or divorce mediation.

These possibilities enabled clients to choose to do a time-limited piece of work in the knowledge that they could return to the service at a later juncture when and if necessary (Family Focus 2005). This model has been taken further and funded by various bodies in other family mediation services in England.

Parent information programmes are well developed in Australia and North America. In recent years, there has been a gradual growth of theses programmes in England and Scotland.

Research is showing that, again, one model does not fit for everyone and that different programmes may be needed to address different levels of conflict. In California, the Alameda group model is a programme specifically devised for high-conflict families and offers parents and children concurrent sessions (Johnston 2004). Another well-established group model developed in America called Kids' Turn offers parents and children the opportunity to work in groups and is well described in a guidebook made available for all (Hannibal 2007). A group model for children called 'Time to Talk' is offered in Scotland (Relationships Scotland). There is great scope to offer children and young people the opportunity to attend a group and to make sense of their family changes with others in the same position.

The wider systems of family, friends and school must be actively considered in promoting positive outcomes for children. Relationships can be lost at worst or overlooked in the emotional chaos. Often, children intimate that a teacher, a grand-parent or a friend offered a safe haven in times of upheaval. Practitioners, as a matter of course, will have this important framework in mind when working with families through separation. An interesting peer group education programme, 'Seasons for Growth' (see website), deals with loss, death, family breakdown and other forms of separation. It is now well established in Australia, New Zealand, Ireland and the UK. Its main advantage is that it is delivered through schools, and is therefore supporting the World Health Organization's aim that schools play a key role in psychosocial development.

7.12 Concluding Remarks

In a review of services and interventions for children of divorcing and separating parents supported by the Joseph Rowntree Foundation, Hawthorne et al. (2003) suggested that provision designed to support children through family change should ensure that children had someone to listen to their views and help them understand the processes that they and their parents were going through. Parents should be supported to reduce stress, and both parents and children should be helped to understand and manage conflict. The survey identified numerous useful programmes but noted that few had been effectively evaluated. The challenge therefore continues as research is showing what parents and children need and request. The review also suggested that a mixed strategy of interventions might be required, given the variety of needs and situations for families.

At the time of publication in England of the research undertaken by the organisation One Plus One (Coleman and Glenn 2009), the Director of the organisation, Penny Mansfield, wrote an article in the Times newspaper, October 8th 2009, entitled 'To help children, start first with the parents'. She stated that the relationships of modern parents are 'more fragile'. The research shows that 'the most effective time to get parents to look at their relationships and parenting is when they are having a baby: this is the moment when Health Visitors and others routinely in touch with new parents could offer more effective help'. This is important information for practice and policy.

Ongoing research and practice innovation continue to promote positive outcomes for children experiencing change in family relationships. It is essential that effective evaluation takes place and that policy and practice should be coherent with research evidence.

The challenge for us all is to hold on to uncertainty in a time of chaos and to help families through that transition ensuring that all voices are heard at a time when forceful stories demand precedence.

References

Blow, K., & Daniel, G. (2002). Frozen narratives? Post-divorce processes and contact disputes. *Journal of Family Therapy, 24*, 85–103.

Blow, K., & Daniel, G. (2005). Whose story is it anyway? In A. Vetere & E. Dowling (Eds.), *Narrative therapies with children and their families*. London: Routledge.

Bowlby, J. (1977). The making and breaking of affectional bonds. *The British Journal of Psychiatry, 130*(201–10), 421–431.

Bowlby, J. (1988). *A secure base – Clinical applications of attachment theory*. London: Routledge.

Burck, C. (1997). Language and narrative. In R. K. Papadopoulos & J. Byng-Hall (Eds.), *Multiple voices: Narrative in systemic family psychotherapy* (Tavistock clinic series). London: Duckworth.

Campbell, D. (2000). *The socially constructed organization*. London: Karnac.

Cockett, M., & Tripp, J. (1994). *The exeter family study, family breakdown and its impact on children*. Exeter: Joseph Rowntree Foundation, University of Exeter Press.

Coleman, L., & Glenn, F. (2009). *When couples part: Understanding the consequences for adults and children*. London: One Plus One.

Dowling, E., & Gorell Barnes, G. (2000). *Working with children and parents through separation and divorce*. London: Macmillan.

Dunn, J. (2008). *Family relationships – Children's perspectives*. London: One Plus One.

Family Focus. (2005). *Family Focus report 2005*. http://www.dcsf.gov.uk/pns/pnattach/20040097/1.htm. Accessed June 14, 2010

Gorell Barnes, G. (2005). Narratives of attachment in post-divorce contact disputes. In A. Vetere & E. Dowling (Eds.), *Narrative therapies with children and their families*. London: Routledge.

Gorell Barnes, G., & Dowling, E. (1997). Re-writing the story: Children, parents and post-divorce narrative. In R. K. Papadopoulos & J. Byng-Hall (Eds.), *Multiple voices: Narrative in systemic family psychotherapy* (Tavistock clinic series). London: Duckworth.

Hannibal, M. E. (2007). *Good parenting through your divorce*. New York: Marlow and Company.

Hawthorne, J., Jessop, J., Pryor, J., & Richards, M. (2003). *Supporting children through family change: A review of interventions and services for children of divorcing and separating parents*. London: Joseph Rowntree Foundation.

Hetherington, E. M., & Kelly, J. (2002). *For better or for worse*. New York: Norton.

Irving, H. H., & Benjamin, M. (2002). *Therapeutic family mediation*. Thousand Oaks: Sage.

Johnston, J. (2004). *The Alameda model*. http://www.justice.gc.ca/eng/pi/fcy-fea/lib-bib/rep-rap/2004/2004_1/p5.html. Accessed June 14, 2010.

Kelly, J. (2009). *Ten top ways to protect your kids from the fallout of a high conflict break-up*. www.mediate.com/Articles/kelly.j./.cfm. Accessed June 14, 2010.

Kelly, J. B., & Emery, R. E. (2003). Children's adjustment following divorce: Risk and resilience perspectives. *Family Relations, 52*, 352–362.

Kent Family Mediation Service (updated 2010). *What most children say: Creating positive outcomes from your children. Pocket guide for parents who live apart*. Sittingbourne: KFMS. www.kentfms.co.uk

King, M., & Trowell, J. (1992). Children, welfare and the law: The limits of legal intervention. In M. Robinson (Ed.), *Family transformation through divorce and re-marriage* (p. 348). London: Routledge.

Mayer, B. (2009). *Staying with conflict*. San Francisco: Jossey Bass.

McIntosh, J. (2007). Child inclusion as a principle and as evidence based practice: Applications to family law services and related sectors. *Australian Family Relationships Clearing House Issues, 1*, 1–23.

Mitcham, M., & Henry, W. J. (2007). High-conflict divorce solutions: Parenting coordination as an innovative co-parenting intervention. *Family Journal: Counselling and Therapy for Couples and Families, 15*(4).

Ogus, A., Walker, J., & Jones-Lee, M. (1989). *Costs and effectiveness of conciliation in England and Wales*. Newcastle upon Tyne: Relate Centre for Family Studies, University of Newcastle, Conciliation Project Unit.

Relationships Scotland. *Family mediation*. www.relationships-scotland.org.uk/family_mediation_other_support.shtml#1. Accessed June 17, 2010.

Rivett, M., & Street, E. (2003). *Family therapy in focus*. London: Sage.

Robinson, M. (Ed.). (1991). *Family transformation through divorce and re-marriage*. London: Routledge.

Rodgers, B., & Pryor, J. (1998). *Divorce and separation: The outcomes for children*. York: Joseph Rowntree Foundation.

Seasons for Growth. www.seasonsforgrowth.co.uk. Accessed July 28, 2010

Smart, C., & Neale, B. (2000, September). It's my life too – Children's perspectives on post-divorce parenting. *Family Law, 30*, 163–169.

Vetere, A., & Dallos, R. (2003). *Working systemically with families: Formulation, intervention and evaluation*. London: Karnac.

Vetere, A., & Dowling, E. (2005). *Narrative therapies with children and their families – A practitioner's guide to concepts and approaches*. London: Routledge.

Young Voice. *When parents part – A film*. www.whenparentspart.org.uk. Accessed June 14, 2010.

Emilia Dowling is a Chartered Clinical Psychologist and Family Psychotherapist in private practice and a member of the Institute of Family Therapy. She worked for many years at the Tavistock Clinic in London where she was head of Child Psychology. She was also a visiting professor at Birkbeck College, London University. She has published widely and is co-author of *Working with Children and Parents through Separation and Divorce*, 2000.
Contact: emilia@dowling2901.plus.com.

Diana Elliott is a trained Social Worker and Systemic Psychotherapist and a member of the Institute of Family Therapy. She set up an independent family mediation service where she practised and trained family mediators for many years.

Emilia and Diana were involved in an innovative project for separating parents and their children at the Institute of Family Therapy in London.
Contact: di_elliott23@hotmail.com.

Chapter 8
Friendships: The Power of Positive Alliance

Karen Majors

8.1 Introduction

As Diener and Diener (2009) comment, positive psychology has had a focus on adulthood and only relatively recently has turned its attention to child development. They acknowledge past research which now makes a valuable contribution to positive psychology concepts. In this chapter on friendships, I will draw on relevant research from child and adolescent development.

Friendships serve a range of important purposes. Mendelson and Aboud (1999) have categorised these as: companionship, intimacy, support, reliable alliance, self-validation and emotional security. There are long-term consequences for children who do not establish friendships and positive peer relations. Several longitudinal studies have found that children with poor peer relations and lack of friends go on to experience maladjustment in terms of life status, perceived competence and mental health difficulties in adulthood (e.g. Cowen et al. 1973; Bagwell et al. 1998). There is evidence to indicate that having friends is associated with good academic performance and school adjustment, and correspondingly not having friends predicts poor academic performance and school adjustment (e.g. Ladd 1990; Wentzel et al. 2004). School adjustment is usefully defined by Ladd and Kochenderfer (1996): 'the degree to which children become interested, engaged, comfortable and successful in the school environment' (p. 324).

Providing individual support for the child who lacks friends and is rejected by classmates is not enough in itself. There is a need not only to help them to develop new skills but also to address the perceptions and behaviours of others in the class (Frederickson 1991).

K. Majors (✉)
Department of Psychology and Human Development, Institute of Education,
University of London, UK
e-mail: k.majors@ioe.ac.uk

S. Roffey (ed.), *Positive Relationships: Evidence Based Practice across the World*,
DOI 10.1007/978-94-007-2147-0_8, © Springer Science+Business Media B.V. 2012

The qualities of friendship for young children differ in some respects from qualities of adult friendships. It should be acknowledged that children of school age are entering a complex social arena where they need to gain peer acceptance and learn to initiate and maintain friendships. They may often need to deal with rebuffs, rejection and the frequent breaking up of friendships in ways that are not typical of adult friendships (Besag 2007).

Not all children initially have the social competence, confidence and emotional capacity needed to negotiate these relationships in a fulfilling way. Also, classmates can vary significantly in terms of how friendly and inclusive they are. A UNICEF report (2007) indicated considerable variation between countries on how helpful and friendly classroom peers were perceived to be. Research has shown that how schools organise and group pupils in schools can act to promote friendships and inclusion across, for example, different racial groups (Hallinan and Williams 1989).

Knowledge and understanding of the developmental tasks of friendships at particular ages supports the identification of effective interventions. Indeed, there are numerous resources now available to help children and whole classes develop friendly relationships. This chapter includes sections on friendship development in the early years, middle childhood and adolescence. Each of these sections outlines research on the psychological significance of each developmental phase and concludes by providing examples of effective interventions and resources available.

8.2   Friendship in Social and Cultural Contexts

Friendship can be defined as a reciprocal relationship where there is mutual liking and enjoyment spent in each other's company.

Whilst we may feel that we make our own choices of friends in what are generally regarded as voluntary relationships, the social and cultural context can influence friendship choice and opportunities for friendship (Chu 2005; Way et al. 2005). Frean (2003) cites the work of Graham Allan, a Professor of Social Relations, who pointed out that whilst these relationships are perceived to be personal and voluntary, they are still determined, to a large extent, by ethnicity, class, age, gender and geography. I would suggest that this might indicate that there are unnecessary constraints that restrict possibilities for friendship.

With regard to gender, for example, most people agree that there are some gender differences observable in the friendships and social networks of both children and adults. Typically, the friendships and social network of boys and men might be centred on activities such as football or other sports. For girls and women, the focus might be on opportunities for conversation and the specific activity, if there is one, of less importance.

The relationships described above might be viewed as stereotypical and a reflection of the influence of society and culture on the gendered expectations of girls and boys in respect of toys, play companions and friendships and women and men in terms of leisure activities and acceptable patterns of friendship. With regard to the former, for example, a parent of a young boy might be perfectly happy that he enjoys using the dressing up box for imaginative play. She might have more concerns when her son requests to be an Angel in the Christmas play alongside female peers rather than as a shepherd with his male peers! As noticeable gender patterns in friendships would seem to be determined, at least in part, by social and/or cultural expectations, we need to avoid making assumptions based on such expectations in order not to impose restrictions on the possibilities for friendship. Not all boys and men like football, and the fact that we now have girls and women's football teams is testament to the fact that some girls and women very much enjoy football!

This chapter is primarily focused on the many positive aspects of friendship. It needs to be acknowledged, however, that some friendships/aspects of a friendship are not so positive. In most friendships, there is a feeling of reciprocity and of being on an approximately equal footing with each other. Qualities of each person may be perceived as different though complement each other's needs and aspirations. Some friendships, however, may contain more negative qualities. They might be perceived to be less equal and reciprocal; there may be an uneven balance of power. A friend who perceives themselves to be less powerful in this situation may at times feel put upon and not valued.

Other less-than-positive friendships may encourage participation in undesirable behaviours such as exclusion, bullying, risk taking and other antisocial behaviours. Leather (2009) found that adolescents who had been excluded from school were more likely to form associations with others and participate in unsociable and risky behaviours in the community. Roffey (2011) asserts that more inclusive environments where students feel connected to school and community are likely to discourage the development of negative groupings, such as gangs. Providing opportunities in schools and in the community where friendships and positive relationships can be sustained amongst diverse life styles and cultures is of benefit to all. The suggested strategies, interventions and resources in this chapter show how more inclusive environments for children and young people can be developed where friendships and positive social relationships are enhanced.

8.3 Friendship, the Peer Group and Social Networks

Researchers have defined friendship as distinct from acceptance by the peer group (people of similar age and status) although both involve perceptions of likeability. Wentzel, Baker and Russell (2009) define the distinction: 'The central distinction between having friends and involvement with larger peer groups is that friends reflect relatively private, egalitarian relationships often formed on the basis of idiosyncratic criteria' (p. 231). Whereas in peer groups, there are publicly known and readily identified and valued group characteristics.

Being accepted by peers may be a first step for many children in friendship formation. Whilst peer acceptance does provide a threshold for friendship, there is evidence that some children who are not generally accepted by peers are still able to form and maintain friendships. Ladd (2005) reviewed research which found that children with social difficulties, those with a tendency towards aggression, abused children and rejected children were able to form friendships. However, he also found that these friendships could have both positive and negative qualities, for instance containing higher levels of conflict.

Whilst research has historically explored and compared friendship and the peer group, recent research has highlighted the complexity of children's friendships and peer relations (Howe 2010). It has been noted that children have social relationships in a variety of social contexts which are dynamic and subject to change. Recent research has investigated children's social networks, which, as Baines and Blatchford (2009) describe, is a term that covers a range of relationships including 'the group of peers they most often hang about with' and friendship networks. A child may have social networks at school and outside of school. There may be a social network connected to a particular activity. Within these groups, some children will have a hierarchy of best friends, friends and network members to play with when the best friend is not available, whilst others prefer to have a group of friends rather than designated best friends.

8.4 The Developmental Significance of Friendships

Newcomb and Bagwell (1996) conducted a quantitative meta-analysis of studies comparing reciprocal friends and acquaintances. The studies covered children from preschool years up to and including early adolescence. Significant differences were found. Friendship relations were characterised by more positive engagement, conflict management, task activity and relationship properties than did acquaintances. Interestingly, there was no difference in the instances of conflict, but friends were then motivated to problem-solve to overcome the conflict, leaving the friendship intact. They conclude: 'The developmental significance of these friendship features may rest in the opportunity they afford children to experience and to practice these critical components of effective interpersonal relations'. (p. 298)

Friendships have a role to play in supporting transitions at various developmental stages throughout the life cycle. In a longitudinal study, Ladd (1990) found that young children showed better adjustments to school and educational attainments if they already had friends in their class when starting school and kept these as well as making new friends. Berndt and Keefe (1992) found that having friends when transferring to different grades and schools was associated with less psychological disturbance in adolescence. Hartup and Stevens (1999) conclude that friendships throughout the life cycle are of developmental significance, but caution that: 'Whether friendships are developmental assets or liabilities depends on several conditions, especially the characteristics of one's friends and the quality of one's relationships with them' (p. 79).

8.5   Friendships Throughout the Life Cycle

Friendships are an important feature of our lives from the early years into adulthood. The nature and quality of these friendships change over time. A developmental perspective of friendships throughout the life cycle helps us to understand the significance and purposes served by friendships at different developmental phases.

Sullivan (1953) theorised that we have distinct social needs that could also be conceptualised as developmental tasks to accomplish at key phases in our development. In infancy, we have a need for security and nurturing from those that are close to us. In the early years (2–6 years), children need to join in play and activities with others. In middle childhood (7–12 years), children have a need to make friends and gain acceptance from their peers. As they move towards adolescence (13–19 years), children have a need for intimacy in their friendships, and in later adolescence, a desire to develop more intimate relationships including sexual relationships. Subsequent research over the years provides evidence to support this theoretical framework. I will draw on some of these research studies in this chapter. As Buhrmester (1996) comments, developmental researchers view the progressive accomplishment of these developmental tasks as enabling the formation of satisfying and fulfilling relationships in adulthood. Thus, friendships in childhood not only have an immediate ongoing impact but also have a formative impact on friendships in adulthood.

8.6   The Early Years

As Rubin (1980) notes, these early friendships provide opportunities for participating and learning about self and relationships in ways that cannot be met in other relationships such as the parent–child relationship.

Studies by psychologists provide evidence that, whilst there is much variation at this age, even young children can show preferences for particular playmates, seeking them out, playing cooperatively with them and showing the beginnings of empathy (e.g. Dunn 2004; Howes 1996). As Dunn (2004) points out, these findings challenge conventional notions that children are not able to form significant friendships until they are 7 or 8 years of age. Qualitative ethnographic studies where young children's interactions in early years settings have been carefully observed over extended time periods have also documented a wide range of skills, behaviours and understandings that children draw on in establishing and maintaining their friendships (Rubin 1980; Meyer 2003; Meyer and Driscoll 1997; Rizzo 1989). Meyer and Driscoll (1997) identified ten categories of strategies used by young children in a day care centre to establish, maintain and terminate friendships. These included proximity, listening, touch, expressing feelings, making jokes, using humour or teasing, making statements about the friendship, engaging in conflict, directing/controlling others, invoking rules and participating in pretend role play where there were shared expectations.

Rubin (1980) provides an example of two 4-year olds, where in a conversation one child becomes aware that he has hurt his friend's feelings and is able to take steps to successfully redress the situation:

David: I'm a missile robot who can shoot missiles out of my fingers. I can shoot them out of everywhere – even out of my legs. I am a missile robot.
Josh: (tauntingly) No, you're a fart robot.
David: (protestingly) No, I'm a missile robot.
Josh: No, you're a fart robot.
David: (hurt, almost in tears) No, Josh!
Josh: (recognizing that David is upset) And I'm a poo- poo robot.
David: (in good spirits again) I'm a pee-pee robot (p. 58).

Developmental psychologists have highlighted the importance of play in these early years, and particularly role play/pretend play between friends, as being crucial to developing social and emotional understanding and cognitive skills (Dunn 2004; Harris 2000). Harris' research demonstrates that when children use their imagination in shared pretence role plays with others, they are able to further their understanding of the real world and to distinguish it from fantasy, and to appreciate perspectives of others. In fact, as Harris points out, it is when children have difficulty in using their imagination in this way, as is the case for children on the autistic spectrum for example, that children experience difficulties in social and cognitive understanding and relating successfully with others.

Dunn (2004) comments that young friendships can be a means of emotional support. She gives the examples of a close friendship being supportive when there are significant life events, e.g. at a time when a sibling is born or on transferring from nursery to school. As Dunn notes: 'It is with the development of the features of shared feelings and ideas, of mutual affection and attachment, of concern for the other, which lead eventually to commitment and loyalty ...' (p. 3).

Like Harris, Dunn also comments on the significance of shared role play with friends. Findings reveal that pretend play between friends is more sustained and harmonious and more complex than play with acquaintances. She concludes that the shared fantasies are important in the development of the friendship: 'Sharing that pretend world can be a key setting for the growth of intimacy, and sharing the excitement generated by the fantasy; it may also perhaps be an important context for sharing what is worrying, as well as exciting' (p. 28).

It is important to consider that, as Smith (2010) notes, children who have experienced disadvantaged environments often do show impoverished pretend play. Early interventions are required to support play and communication skills in order to promote optimal conditions for friendship formation and educational progression.

8.6.1 Implications for Positive Practice

- In early years settings, aim for a small group size (up to 12 children). This provides optimal conditions for pretend play and the development of quality friendships (Smith and Connolly 1980).

- Provide a space and props to encourage creative shared role play. So in addition to a themed home corner, have alternative periods where space is available with a variety of materials, e.g. dressing up clothes, boxes, screens, sheets of material etc., for children to develop their own shared themes. Broadhead (2004) uses the term the 'Whatever you want it to be' place for this resource.
- Where children are having difficulties in peer relations and friendships, carry out observations to clarify their skills and highlight areas for development. A useful tool for observing play is 'The Social Play Continuum' in Broadhead's (2004) book, *Early Years Play and Learning*.
- Provide guidance, model and comment on friendly behaviour.
- Supervise at a distance. Give children time to learn to sort out conflicts and support where needed.
- Provide opportunities to talk things through with a child when there has been upset and conflict. This helps the child understand their own feelings and those of others (Dunn 2004).
- Use role play with puppets where the children can practise a wide range of friendship skills, including how to gain entry to a group or deal with being turned down (Webster-Stratton 2009).
- Encourage parents to invite playmates home and support this by providing information on friendships in the playgroup/class room and with ideas for activities if required (Webster-Stratton 2009).
- Provide activities and opportunities which invite children to take turns and share, e.g. dressing up clothes and props, and wheeled toys designed for two children to ride (Dowling 2010).
- Use storybooks on friendships to raise awareness and discuss features of friendships.
- For children transferring to school and needing to develop language/communication and social and early learning skills, set up friendship groups. In this approach, an adult such as a teaching assistant works with a group of up to four children for half an hour a day. The emphasis is on participating in enjoyable activities rather than more structured educational activities. Cooking, art activities and growing plants and gardening are ideal activities. This safe space can be used to facilitate verbal and non-verbal communication, interactive play and friendly behaviours.
- A useful resource with activities for very young children and up to age 5 years is: *100 ideas for teaching personal, social and emotional development* (Thwaites 2008).

8.7   Friendship in Middle Childhood

As children move into middle childhood, play with others continues to be an important factor in developing social networks and friendships. The form of play is in pretence games and also physical, rule-based games, e.g. ball games, chase, skipping with elastic etc., often with a competitive element.

Blatchford (1998) researched children aged 8–9 years transferring to junior school and monitored their friendship formation and the stability of friendship groups over the year. He observed that games played at break time in the school served two important functions. First, the variety of games played at break time provided a structure to enable children to have contact with other children on transfer to the junior school, and this social networking supported friendship formation. Blatchford noted that initially there was a flurry of activity as children sought out friendships. Later on in the school year, however, friendship groups stabilised, and entry to games was more exclusive as they were entwined with particular friendship groups.

Interestingly, some of the children interviewed about why children had particular friends spoke of best friends transcending the game connection: Their best friends were those that were always available to play with – e.g. John told the researcher that best friends were always available to play with and there when needed, so that: 'sometimes Graham doesn't play with me and sometimes Shawn doesn't but Tim always does though we play different games' (p. 79).

This view of friendship was also apparent in the interviews carried out by Wordley (2010), who carried out in-depth interviews with a small sample of 8-year-old children regarding their classroom friendships and learning.

Guy: '…Anthony is a good friend cos like if you don't have anyone to play with or something, he'll always be willing to come and play with you or stop what he's doing, or maybe ask you if what he was doing, you might want to go and play with him with some of your friends'.

In another interview with Mia:

Claire: So what's a difference between a friend and a best friend?
Mia: Well, 'cos like Gemma and Holly mostly play with me and like Amelia plays with someone else but occasionally she plays with me.

Baines and Blatchford (2011) highlight the importance of school break times or recess as being one of the main opportunities for children to play with friends and develop friendships. They note that break times are particularly valuable as children today have less opportunity for unsupervised activities and contact with others outside of school. This situation, they suggest, may be due at least in part to increasing parental concerns about child safety and heightened parental supervision as a result. Baines and Blatchford are therefore concerned to note that these periods in the school day are increasingly being abolished or shortened in countries such as the USA, Australia and the UK. School staffs frequently cite problem behaviour and needing time for teaching the curriculum as reasons for reducing break times. Baines and Blatchford comment that whilst there are substantial campaigns across many countries to enhance play facilities outside of school, there are few such campaigns to protect break time/recess.

At this stage of development, as parents and teachers are often aware, there may be frequent making and breaking of friendships as children develop their social and communication skills and their ability to manage their emotions. Wordley's (2010) interview with Laura, aged 8 years, gives a flavour of the ebb and flow in these relationships and Laura's awareness of the process:

> Lisa, Carmel and Jacinta they do normally have fall outs but they're like one day Jacinta and Carmel are friends and they leave Lisa out because they all have an argument and then the next day Jacinta and Lisa and then the next Carmel and Lisa and Jacinta gets left out and it goes all around like that…

This quote also serves to illustrate a distinctive feature of this developmental phase in that children tend to form same-sex social networks and friendships. It is thought that children seek same-sex social networks because they share similar interests and play styles (Maccoby 1998). Baines and Blatchford (2009) carried out research comparing girls' and boys' social networks and friendships in the playground. They found, as has previous research, that boys tended to form larger social networks than girls, consisting of both friends and non-friends. Girls' social networks were smaller and consisted mainly of best friends and friends.

8.7.1   Social Networks Outside of School

Most research on children's social networks has been carried out in the school context, and there is a need to research on children's social networks and friendships outside of school. This is particularly as there have been significant changes in children's opportunities to spend time with their friends and in the nature of communicating and maintaining friendships. Thus, with regard to the latter, children frequently maintain friendships through texting and using their mobile phones and online 'chat forums'.

Layard and Dunn (2009) view the pace and change of this decade, of society in general and of experiences of childhood in particular, as unprecedented, and that we need to consider the impact on children and young people. Friendship was one of the seven themes explored by The Good Childhood Inquiry panel. This Inquiry set out to consider experiences of all children in the United Kingdom and made comparisons with research findings from other countries. Layard and Dunn note that there are fewer areas for safe play and that children have much less freedom to go out with friends unsupervised. Thus, some parents spend much of their time ferrying their children to supervised activities and parties. Other parents may not have the resources to do this, and children remain at home, sometimes spending large amounts of time on the computer.

To conclude, in the middle school years, children recognise and develop a range of friendships with differing qualities according to whether they are casual friends, good friends or best friends. Towards the end of middle childhood, children are increasingly making friendship choices based on personality, and there is a level of intimacy in a growing awareness of sharing and supporting. As Doll (2010) points out, these friendships involve a degree of loyalty, and children need to balance their own interests with the needs of their friend. They therefore need to be able to see a situation from their friend's perspective and to make small compromises.

8.7.2   *Implications for Positive Practice*

- Children need increased access to recreation spaces in the community, including playgrounds and playing fields for unsupervised play (Layard and Dunn 2009).
- Children need to have opportunities to participate in a range of activities outside of school to sustain interests and friendships with others.
- Interventions should make optimal use of the school playground to provide enjoyable play space and opportunities to make and consolidate friendships. Involve the children in designing an exciting school playground that meets the diverse needs and desires of the children. Children could survey classmates to find out what they would like. The playground needs to provide places for physical activities such as football and chase games, and also quieter activities. Include a signposted friends meeting place where children can go to if they want someone to play with or talk to.
- Some schools have trained and supported a team of children (squad) to befriend others in the playground and help sort out disputes over games.
- An excellent resource for developing the play ground is *Resilient Playgrounds* by Beth Doll with Katherine Brehm (2010).
- Discuss friendships and friendly behaviour as a class. Agree on class principles which would aim to ensure that individuals are valued, difference is accepted and that all are included in play and work activities.
- Use Circle Time to talk through and resolve friendship issues/unfriendly behaviour as they arise. A useful book is *Circle Time Resources* (Robinson and Maines 2004).
- Provide activities in the classroom that invite collaboration, e.g. solving a science problem or shared story writing. Provide adult commentary on helpful and friendly behaviour.
- Provide opportunities for children to work with their friends on problem tasks.
- Provide opportunities at other times for children to get used to working with different members of the class.
- This is probably the best time for group work to develop the skills and social understanding of children who are finding it difficult to gain peer acceptance and establish friendships. Three useful resources for middle childhood are:
  - *The Friendship Formula: A Social Skills Programme to Develop an Awareness of Self and Others* (Schroeder 2008).
  - *How to Promote Children's Social and Emotional Competence* (Webster-Stratton 2009), particularly Chapter 10: *Peer Problems and Friendship*.
  - *Developing Children's Social, Emotional and Behavioural Skills* (Costi 2009).

- Parents and teachers need to value children's friendships. They need to encourage children to make friends and maintain friendships, e.g. following a change of school and moving house. Children need opportunities to have their friends stay with them for both play and study (Layard and Dunn 2009).

8.8 Adolescent Friendships

At this phase of development, friends and the social networks they are contained within become increasingly important and enable a range of developmental needs to be met. Young people have a need for companionship and a growing intimacy alongside meeting the challenge of new life experiences including transition to high school and later transitions to university and/or work involving changes in friendships and social networks.

School continues to be an important source of friends. Hamm and Faircloth (2005) found that these friendships played a vital role in enabling adolescents to develop a sense of belonging to the school. They describe such a sense of belonging as relating to: 'students' perceptions that they are liked, respected, and valued by others in the school' (p. 61).

Hamm and Faircloth found that school friendships provided a secure base that helped adolescents to cope with the social context of the high school.

Researchers of peer relations, friendships and school break time have commented that in contrast to early years and middle childhood, adolescent friendships are characterised by a lack of play, games and physical activities at break time, and there is more emphasis on opportunities to talk and to 'hanging around' together (Blatchford 1998). He comments that break times for older students in secondary schools provide an important function in providing loosely supervised areas where adolescent girls and boys can socialise.

At this time, adolescents need to develop their sense of identity and belonging, and interactions with friends and friendship groups facilitate this. As Cotterell (2007) notes: 'Two particular social provisions that are supplied by friends as a group are social integration into a friendship network and reassurance of worth through the social validation of friends' (p. 80).

Adolescent friends serve a very important purpose in providing acceptance and emotional support at a time when they are becoming more independent and less reliant on parents. The level of intimacy in a friendship is an indicator both of the maturing quality of friendship and, indeed, predicts wellbeing and self-esteem in adolescence (Buhrmester 1990). Loyalty also distinguishes adolescent friendships from other relationships. There may be gender differences here in that girls and women's friendships are often characterised as having a greater level of intimacy and self-disclosure. Thus, it could be argued that this facilitates more emotional support than that available within male friendships.

There is, however, a need to challenge assumptions made about male friendships. Recent qualitative research studies challenge assumptions that boys do not want close friendships (Chu 2005; Way et al. 2005). Chu (2005) found that adolescent boys interviewed in this study actually did want to have close male friendships, though some felt that needing to prove masculinity and protect vulnerability were barriers to such friendships.

Optimistically, Chu notes that despite these barriers, some adolescent boys did form close friendships, and these friendships actually supported them in dealing with male peer pressure to conform:

> Ethan: When I was thirteen, I met my closest friend right now, and he really helped me to become who I want to become. I felt like we both kind of helped each other grow into, like, who we want to be right now. Up until that time, I'd kind of been thinking, 'Well, I don't really like this, so why am I doing it?' but continued to do it, like just dressing all neat and trying to impress everyone I met and trying to be, like, the perfect kid. But in meeting my friend, he really helped-we both helped each other a lot to become who we are right now. And we both like who we are right now, to some extent (p. 16).

Way et al. (2005), in a study of ethnic-minority urban adolescents, found that both girls and boys desired close friendships, and they did not differ in emphasising the keeping of secrets and self-disclosure as important features of their closest friendships. Cotterell (2007) cautions about making assumptions about gender differences in intimacy and communication and urges that there should be a closer examination of gender differences in styles of intimacy and communication to enhance a greater understanding.

As Scholte and Van Aken (2008) comment, friendships are formed where 'common ground' and 'affirmations' about the friendship are made. Whilst perceived similarities might be important in establishing the common ground, they become less important as the friendship becomes established. Maintenance of the friendship is dependent on the quality of the friendship. Thus, friendships which are emotionally supportive, and where there is trust and intimacy, may well survive for many years. Other friendships which may have these qualities to a much lesser degree are unlikely to survive in the long run.

Outside of school, young people continue to develop a range of interconnected friendship groups or cliques, within a larger peer crowd or social cluster (Cotterell 2007). Membership of these groups is fluid and changeable. As in middle childhood, within these groups, adolescents are likely to have some close friendships and more casual friends and acquaintances. Whilst most adolescents will still enjoy spending time with a small group of same-sex friends, they also seek opportunities and are excited to be part of large mixed sex crowds, e.g. at parties, or music concerts, or simply at the beach, park or street corner. This wider social cluster provides opportunities for mixed sex friendship groups or cliques in later adolescence and for romantic relationships.

There is a need for communities to consider activities, spaces and resources to meet the social and leisure needs of adolescence, some of whom report that there is nothing for them to do or go to. It is also apparent that in early adolescence, some who might have confidently tried new activities as a child lack social confidence to go to clubs and activities unless accompanied by a friend and are also much influenced by what their peer group might consider to be 'cool' or 'un-cool'.

8.8.1   Implications for Positive Practice

- There is a need to work with young people to identify stimulating and supportive areas where young people can meet.
- Layard and Dunn (2009) recommend the setting up of Young People's Centres which offer high-quality activities such as IT, music, drama and dance, sport and volunteering as well as psychological support and careers advice.
- Interventions should aim to support transitions to establish positive peer relations and to provide new friendships to flourish: *B.E.S.T. Buddies Bettering Everyone's Secondary Transition: A comprehensive training programme introducing a peer buddy system to support students starting secondary school* (Smith 2003).

8.8.2   Friendship Transition Groups

Short-term group work during transition for adolescents who lack confidence and might be overwhelmed by the social and organisational expectations of secondary school can be very effective. For example, a summer project could involve 1 week of the summer holiday. In this time, staff from Education Support Services could run an orientation group in the secondary school. Activities could include games that enable the young people to find their way around the school and activities to raise self-esteem and promote positive interactions and involvement in social and leisure activities. These young people start school feeling knowledgeable and confident, already knowing some new people.

Other schools have run Friendship Groups for socially vulnerable pupils on transfer to secondary school. These could be run weekly by staff from Education Support Services for the first term. The aim is to provide a secure base to develop trusting relationships, in order to express feelings and worries. Activities are provided to develop communication and assertiveness skills, friendship, self-esteem and problem-solving skills. Initially, the sessions need to be structured and contain several activities. As the young people develop trust and confidence and communication skills, they are able to use the group to discuss their situations and problem solve and to support each other. Experience of running these groups has shown that adolescents are not looking to adults to sort out problems. Group members often do have the resources amongst themselves to support each other and problem solve given appropriate opportunities to do so.

Interventions should develop a sense of belonging by offering a wide range of after-school clubs catering for a diversity of interests. They should also provide a range of activities for boys as this provides a focus for their relationships.

Peer support improves both learning and positive interactions: *Peer Support Works: A Step by Step Guide to Long Term Success* (Cartwright 2007).

8.9   Friendships in Adult Life

In later adolescence and into adulthood, friendships are important though time is also increasingly spent with romantic partners. Most adults will also go on to become parents. The traditional view of family and social relations puts family ties before friendships. Pahl and Spence (2003-4) assert that this does not reflect the reality of people's lives and the complexity of social relationships. They put forward a model of 'personal communities' to describe an individual's commitments to family and friends. Thus, an individual will have a high commitment to specific family members ('given' relationships in the sense that blood ties are not chosen) and friends ('chosen' relationships in the sense that friendships are primarily voluntary relationships). A lower level of commitment will be shown to other given (family) and chosen (friends) relationships. This model allows for the power of informal support structures to be recognised.

Close friendships, sometimes formed at school, may endure over years and may well last into adulthood. These would constitute high commitment 'chosen' relationships in Pahl and Spence's model. Cotterell (2007) lists the 'distinctive qualities' of sustaining a friendship as: 'sharing enjoyable activities, being loyal and available, being ready to assist, being sensitive to friend's feelings, expressing confidence in the friends, and providing comfort and optimism in times of difficulty' (p. 80).

A small-scale study for this publication was conducted in order to shed light on the defining features of long-lasting friendships. Questionnaires on best friends were completed by 30 adults aged between 24 and 59 years. This included men and women, predominantly white British; 33% were from different nationalities. Whist the sample was small, some clear patterns emerged. 94% of friendships were same sex, and 87% of friendships were same age or within 1 year. Most had met their friend at school or university (73%). The length of friendship was between 5 and 49 years. The questionnaire asked an open-ended question on why people thought the friendship with their best friend had endured. The following themes were identified:

- Shared experience/interests/values
- Good company/humour/fun/get on well/relaxed
- Trust/loyalty/open/talk about anything/acceptance
- Reciprocity/both make time/bond

Some friendships had endured despite those friends not living nearby: 44% said that their friend did not live nearby and in some cases lived in a different country.

8.10   Conclusion

Having a range of social networks and fulfilling friendships is important to our wellbeing. An understanding of the complexity of social interactions to be negotiated over the life cycle is a prerequisite for adults aiming to promote an environment for others where friendships can begin and flourish. Positive interventions can be designed that are helpful in ensuring optimal conditions for the development of friendship skills.

References

Bagwell, C., Newcomb, A., & Bukowski, W. (1998). Preadolescent friendship and peer rejection as predictors of adult adjustment. *Child Development, 69*(1), 140–153.

Baines, E., & Blatchford, P. (2009). Sex differences in the structure and stability of children's playground social networks and their overlap with friendship relations. *British Journal of Developmental Psychology, 27*, 743–760.

Baines, E., & Blatchford, P. (2011). Playground games and activities in school and their role in development. In A. Pellegrini (Ed.), *Oxford handbook of the development of play*. New York: Oxford University Press.

Berndt, T., & Keefe, K. (1992). Friends' influence on adolescent's perceptions of themselves in school. In D. H. Schunk & J. L. Meece (Eds.), *Students' perceptions in the classroom* (pp. 51–73). New York: Lawrence Erlbaum Associates.

Besag, V. (2007). *Understanding girls' friendships, fights and feuds*. Berkshire: London University Press.

Blatchford, P. (1998). *Social life in school: Pupils' experience of break time and recess from 7 to 16 years*. London: Falmer Press.

Broadhead, P. (2004). *Early years play and learning*. London: RoutledgeFalmer.

Buhrmester, D. (1990). Intimacy of friendship, interpersonal competence, and adjustment during preadolescence and adolescence. *Child Development, 61*, 1101–1111.

Buhrmester, D. (1996). Need fulfilment, interpersonal competence, and the developmental contexts of early adolescent friendship. In W. Bukowski, A. Newcomb, & W. Hartup (Eds.), *The company they keep: Friendship in childhood and adolescence* (pp. 158–185). New York: Cambridge University Press.

Cartwright, C. (2007). *Peer support works: A step by step guide to long term success*. London: Network Continuum Education.

Chu, J. (2005). Adolescent boys' friendships and peer group culture. *New Directions for Child and Adolescent Development, 107*, 11–20.

Costi, M. (2009). *Developing children's social, emotional and behavioural skills*. London: Continuum.

Cotterell, J. (2007). *Social networks in youth and adolescence*. London: Routledge.

Cowen, E., Pederson, A., Babgian, H., Izzo, L., & Trost, M. A. (1973). Long-term follow up of early detected vulnerable children. *Journal of Consulting and Clinical Psychology, 41*, 438–446.

Diener, E., & Diener, C. (2009). Foreword. In R. Gilman, E. S. Huebner, & M. Furlong (Eds.), *Handbook of positive psychology in schools* (p. xi). New York: Routledge.

Doll, B. (2010). *Resilient playgrounds*. London: Routledge.

Dowling, M. (2010). *Young children's personal, social and emotional development*. London: Sage.

Dunn, J. (2004). *Children's friendships. The beginnings of intimacy*. Oxford: Blackwell Publishing.

Frean, A. (2003). Friends like these: The relationships that shape our lives. *The Edge, Economic and Social Research Council, 13*, 8–10.

Frederickson, N. (1991). Children can be so cruel: Helping the rejected child. In G. Lindsay & A. Miller (Eds.), *Psychological services for primary schools*. Harlow: Longman.

Hallinan, M., & Williams, R. (1989). Interracial friendship choices in secondary schools. *American Sociological Review, 54*(1), 67–78.

Hamm, J., & Faircloth, B. (2005). The role of friendship in adolescents' sense of school belonging. *New Directions for Child and Adolescent Development, 107*, 61–78.

Harris, P. (2000). *The work of the imagination*. Oxford: Blackwell.

Hartup, W., & Stevens, N. (1999). Friendships and adaptation across the life span. *Current Directions in Psychological Science, 8*, 76–79.

Howe, C. (2010). *Peer groups and children's development*. Chichester: Wiley-Blackwell.

Howes, C. (1996). The earliest friendships. In W. Bukowski, A. Newcomb, & W. Hartup (Eds.), *The company they keep: Friendship in childhood and adolescence* (pp. 66–86). New York: Cambridge University Press.

Ladd, G. (1990). Having friends, keeping friends, making friends, and being liked by peers in the classroom: Predictors of children's early school adjustment? *Child Development, 61*, 1081–1100.

Ladd, G. (2005). *Children's peer relations and social competence: A century of progress*. London: Yale University Press.

Ladd, G., & Kochenderfer, B. (1996). Linkages between friendship and adjustment during early school transitions. In W. Bukowski, A. Newcomb, & W. Hartup (Eds.), *The company they keep: Friendship in childhood and adolescence* (p. 324). New York: Cambridge University Press.

Layard, R., & Dunn, J. (2009). *A good childhood: Searching for values in a competitive age*. London: Penguin.

Leather, N. (2009). Risk-taking in adolescence: A literature review. *Journal of Child Health Care, 13*, 295–304.

Maccoby, E. (1998). *The two sexes: Growing up apart, coming together*. Cambridge: Harvard University Press.

Mendelson, M., & Aboud, F. (1999). Measuring friendship quality in late adolescents and young adults: McGill friendship questionnaires. *Canadian Journal of Behavioural Science, 31*, 130–132.

Meyer, J. (2003). *Kids talking: Learning relationships and culture with children*. Oxford: Rowman and Littlefield Publishers.

Meyer, J., & Driscoll, G. (1997). Children and relationship development: Communication strategies in a day care centre. *Communication Reports, 10*, 75–85.

Newcomb, A., & Bagwell, C. (1996). The developmental significance of children's friendship relations. In W. Bukowski, A. Newcomb, & W. Hartup (Eds.), *The company they keep. Friendship in childhood and adolescence* (pp. 289–321). New York: Cambridge University Press.

Pahl, R., & Spence, L. (2003-4). *Personal communities: Not simply families or 'fate' or 'choice'* (Working paper, ISER paper 2003-4). Colchester: University of Essex.

Rizzo, T. A. (1989). *Friendship development among children in school*. Norwood: Ablex Publishing Corporation.

Robinson, G., & Maines, B. (2004). *Circle time resources*. Bristol: Lucky Duck Publishing.

Roffey, S. (2011). Enhancing connectedness in Australian children and young people. *Asian Journal of Counselling, 18*(1), 1–25.

Rubin, Z. (1980). *Children's friendships*. Glasgow: Fontana.

Scholte, R., & Van Aken, M. (2008). Peer relations in adolescence. In S. Jackson & L. Goossens (Eds.), *Handbook of adolescent development* (pp. 175–199). Hove: Psychology Press.

Schroeder, A. (2008). *The friendship formula: A social skills programme to develop an awareness of self and others*. Cambridge: LDA.

Smith, C. (2003). *B.E.S.T Buddies Bettering Everyone's Secondary Transition: A comprehensive training programme introducing a peer buddy system to support students starting secondary school*. Bristol: Lucky Duck Publishing.

Smith, P. (2010). *Children and play*. Chichester: Wiley-Blackwell.

Smith, P., & Connolly, K. (1980). *The ecology of preschool behaviour*. Cambridge: Cambridge University Press.

Sullivan, H. (1953). *The interpersonal theory of psychiatry*. New York: Norton.

Thwaites, J. (2008). *100 ideas for teaching personal, social and emotional development*. London: Continuum.

UNICEF. (2007). *Child poverty in perspective: An overview of child well-being in rich countries: A comprehensive assessment of the lives and well-being of children and adolescents in the economically advanced nations.* Geneva: UNICEF Innocenti Research Centre Report Card 7.

Way, N., Gingold, R., Rotenberg, M., & Kuriakose, G. (2005). Close friendships among urban, ethnic-minority adolescents. *New Directions for Child and Adolescent Development, 107*, 11–20.

Webster-Stratton, C. (2009). *How to promote children's social and emotional competence.* London: Sage.

Wentzel, K., Barry, C., & Caldwell, K. (2004). Friendships in middle school: Influences on motivation and school adjustment. *Journal of Educational Psychology, 96*, 195–203.

Wentzel, K., Baker, S., & Russell, S. (2009). Peer relationships and positive adjustment at school. In R. Gilman, E. Scott Huebner, & M. J. Furlong (Eds.), *Handbook of positive psychology in schools.* New York: Routledge.

Wordley, C. (2010). *Friendship and learning: A study of Year Four's perceptions of friendship and whether their friends help them to learn.* Unpublished PGCE assignment, Faculty of Education, University of Cambridge.

Karen Majors is a tutor on the educational psychology training course at the Institute of Education, London University. She has written on friendship in the school context and completed her doctorate on Imaginary Friendships in children. Contact: k.majors@ioe.ac.uk

Chapter 9
Developing Positive Relationships in Schools

Sue Roffey

9.1 Introduction

Schools play a significant part not only in the formal and informal education of young people but also in their wellbeing – and hence the wellbeing of families and communities of the future. In 1995, the World Health Organization introduced the Global School Health initiative (WHO 1995) and brought the concept of education for wellbeing into the foreground. Related initiatives have since been adopted or developed by governments and education authorities in many parts of the world. In 2003, the Wingspread Declaration: A National Strategy for Improving School Connectedness was issued in the USA. This is based on a detailed review of the relevant research as well as in-depth discussions amongst leaders in health and education in the USA. It summarises the evidence for positive relationships across education (Blum and Libbey 2004).

Wellbeing comprises not only physical but also psychological health. This is demonstrated by both optimal functioning and predominantly positive feelings (Noble et al. 2008). It is where people are flourishing rather than languishing in their everyday lives (Keyes and Haidt 2003). Although acknowledging a responsibility to respond to individual needs and specific issues, this broader concept of health has increasingly incorporated a whole-school approach in which all aspects of the school system are targeted to establish a health-promoting environment for all (Wyn et al. 2000; Leger 2005).

S. Roffey (✉)
School of Education, University of Western Sydney, Sydney, Australia

Department of Clinical, Educational & Health Psychology, University College, London, UK
e-mail: sue@sueroffey.com.

S. Roffey (ed.), *Positive Relationships: Evidence Based Practice across the World*,
DOI 10.1007/978-94-007-2147-0_9, © Springer Science+Business Media B.V. 2012

The Organization for Economic Cooperation and Development, comprising 30 nations, issued its first report in 2009 on indicators of child wellbeing (OECD 2009). The six dimensions identified are material wellbeing, housing and environment, health and safety, risk behaviours and quality of school life. How 'quality' is defined and developed goes beyond material resources and the curriculum to the heart of the teaching endeavour. Emotions and relationships exist all day, every day in the classroom, staffroom and throughout the school. Sometimes these feelings and relationships, especially for more vulnerable students, can be overwhelmingly negative. The quality of the learning environment therefore depends, not only on curriculum content, but also how accessible this is to students. The active promotion of positive feelings – enjoyment, achievement, optimism, safety and a sense of belonging – alongside positive and healthy relationships facilitate an environment in which everyone is able to flourish and learn (Fredrickson 2009; Roffey 2011a).

The ethos of schools and the quality of the learning environment has been a focus of research for several decades, particularly in relation to behavioural issues. The Elton Report on Discipline in Schools in the UK (DES 1989) advocated a coherent whole-school approach to behaviour based on good relationships between all members of the school community. The Steer Report on Learning Behaviour (DfES 2005a), nearly 30 years later, says that despite the differences in educational practices, this still holds true. The difference now is how much more we know about what constitutes good relationships in schools and the multiple and interrelated outcomes, not only for behaviour, but also for academic achievement (Hattie 2009; Hearn et al. 2006) and mental health (Spratt et al. 2006; Murray-Harvey 2010). Most importantly, researchers and practitioners have discovered and developed ways in which these relationships might be brought about.

9.2 Social Capital in Schools

Physical capital comprises hardware resources, such as buildings and equipment, human capital comprises knowledge and skills and social capital refers to the quality of relationships within an organisation or community. Social capital can be defined as the levels of trust, mutual responsibility and reciprocity that people experience in their interactions with each other and their sense of belonging to a particular community with a shared identity and shared values (Putnam 2000). Social capital not only enhances feelings of safety and wellbeing, but also enables groups of people to work together towards shared goals. It enhances the resources of an organisation in multiple ways by increasing the flow of information, ideas, advice, help, opportunities, contacts, emotional support and goodwill (Adler and Kwon 2002). Baker and Dutton (2007) talk about the importance of developing positive social capital where this is developed for the benefit of the greater good rather than increasing connections for one group at the expense of others. It is the difference between inclusive and exclusive belonging, the latter being where group members maintain their sense of wellbeing by keeping 'inferior' others out. Positive social capital helps everyone in an organisation flourish.

You can determine the level of social capital within a school by the way people talk to and about each other, the quality of the 'emotional' climate, and the extent to which this appears to be calm, supportive and purposeful. There is evidence that interventions that add to the levels of social capital can help protect against the adverse effects of psychosocial stressors (Phongsavan et al. 2006), as well as promote prosocial behaviour and engagement (Jennings and Greenberg 2009).

Participation, empowerment and a sense of connection are central to a high level of social capital. Schools that are less hierarchical and didactic are more likely to involve all members of the school community in respectful interactions. Onyx and Bullen (2000) identified the following factors for measuring social capital in schools:

- Levels of participation in the community
- Proactivity in a social context and a sense of personal and collective efficacy
- Feelings of trust and safety
- Tolerance of diversity
- Feeling part of a team

The quote below (cited in Roffey 2008) illustrates several of these elements:

I'm just blown away by how kind the teachers are to students here... but I think that's just a follow-on of the whole culture. You sit in the dining room and you never have to be mindful of what you're saying, because everyone's on the same side ... the staff are supportive of each other, and I think that carries across into the classroom (teacher, high school).

The health-promoting school aims to promote change in three broad areas:

- Formal curriculum in health education
- Connectedness and caring relationships between all stakeholders
- Recognition of the important role the school has to promote health and development of links with the wider community to support this role

One study (Sun and Stewart 2007) found that the health-promoting school approach had the capacity to substantially affect the relationships that people had with one another and the school psychosocial environment. Intervention activities were developed in ten primary schools around issues identified by each school community, such as resilience, anti-bullying and communication skills. The findings suggest a strong link between taking action on these issues and the promotion of social capital with specific regard to feelings of trust and safety, tolerance of diversity and work relationships with colleagues. This matches the experience of Antidote (Tew 2010), who discovered that open, safe and equal debate around issues of improving the school environment impacted on relational dynamics and how people felt about themselves and their colleagues. The collection of data gathered multiple views, avoided blame and generated a wide spectrum of ideas. This process in itself increased the level of social capital and fostered creative solutions in which everyone felt they had ownership.

9.3   The Ecology of Student and School Wellbeing

There is rarely a straight line between cause and effect in human behaviour. Outcomes at any one time are the result of interactive, circular and accumulative causation. Relationships are rarely established or broken in an instant. Beliefs determine actions that influence responses from others. This builds a history that leads to expectations and repeated cycles of interaction. Relationships are, however, not only rooted in personal constructs of the world, but also in the social and cultural milieu in which individuals are living. These offer a set of beliefs about how things 'should' be as well as impacting on the resources available.

Bronfenbrenner (1979) first gave prominence to an ecosystemic view of human development and others have taken and applied this model to related issues (de Jong 2003; Felner 2006; Friesthler et al. 2006). This model says that the most important influence on a child's development is what happens at the 'micro-level' and the interactions that individuals have with those in their immediate world. In schools, this is reflected in a school's mission to have as a central focus the 'whole child' and all their experiences in order to optimise each student's development in all domains. This 'whole child' focus appears to extend to the 'whole person' and the acceptance of diversity across staff and families as well as students. The next level, the meso-system, comprises the beliefs, values and skills that determine the quality of relationships throughout the school. At the exosystem are procedures and policies that impact on what happens at the microsystem and mesosystem. This includes resources that are available and access to these, working schedules and organisational expectations. At the macro-system are cultural norms, values and laws. These have a cascading influence throughout the other systems. The chronosystem recognises that systems are forever interacting and changing over time. Although elements of relationships within a school ecology may be addressed separately, none stands alone. Influences and actions are bidirectional both within and between levels of the system. Conversations in the staffroom impact on what happens in the classroom, how welcome a parent feels will, in part, be determined by policies and procedures that determine how families are 'positioned' in the school.

In a qualitative study exploring the development of emotional literacy in two secondary and four primary schools in Australia, this ecology became apparent. See Fig. 9.1 below (Roffey 2008). Unless stated otherwise, all quotes in this chapter are taken from this research. All the schools in this study had been identified as having actively raised awareness of emotional literacy and relational quality throughout the school. Teachers, students, school counsellors and school principals were interviewed to explore what had happened in this development, what difference it made to them and what they thought had influenced these outcomes. It became clear in the analysis that how students felt about their school and the relationships they experienced with teachers was mirrored by how teachers felt about their relationships with colleagues and with management. School culture and expectations filtered down to the interactions that took place.

> … if you have a happy staff, then I think that leads to you being happy in your own classroom, and leads to happy relationships with the children, and the children with each other. (teacher)

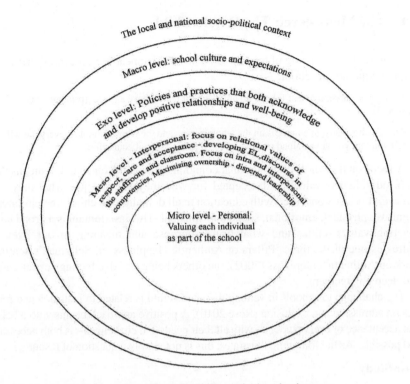

The local and national socio-political context

Macro level: school culture and expectations

Exo level: Policies and practices that both acknowledge and develop positive relationships and well-being

Meso level - Interpersonal: focus on relational values of respect, care and acceptance - developing EL discourse in the staffroom and classroom. Focus on intra and interpersonal competencies. Maximising ownership - dispersed leadership

Micro level - Personal:
Valuing each individual
as part of the school

Fig. 9.1   An eco-systemic analysis of emotional literacy in the school context

A related project in the UK explored the factors that enabled staff and students to engage most effectively with teaching and learning (Haddon et al. 2005). This took place in two schools over 3 years. The researchers found that five aspects of a school were linked to people's capacity to fully engage. These are encapsulated in the acronym CLASI – how Capable, Listened to, Accepted, Safe and Included each person felt. These aspects impacted on the emotional climate of the school, formal and informal communications, day-to-day practices and the way relationships were experienced.

This study also identified factors critical to the development of positive relationships throughout the school for both students and staff. Again there is significant overlap between what happens for students and what happens for teachers in terms of emotional safety; time, space and permission given by the school for relationship building and the sense of feeling connected not only to friends but also to others in the school context.

A focus on relationships throughout the school has a positive ripple effect impacting on not only on wellbeing, but also the motivation and performance of both students and their teachers (Martin and Dowson 2009). The development of a whole school approach that enhances social capital is effective in many dimensions.

9.4   The Micro-level: The Whole Child

A vision for the wellbeing of the whole child would appear to be a central driver for relational quality in school.

> We build an acceptance of others, all are different but all have a place. (principal, primary school)

> There's absolutely an emphasis on the whole person and the whole school ... everyone will tell you that you are a valued member of the team ... (school counsellor)

A focus on the whole child has dual connotations. On the one hand, it means that each individual is valued and accepted for who they are, not just what they can achieve. It is also concerned with education in all domains of a child's development, cognitive, physical, emotional, social and spiritual. This last domain is a broad term covering values, ethics and what brings purpose and meaning to our lives. It addresses one of the three 'Pillars of Authentic Happiness' in Seligman's seminal work on Authentic Happiness (2002), the others being positive feelings/experiences and deep engagement.

The challenge to schools in valuing the whole child is related to inclusion and policies on admission and exclusion (Rose 2010). A positive approach begins with a belief that acceptance of every student – with all their needs and challenges – is both necessary and possible. As the following illustrates, this is not simply a question of resources.

Case Study

As part of her work for the United Nations Convention on the Rights of the Child, Gerison Lansdown has visited schools around the world. She was particularly impressed by a government primary school in Nepal. The far-sighted head teacher had decided to include 12 blind children alongside his mainstream pupils. He had minimal resources but a determination and belief, apparently shared by his staff, that these children deserved an education. Disability is seen as 'bad karma' in Nepal and children are often marginalised or even rejected if they are not 'normal'.

These pupils, from across the country, lived in very basic accommodation attached to the school. Their hostel would be unlikely to meet any Western standard of health and safety. They were first taught Braille and then integrated into classrooms with other pupils, paired with sighted children so they could help each other. The sighted students were often astonished to find that their visually impaired classmates were often as able, and sometimes more capable, of achieving than they were.

Gerison was invited to speak with the blind children about their experiences. This in itself was unusual in a country where the child's voice is rarely encouraged. The young students said it was the first time they had friendships, that the teachers were kind to them. One young boy, aged about eight, said that coming to school had been the best and possibly the only positive experience of his life. He had been kicked by a drunken father, told he was useless and should never have been born – but when he came to school he realised that not only could he learn but also he could be loved – he felt included and part of something. His life was 'going somewhere' and wasn't just being kicked aside.

In another example, the Catholic Education Office in Melbourne has made Student Wellbeing a central platform of policy. The aim is to promote school communities where the whole person is valued.

> ... students (and staff) are given every opportunity to be affirmed in their dignity and worth, confirmed in their personhood and assisted to grow to their full potential (CECV 1994:2)

Student Wellbeing Coordinators in primary schools have regular professional development to enhance their knowledge base and confidence in developing the practical applications of their role. Many have taken a Master's course at the University of Melbourne where their research projects are building a strong evidence base about the development of wellbeing in the school context.

> Key elements of student wellbeing are positive self-regard, respect for others, positive relationships, responsible behaviours and personal resilience. Alongside this comes the active promotion of the values of love, respect, compassion, tolerance, forgiveness, repentance, reconciliation and justice.

Many of these values are implicated in the development of positive relationships. The next section explores both specific interactions and the impact of these interactions across the whole school system.

9.5   The Meso-level: Relational Values and Skills Across the School

9.5.1   Teacher–Student Relationships: High Expectations, Care and Participation

According to a meta-analysis by Cornelius-White (2007), learner-centred teacher–student relationships are effective in many dimensions. Relationships that are non-directive, empathic, warm and encourage thinking and learning have correlations with the following: increased participation, critical thinking, student satisfaction, perceived and actual achievement, self-esteem, positive motivation, social connection and attendance. There are also correlations with low drop-out rates and reduction in disruptive behaviour.

Hattie's meta-analysis of over 800 meta-analyses relating to effective education (Hattie 2009) also says that schools need to create environments where students can feel safe to learn and explore their understanding. Mistakes must be welcomed as part of this process. As each student constructs their learning differently, teachers need to have feedback from their pupils so they know how to make learning meaningful. Feedback is commonly one-way, where teachers tell students how they are doing rather than students telling teachers how they have made sense of what has been taught. Hattie's findings also show that too often students are written off. He maintains that high expectations for all students are essential for effective education. This is synonymous with one of the major protective factors for children at risk.

Many researchers, including Hattie, have commented on the need for adults to care for children. This has been succinctly and powerfully articulated by Bronfenbrenner (2004): 'In order to develop, a child needs the enduring, irrational involvement of one or more adults in care and joint activity with the child. Somebody has to be crazy about that kid'.

Many teachers go into their profession with a passion both for teaching and a determination to do their best for their students. They often become disillusioned because of overwhelming workloads, pressure to 'teach to test' and the challenges of managing difficult behaviour (Galton and McBeath 2008; Roffey 2011b). The ethic of care can become lost in the day-to-day demands. This can lead to teachers saying that they care about their students but young people not experiencing this. What students say does help them feel they matter are the following teacher attitudes and positive behaviours, many of which take little additional time but a high level of awareness: The following quotes are from students cited in Robertson (2006) in the USA and the NSW Commission for Children and Young People (2009) in Australia; ages range from kindergarten to undergraduate:

- *If you know our names it helps*!
- *They smile at me.*
- *They will be nice to you.*
- *Don't say one student is better than another.*
- *The best teachers are hopeful that we will succeed. They believe in us.*
- *My favourite teacher was a good listener, she let me explain. She didn't embarrass me in class when I didn't know the answer.*
- *I think they should relate lessons to our lives, society, and maybe even laugh once in a while?*
- *A good teacher knows how to control students without screaming at them.*
- *He makes people feel good about themselves, because they've achieved something. 'Cos he sort of helps you achieve it.*

Caring teachers can provide a motivational trigger for both engagement with learning and prosocial behaviour. The educational philosopher Nel Noddings, who has written extensively on the moral imperative for an ethic of care in education, sums this up.

> It is obvious that children will work harder and do things – even odd things like adding fractions – for people they love and trust. (Noddings 1988)

Students associate their own and their teachers' positive emotional states with good teaching and good learning (Moore and Kuol 2007). Pupils warm to teachers who are usually cheerful and optimistic.

> Teachers here are focused on your life – so you don't bring home stress to school. They really care for us. (student)

Article 12 in the United Nations Convention on the Right of the Child says that children have a right to an opinion, and for that opinion to be heard in all matters concerning the child. Children's ability to make decisions and to be experts in their own lives is often underestimated. When given the opportunity and encouragement children and young people can show surprising insight. This is illustrated below.

Case Study

Account of a conference presentation by 9–12 year olds on their study of maturity
(Yardley 2009, cited with permission)

We listen as the group considers whether maturity necessarily makes you happy, and whether it can also make you sad – 'the idea of it makes you happy' says one child 'the reality of it can sometimes make you unhappy', 'because' – offers another child – 'of the responsibility you might not want'. As these thoughts begin to excite our own synapses into action, the group then moves on to discuss the 'being' and 'doing' aspects of maturity as they have encountered them in their lives, including those responsibilities they willingly accept and feel comfortable with, and the responsibilities that they fear, feel ill-equipped to shoulder or simply find irritating or 'unfair'.

In the same session we hear the students consider whether maturity can help people cope when life is painful – or when they have a broken heart. We might feel some sympathetic shivers of recognition as we listen to these 9–12 year olds talk about what kind of things break their own and other people's hearts – 'when you are betrayed', 'when you lose your friends, or someone special that you love', 'when you lose your home or your country', 'when you are humiliated', 'when someone dies'.

Eliciting and hearing student views has implications for the relationship that teachers have with their students. It shows interest and respect. The NSW Commission (2009) study found that children want adults in the school community to take them seriously and act on issues that concern them. When that doesn't happen they feel misunderstood and powerless. Students said that not only do children and young people have good ideas but also bring a different perspective. They felt that all children should have a right to be involved, not just a select few.

9.5.2   Relationships Between Students

Relationships between students are often a focus of discussion on issues related to bullying and rejection. A positive psychology view, however, explores the factors that contribute to inclusion, friendship and support between pupils. Once in place these reduce the incidence of negative social behaviours. McGrath and Noble (2010) explored commonalities between six primary and five secondary schools that enjoyed low levels of bullying. In these, they found the following:

- An effective leadership working constructively with teachers to implement a whole school vision for safety and wellbeing
- An effective behaviour policy
- Planning for a 'relationship culture' which adopted strategies such as cooperative learning, cross age social activities and actively teaching prosocial skills and values
- A high priority placed on student wellbeing

The social dimensions of school and how connected students feel are increasingly acknowledged as central to their engagement and wellbeing. When children are asked about school, friendship figures significantly. This is from their earliest days at school throughout high school (NSW Commission 2009).

Children need to know how to interact well with others, what is involved to establish and maintain friendships, how to operate in a group and what is involved in resolving conflicts. The introduction of social and emotional learning programmes has been increasing with some positive outcomes for students in many dimensions. In the UK, the Social and Emotional Aspects of Learning (SEAL) programme was introduced to primary schools in 2005 and secondary schools in 2007 (DfES 2005b). Evaluation in 84 primary schools in Sheffield between 2005 and 2007 indicated high levels of success (Pullinger 2008), including improvements in behaviour and the way children were able to express feelings. Some pupils had learnt to sort out low-level conflict on their own and incidents of bullying were reduced. Payton et al. (2008) analysed three large-scale reviews of research on the impact of social and emotional learning (SEL) programmes on elementary and middle school students from Kindergarten to Grade 8 in the USA. The reviews included 317 studies and involved 324,303 children. The researchers found raised achievement scores, increased social and emotional skills in test situations, improved social behaviours, more positive views about the self, others and school and reduced anxiety and depression.

The delivery of programmes is relevant to their effectiveness. High levels of control and didactic pedagogy do not change behaviour from the inside out. Circle Solutions is a framework for group interaction, based in positive psychology, which aims to promote relationship skills and a caring classroom ethos. It is a pedagogy based in the principles of inclusion, respect, safety and democracy (Roffey 2006). An evaluation of its implementation in eight primary schools indicated that positive outcomes require teachers to believe that relationships are important and facilitate circles in a way that is congruent with the principles and intended outcomes (McCarthy 2009). When this happens, it facilitates both self-awareness and positive relationships between students and also between teachers and students.

> ... the children that I had been working with since March (were) working together as a team and creating friendships and bonds ... No longer were they being disruptive and not talking to one another ... (Undergraduate student facilitator of Circle Solutions)

9.5.3 Staff Relationships

Positive interactions amongst staff are strongly associated with teacher wellbeing on several fronts.

When teachers are burnt out they feel a lack of competence and often distance themselves from their peers. Pillay et al. (2005) refer to this as 'depersonalisation'. This negative spiral can be interrupted by fostering positive relationships where colleagues are helped to identify their strengths and provided with emotional and practical support to deal with what may seem to be overwhelming issues. It helps when others acknowledge that they too have struggled. When teachers felt able to seek support from their colleagues, especially the school executive, they were better able to manage stress (Howard and Johnson 2002).

When teachers talk about what helps them feel they belong to their school, they say that being greeted, especially by name and with a smile, being asked their opinion, having their efforts acknowledged and strengths valued, all make a difference to how they feel about themselves and their colleagues. Their relational needs are just the same as their pupils!

Many teachers appear to feel that despite putting their hearts and backs into what they do, few notice or comment. This decreases motivation and can lead to a toxic environment with low social capital. When the opposite happens it provides a building block for developing both individual wellbeing and school culture.

> My confidence has increased... it could be a product of this different energy at the school... Even receiving a compliment, like 'you're doing a great job'... (school counsellor, high school)

The way staff relate to each other also provides a model for how students behave.

> It comes from the staff first - you can see the staff getting on, and having a bit of fun...so (students) know that we're all friends, and that's an example of good behaviour (teacher, primary school)

9.5.4 Home–School Relationships: Positive Partnerships

The rationale for positive home–school relationships is far reaching and congruent with the multiple stakeholder perspective of health-promoting schools. Positive interactions with families motivate children in school (Hoover-Dempsey et al. 2005). When parents feel comfortable and valued, they will pass on messages to their children about the value of school and this increases the respect that students have for staff (Pianta and Walsh 1996). Supportive relationships may also increase parental confidence in their role and give them strategies to parent more effectively (Roffey 2004). It may also support the educative process when families become involved in backing up what teachers are doing in school. There is now a substantive literature on school–community relationships and the need for all stakeholders to work together. This requires awareness of both the formal and informal power structures in schools and ways in which these may promote or inhibit constructive relationships.

It is often the families of younger children and those with special educational needs that have most to do with the school, together with aspirational parents who want to ensure their child gets the best possible education. The challenge is to engage with as many families as possible.

Teachers may, however, be wary of parents and concerned about the potential for criticism. They may perceive them as demanding or unreasonable or alternatively inadequate or uncaring. There can be a power struggle between parents who 'know their rights' and educators who 'know what's best'. It is usually incumbent on schools to be highly professional in their approach to parents and behave in ways to support collaborative relationships. Partnership is often used to describe this process but this requires an approach from school that sees parents as equal and acknowledges the expertise of the parent on their child (Roffey 2002). It can require high levels of emotional literacy from the professionals.

9.6 Exo-level

This comprises the structural elements of policy, resources and organisation. It is exemplified in the congruence of policies, the ways in which these policies are developed, and the communication practices that keep everyone well informed without being overwhelmed. A behaviour policy based in rules, rewards and sanctions – including exclusion – does not fit comfortably with a school ethos in which relationships have a high profile. A restorative approach, which emphasises responsibility to the community and repairing of 'harm', is a better fit. It fosters the sense of connection that vulnerable and often challenging young people need.

The way resources are prioritised demonstrates the vision of the school. Time is a prime example of this. Teachers who say 'there is no time' available for building relationships because of the need to cover curriculum content are making a statement about what is seen as important. When social and emotional learning is figured into the timetable, there are expectations on everyone to reflect on how they interact with each other.

9.7 The Macro-level: School Leaders and School Culture

As the job of leaders is to develop a shared culture (Fullan 2003), this requires a leadership style that both trusts and empowers others. Transformational leaders (Leithwood et al. 1999) are said to manifest values of collaboration and a commitment to democratic processes. Everyone being involved in the process of change in itself builds social capital.

> First and foremost, it has to be collaborative. You can't have someone from the top saying: 'this is what we're going to do'. You need to give everyone the opportunity… to have ownership of it and to put their thoughts to it (teacher, high school)

> I guess there's a real acceptance of each other's roles, and a feeling that we're all equal in this, we're all in this boat together, let's work as best as we can together. I think that does increase confidence levels within staff … (school counsellor, high school)

The most powerful influence on relational quality in a school is found with the school leader and the leadership team. Their vision of the school and how well they are able to both communicate this effectively to others and also inspire their endorsement is fundamental to positive change (Roffey 2007).

Channer and Hope (2001) found that transformational leaders demonstrated a strong belief in other people. Although their instinct was to take charge, they used the team around them to deliver a goal and valued excellence in others as well as themselves.

Where relationships are a core feature of the school's vision, it is incumbent on leaders that they be seen to 'walk the talk'. Although the possession of both generic and job-specific knowledge and skills is necessary, emotional intelligence, both personal and interpersonal, is central to being an effective principal. Scott (2003) found that, out of 11 core competencies of effective principles, eight are related to their levels of emotional intelligence. He summarised the qualities and approaches that enable leaders to develop child friendly school communities (Scott 2005). Such leaders:

- Have a clear vision for their school
- Have a commitment to making a positive difference for all students
- Are able to stay calm and keep things in perspective when things don't go well
- Have a sense of humour
- Are flexible and responsive to changing demands
- Are self aware and know their strengths and limitations
- Reserve hasty judgement but make tough decisions when necessary
- Demonstrate empathy
- Have a positive outlook
- Are able to listen, empower others and work as a team member as well as take initiative and be authoritative
- Keep the 'big picture' in focus in analysing problems
- Are open to learning and to support
- Are resilient and able to persevere in the face of challenges

Singh and Billingsley (1996) found that school leaders who gave feedback, encouragement and were in favour of participatory decision making fostered commitment within their staff. A further factor less evident in the educational literature but increasingly in positive psychology research is the importance of a positive, 'can do' attitude by leaders. There is a body of evidence that shows that an upbeat mood and optimistic outlook is infectious and can support the development of positive relationships and associated change (Avolio and Gardner 2005).

There is a synergy between the qualities of effective principals and the features of a both learner centred and health-promoting school. School leaders have a critical role in ensuring an effective learning environment for every student – from the most able and compliant to the most disadvantaged and difficult. To do this they need to attend to the quality of their interactions with staff but also ensure that policies within the school are congruent.

9.8 Conclusion and a Word About Sustainability

Although academic outcomes are still the primary measure of school success, there are indications that there is increasing attention being paid by governments to the levels of social capital within schools and the positive differences that a school can make for all its students, especially the more disadvantaged. Keeping the evidence at the forefront of political debate is necessary in order for future policies to reflect effective practice.

We have a crisis in many communities with increased antisocial behaviour and a strong focus on individual rights rather than community wellbeing. If society is going to thrive in the future, then there needs to be greater understanding and skills in building positive relationships. These need to focus on the 'we', what is best for all of us, rather than the 'me', what is in my interest alone. Even though many may say that it is parents who should be supporting the social and emotional development of children, not all can manage this. If our children do not have the opportunity to learn about positive healthy relationships in their communities they need to learn these in school, in the social world set up for learning and teaching. This learning requires both a specific knowledge content and a context and school environment that is congruent. This includes the examples set by teachers (Roffey 2010).

Current teacher education programmes and professional development programmes often fail to address the ethic of care and its impact on the educational process (Owens and Ennis 2005). Where teacher education courses raise awareness of the impact that relationships in schools have on academic and behavioural outcomes they help to ensure that new entrants learn what is involved in establishing and maintaining the relationships that facilitate an effective learning environment. The Hunter Institute of Mental Health fosters this for teacher education courses around Australia with their publication *Connections*.

School leaders can be powerful initiators and drivers of relational quality in school and need support from their own managers to encourage a whole school, whole child approach. There also needs to be an expectation that leaders will access professional development to foster their emerging knowledge and skills.

Nothing succeeds like success. Celebrating and sharing good practice and the outcomes gained is effective in inspiring positive change. Doppler (2008) reports on the outcomes of using a relationship and restorative approach in her school. These are the edited highlights (as cited in Roffey 2011a):

- Parents and students have responded positively to the programme.
- Personal accountability for actions has occurred and students have been empowered to 'make things right' both academically and socially.
- Student achievement has increased with results being above average.
- Student suspension rates have dropped to nil in the past 3 terms.
- Staff and students are empowered to repair and rebuild relationships negating the need for children to be referred to the office and executive.
- Mistakes are viewed as opportunities for insight.

- There is a real 'can do' attitude.
- Data indicates a more motivated and engaged student population.
- Student attendance rates are excellent.
- A higher participation rate of students where previously only the 'elite' entered.
- Staff feel more confident, valued and supported.
- Attendance rates at events indicate a community that feels included and valued.

Positive school relationships can make a significant difference on many levels, in many areas and to all stakeholders. It therefore makes sense for all schools to focus on the ecological development of relational quality school-wide, for both educational excellence and authentic wellbeing.

References

Adler, P. S., & Kwon, S. (2002). Social capital: Prospects for a new concept. *Academy of Management Review, 27*, 17–40.

Avolio, B. J., & Gardner, W. L. (2005). Authentic leadership development: Getting to the roots of positive leadership. *The Leadership Quarterly, 16*(3), 315–338.

Baker, W., & Dutton, J. E. (2007). Enabling positive social capital in organisations. In J. E. Dutton & B. R. Ragins (Eds.), *Exploring positive relationships at work: Developing a theoretical and research foundation*. Mahwah: Lawrence Erlbaum Associates.

Blum, R. W., & Libbey, H. P. (2004). Executive summary, issue on school connectedness: Strengthening health and education outcomes for teenagers. *Journal of School Health, 74*(7), 231–232.

Bronfenbrenner, U. (1979). *The ecology of human development: Experiments by nature and design.* Cambridge, MA/London: Harvard University Press.

Bronfenbrenner, U. (2004). *Making human beings human: Bioecological perspectives on. human development*. London/Thousand Oaks: Sage Publications.

Catholic Education Commission Victoria (CECV). (1994). *CECV policy 1.14: Pastoral care of students in catholic schools*. Melbourne: CECV.

Channer, P., & Hope, T. (2001). *Emotional impact: Passionate leaders and corporate transformation*. Basingstoke: Palgrave.

Cornelius-White, J. (2007). Learner-centred teacher–student relationships are effective: A meta-analysis. *Review of Educational Research, 77*(1), 113–143.

de Jong, T. (2003). A framework of principles and best practice for managing student behaviour in the Australian education context. *School Psychology International, 26*(3), 353.

Department for Education and Skills. (2005a). *The Steer report: Learning behaviour: The report of the practitioners group on school behaviour and discipline*. London: DfES.

Department for Education and Skills. (2005b). *Social and emotional aspects of learning*. London: DfES.

Department of Education and Science. (1989). *Discipline in schools report of the committee of enquiry, chairman Lord Elton*. London: HMSO.

Doppler, L. (2008). *Restorative practices at Rozelle public school.* Available on http://www.schools.nsw.edu.au/studentsupport/behaviourpgrms/antibullying/casestudies/

Felner, R. (2006). Poverty in childhood and adolescence: A transactional-ecological approach to understanding and enhancing resilience in contexts of disadvantage and developmental risk. In S. Goldstein & R. Brooks (Eds.), *Handbook of resilience in children* (pp. 125–47). New York: Springer.

Fredrickson, B. (2009). *Positivity: Groundbreaking research to release your inner optimist and thrive*. Oxford: OneWorld Publications.

Friesthler, B., Merritt, D. H., & LaScala, E. A. (2006). Understanding the ecology of child maltreatment. A review of the literature and directions for new research. *Child Maltreatment, 11*, 263–280.

Fullan, M. (2003). *The moral imperative of school leadership.* Thousand Oaks: Corwin Press Inc/ Sage Publications.

Galton, M., & McBeath, J. (2008). *Teachers under pressure.* London: Sage Publications.

Haddon, A., Goodman, H., Park, J., & Deakin Crick, R. (2005). Evaluating emotional literacy in schools: The development of the school emotional environment for learning survey. *Pastoral Care in Education, 23*(4), 5–16.

Hattie, J. (2009). *Visible learning, a synthesis of over 800 meta-analyses relating to achievement.* London: Routledge.

Hearn, L., Campbell-Pope, R., House, J., & Cross, D. (2006). *Pastoral care in education.* Perth: Child Health Promotion Research Unit, Edith Cowan University.

Hoover-Dempsey, K., Walker, M., Sandler, H., Whetsel, D., Green, C., Wilkins, A., & Closson, K. (2005). Why do parents become involved? Research findings and implications. *The Elementary School Journal, 2*(106), 105–30.

Howard, S., & Johnson, B. (2002). *Resilient teachers: Resisting stress and burnout.* In Proceedings of the Australian Association for Research in Education Conference, Problematic Futures: Education Research in an Era of Uncertainty, Brisbane, 1–5. Available from http://www.aare.edu.au/02pap/how02342.htm

Jennings, P. A., & Greenberg, M. T. (2009). The pro-social classroom: Teacher social and emotional competence in relation to student and classroom outcomes. *Review of Educational Research, 79*(1), 491–525.

Keyes, C. L. M., & Haidt, J. (Eds.). (2003). *Flourishing: Positive psychology and the life well lived.* Washington, DC: American Psychological Association.

Leithwood, K., Jantzi, D., & Steinbach, R. (1999). *Changing leadership for changing times.* Buckingham: Open University Press.

Martin, A. J., & Dowson, M. (2009). Interpersonal relationships, motivation, engagement, and achievement: Yields for theory, current issues, and educational practice. *Review of Educational Research, 79*(1), 327–365.

McCarthy, F. (2009). *Circle time solutions: Creating caring school communities.* Sydney: Report for the NSW Department of Education.

McGrath, H., & Noble, T. (2010). Supporting positive pupil relationships: Research to practice. *Educational and Child Psychology, 27*(1), 79–90.

Moore, S., & Kuol, N. (2007). Matters of the heart: Exploring the emotional dimensions of educational experience in recollected accounts of excellent teaching. *International Journal for Academic Development, 12*(2), 87–98.

Murray-Harvey, R. (2010). Relationship influences on students' academic achievement, psychological health and wellbeing at school. *Educational and Child Psychology, 27*(1), 104–115.

Noble, T., McGrath, H., Roffey, S., & Rowling, L. (2008). *A scoping study on student wellbeing.* Canberra: Department of Education, Employment and Workplace Relations (DEEWR).

Noddings, N. (1988). Schools face crisis in caring. *Education Week, 8*(14), 32.

NSW Commission for Children and Young People. (2009). *Ask the children: Children speak about being at school.* Available from http://www.kids.nsw.gov.au/kids/resources/publications/askchildren

OECD. (2009). *Doing better for children.* Accessed August 9, 2010, from www.oecd.org/els/social/childwellbeing

Onyx, J., & Bullen, P. (2000). Measuring social capital in five communities. *The Journal of Applied Behavioral Science, 36*(1), 23–42.

Owens, O. P., & Ennis, C. D. (2005). The ethic of care in teaching: An overview of supportive literature. *Quest, 2005*(57), 392–425.

Payton, J., Weissberg, R. P., Durlak, J. A., Dymnicki, A. B., Taylor, R. D., Schellinger, K. B., & Pachan, M. (2008). *The positive impact of social and emotional learning for kindergarten to eighth-grade students. Findings from Three scientific reviews.* Available at http://www.casel.org/sel/meta.php

Phongsavan, P., Chey, T., Bauman, A., Brooks, R., & Silove, D. (2006). Social capital, socio-economic status and psychological distress among Australian adults. *Social Science & Medicine, 63*, 2546–2561.

Pianta, R. C., & Walsh, D. J. (1996). *High risk children in schools: Constructing sustaining relationships*. New York: Routledge.

Pillay, H., Goddard, R., & Wilss, L. (2005). Wellbeing, burnout and competence implications for teachers. *Australian Journal of Teacher Education, 30*(2), 21–31.

Pullinger, N. (2008). *Evaluation of the Sheffield SEAL program*. Sheffield: Sheffield Education Services.

Putnam, R. (2000). *Bowling alone: The collapse and revival of American community*. New York: Simon and Schuster.

Robertson, J. (2006). 'If you know our names it helps!' Student perspectives on good teaching. *Qualitative Enquiry, 12*(4), 756–768.

Roffey, S. (2002). *School behaviour and families: Frameworks for working together*. London: David Fulton.

Roffey, S. (2004). The home-school interface for behaviour. A conceptual framework for co-constructing reality. *Educational and Child Psychology, 21*(4), 95–107.

Roffey, S. (2006). *Circle time for emotional literacy*. London: Sage Publications.

Roffey, S. (2007). Transformation and emotional literacy: The role of school leaders in developing a caring community. *Leading and Managing, 13*(1), 16–30.

Roffey, S. (2008). Emotional literacy and the ecology of school wellbeing. *Educational and Child Psychology, 25*(2).

Roffey, S. (2010). Content and context for learning relationships: A cohesive framework for individual and whole school development. *Educational and Child Psychology, 27*(1), 156–167.

Roffey, S. (2011a). *Changing behaviour in schools: Promoting positive relationships and wellbeing*. London: Sage Publications.

Roffey, S. (2011b). *The new teacher's survival guide to behaviour* (2nd ed.). Sage Publications: London.

Rose, R. (Ed.). (2010). *Overcoming international obstacles to inclusion*. London: Routledge.

Scott, G. (2003). *Learning principals: Leadership capability and learning research*. Sydney: New South Wales Department of Education and Training, Professional Support and Curriculum Directorate.

Scott, G. (2005). Leadership for a child friendly community. In *Visions of a child-friendly community*. Sydney: National Association for the Prevention of Child Abuse and Neglect and University of Western Sydney.

Seligman, M. E. P. (2002). *Authentic happiness: Using the new positive psychology to realize your potential for lasting fulfilment*. New York: Free Press.

Singh, K., & Billingsley, B. S. (1996). Intent to stay in teaching. *Remedial and Special Education, 17*(1), 37–48.

Spratt, J., Shucksmith, J., Philip, K., & Watson, C. (2006, September). 'Part of who we are as a school should include responsibility for wellbeing': Links between the school environment, mental health and behaviour. *Pastoral Care, 24*(3), 14–21.

St. Leger, L. (2005). Protocols and guidelines for health-promoting schools. *Promotion and Education, 12*, 145–147.

Sun, J., & Stewart, D. (2007). How effective is the health-promoting school approach in building social capital in primary schools? *Health Education, 107*(6), 556–574.

Tew, M. (2010). Emotional connections: An exploration of the relational dynamics between staff and students in schools. *Educational and Child Psychology, 27*(1), 133–146.

Wingspread Declaration. (2003). Published in a special issue on School Connectedness for the *Journal of School Health* (2004), *74*(7), 233–234.

World Health Organisation. (1995). *WHO global health initiative: Helping schools to become 'health promoting schools'*. Geneva: WHO.

Wyn, J., Cahill, H., Holdsworth, R., Rowling, L., & Carson, S. (2000). MindMatters, a whole-school approach promoting mental health and wellbeing. *The Australian and New Zealand Journal of Psychiatry, 34*(4), 594–601.

Yardley, A. (2009). Children as experts in their own lives. *Child Indicators Research*, Special Issue, International ISCI Conference, Sydney.

Sue Roffey is an educational psychologist, Adjunct Associate Professor at the School of Education, University of Western Sydney and an Honorary Lecturer at University College, London. She is a prolific author on behavioural and relational issues, works internationally as an educational consultant, and is a founder member of the Wellbeing Australia network. Sue is on the editorial board of *Educational and Child Psychology* and *a Fellow of the Royal Society of Arts*.

Contact: sue@sueroffey.com

Chapter 10
Positive Relationships at Work

Sue Langley

10.1 Introduction

Most people spend a significant amount of time at work, therefore being employed in an organisation that allows people to experience positive emotions; engagement and meaning can make a considerable difference to overall life satisfaction and individual flourishing. How many people do work in positive institutions that allow them to experience a sense of positive accomplishment every day? What impact does this have on the individual and the organisation? What can individuals and organisations do to create positive relationships at work? This chapter explores answers to some of these questions.

Based on their organisational surveys over the years, Gallup suggests that there are a few key elements that increase employee engagement (Gallup 2008). Their 12 elements are:

1. I know what is expected of me at work.
2. I have the materials and equipment I need to do my work right.
3. At work, I have the opportunity to do what I do best every day.
4. In the last 7 days, I have received recognition or praise for doing good work.
5. My supervisor, or someone at work, seems to care about me as a person.
6. There is someone at work who encourages my development.
7. At work, my opinions seem to count.
8. The mission or purpose of my organisation makes me feel that my job is important.
9. My associates and fellow employees are committed to doing quality work.
10. I have a best friend at work.
11. In the last 6 months, someone at work has talked to me about my progress.
12. The last year, I have had opportunities at work to learn and grow.

S. Langley (✉)
Langley Group Pty Ltd, 1 Gunshot Alley, Suakin Drive, Mosman, NSW, 2088, Australia
e-mail: sue@langleygroup.com.au

S. Roffey (ed.), *Positive Relationships: Evidence Based Practice across the World*,
DOI 10.1007/978-94-007-2147-0_10, © Springer Science+Business Media B.V. 2012

Fig. 10.1 Positive psychology
model © emotional intelligence worldwide pty ltd

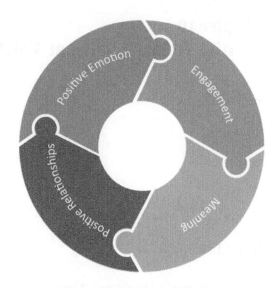

Several of these elements link closely with positive relationships and emotional intelligence, such as 'having a best friend at work', 'getting to do what I am good at' and 'having a supervisor who cares about me'. These elements may come with good leadership, such as encouraging development, valuing opinions and making someone feel important. Positive psychology provides insights into these elements with a flourishing mindset for individuals and organisations.

Kim Cameron, a leader in the field of positive organisational scholarship, believes: 'Evidence regarding the importance of subjective wellbeing, positive emotions, character strengths, and virtues such as gratitude, optimism, and forgiveness has provided leaders in organisations with a great deal of insight regarding the power of the positive'. (Bernstein 2003).

This chapter will explore positive relationships in line with the following framework based on Seligman's four pillars of positive psychology (ABC Australia 2009). Understanding more about positive emotion (and emotions in general), engagement and a strength-based approach, and meaning can help build positive relationships in the workplace (Fig. 10.1).

10.2 Emotions in the Workplace

Human beings are emotional and social creatures. Emotions are a consistent, if ever changing, presence. They provide important data to help both survival and general social functioning. Ekman (1999) says: '... the fundamental function of emotion is to mobilize the organism to deal quickly with important interpersonal encounters'.

All relationships are suffused with emotion, whether this is positive or negative, so understanding more about specific feelings can help improve relationships in the workplace. Specifically, it is helpful to understand how emotions and moods affect others and contribute to or detract from those relationships.

Employee moods and emotions influence several critical elements in organisations – such as job performance, turnover, creativity, decision making. Research supports what may be seen as common sense, although as Voltaire once said, 'Common sense is not so common'.

Consider the following:

> John strides into the office. He's had a rough morning. His two year old had been up half the night sick so he's had little sleep. Due to the chaos in the house he missed his usual train, so he is now stressed, rushing and is late. His routine is messed up. He has a meeting at 9.30 am that he knows he's not prepared for and he's irritable and anxious.
>
> As he strides past two of his colleagues they greet him with a cheery 'Morning John.' He grunts back, thinking, 'How can someone be so annoyingly happy in the morning,' and noisily dumps his stuff at his desk.
>
> As John bangs around getting settled in his colleagues say to each other 'Oh no, better steer clear of John this morning. He's in one of his moods again.'

This type of interaction happens every day in many offices. Does it make John a bad person? Of course not: he is expressing emotions based in a number of challenges in his life. He is unaware of how his emotions are affecting those around him, the impact on his team members and how his mood affects the climate of the office.

This situation may be common in the workplace – one person's negative emotion influences those around them, especially if they have a big personality, high status or are senior in the hierarchy. Does it mean that in order to have positive relationships, we have to be happy all the time; that we have to fake it and pretend to be joyous when we are feeling anxious or down? This is not the case as we will see when we explore negative emotions.

10.2.1 Positive Emotions

People in positive moods are more receptive and open to new ideas. This can assist organisations when they are facing change or when individuals are dealing with negotiations and conflict resolution. People are more creative when experiencing positive moods, which helps organisations come up with new ideas that give them the edge over their competitors (Caruso and Salovey 2004). Dan Pink cites Google as an organisation that allows its team 1 day a week to work on whatever they want, as long as they show what they have done. During this time, employees have come up with numerous new ideas and fixes, including Gmail (Pink 2009). New organisations need staff who do not necessarily fit a conformist mould and trained to obey orders to the letter – many still operate like this despite the fact that research shows that it is to neither the organisation's benefit nor the individuals'. Autonomy is becoming more important in organisations to keep ahead (Pink 2009).

Experiencing and expressing positive emotion would seem to enhance performance in individuals, teams and organisations (Barsade and Gibson 2007).

Positive emotions that are expressed through effective communication influence cooperation and pro-social behaviour, which is more likely to lead to positive performance outcomes.

Positive relationships and positive emotion at work can also help reduce sick leave and absenteeism, as happier, more optimistic people tend to be healthier, have stronger immune systems and recover quicker from illness. Research has found that people who are in the upper reaches of happiness on psychological tests develop about 50% more antibodies than average in response to flu vaccines (Lemonick 2005).

Case Study

One organisation has reduced their sick leave by 40% over a 5-year period by embedding positive psychology tools and techniques into the culture and business practices. These included gratitude lists, best things, using strengths for goal setting, monitoring the positive/negative ratio in meetings and many more. Camp Quality, Sydney, Australia

10.2.2   Negative Emotions

Positive psychology does not suggest that people need to be happy and joyous at work all the time. There is research to suggest that people can be more accurate, more able to find problems and do detailed work more effectively when in a slightly neutral to negative mood (Caruso and Salovey 2004). Negative moods are important for our survival and not to be ignored (Ekman 1999). Positive psychology helps us explore how to ensure our negative emotions do not become destructive.

Reviewing the earlier situation with John, we can see that positive relationships can be undermined if people are experiencing and expressing negative emotions in ways that impact others. John's colleagues recognise the pattern in him and may have a tendency to steer clear of him, when 'he is in one of his moods'. This will impact the performance of the team in several dimensions: maybe others start to shut John out of key discussions because it is easier to do that than to deal with his mood; maybe when they do include him, he is more likely to find fault and be aggressive in his responses and make his colleagues feel belittled or uncomfortable. Over time, the relationships at work may start to break down, cooperation is likely to decrease and the team may end up in a downward spiral.

Alternatively, people who express authentic positive emotions tend to create upward spirals and 'spring outward as well, infusing, connecting and energising whole networks, communicates and organisations' (Fredrickson and Dutton 2008).

A simple example of this is the person on the checkout at the supermarket or the bus driver in the morning. If they are positive, it has a positive influence on customers. Top performing leaders elicited laughter from their subordinates three times as often, on average, than mid-performing leaders (Goleman and Boyatzis 2008).

Negative emotions between individuals can cause conflict, although at a deeper level, this is more often initiated by a clash of values. Negative emotions, however, maintain the conflict and/or prevent individuals dealing with it effectively. We know that positive emotions influence the ability to resolve conflict (Barsade and Gibson 2007) and negative emotions are more likely to exacerbate difficulties.

10.3   Positive Emotions and Relationships

Positive emotion has a significant impact on positive relationships at work. We are drawn to those who are happier and more optimistic. People like to be around such individuals and often feel inspired by them to do better (Carver et al. 2010). Increasing levels of positive emotion in the workplace is therefore a valid aim.

This needs strategic planning and action from different levels of an organisation. Positive psychology research has provided insights that can translate into changes in practice in the workplace – more than just changes in reward and recognition programmes or traditional organisational practices.

Above a certain point, money doesn't increase happiness and wellbeing (Kahneman and Deaton 2010), although organisational psychology and motivational research show that a standard and fair level of remuneration is necessary to avoid de-motivation. Once a person's salary reaches a certain level and these levels change depending on the country, further increases may lead to an improved sense of success but do not necessarily increase day-to-day happiness. There is a big difference in happiness between earning $10,000 and $50,000; whereas there is little difference in happiness between earning $100,000 and $150,000. In the former, the extra money can buy a person out of poverty, poor health and adversity.

> Positive feelings, although perhaps subject to some influence from income, are largely driven by temperament, personal relationships and activities that create interest and flow (Diener and Kahneman 2009).

Case Study

One 'not for profit' organisation, which doesn't have the ability to offer significantly increased salaries, has embedded many ideas taken from positive psychology, including the three blessings and gratitude ideas into their workplace. They have a 'Goofitti' board up in the reception area of each office and each person before they leave the office writes down the best thing that has happened to them today. This has led to some wonderful results in the relationships around the office as well as increasing positive emotion. The board highlights things about work colleagues that were previously unknown, so the team are starting to learn more about each other. This in turns helps them understand each other better and therefore able to handle conflict and difficult situations more clearly. It also helps team members go home in a better mood, which apparently is contributing to nicer home lives for their partners – instead of going home ruminating on the worst aspects of the day they go home focused on the best things. Camp Quality, Sydney, Australia

10.4   Positive Emotions and Collaboration

Happier people are more altruistic and therefore more likely to help each other – cooperation produces results. Altruistic emotions and behaviours are also associated with higher levels of flourishing both physically and psychologically (Post 2005). Less cooperation can lead to greater conflict, and more importantly for organisations, poorer financial performance (Barsade et al. 2000).

Positive emotions also help broaden people's feeling of self/other overlap in the beginning of a new relationship (Fredrickson 2001). Regular positive, in-the-moment connections increase feelings of inclusion in a team and a sense of belonging. This links to Maslow's motivation theory (Maslow 1943) and also in turn builds more positive relationships and more chances of cooperation.

Buckingham and Coffman (1999) found that strong relationships with co-workers increase commitment between each other. For Camp Quality, in the case study above, the 'Goofitti' board helps build those strong relationships.

With a different culture, an organisation can find that team members are encouraged to be so individualistic that collaboration and positive relationships are hampered.

Case Study

One organisation has a culture of driving for results – everything is about hitting the numbers, which is the focus of every individual in the organisation. This culture provides a toxic environment as in the pursuit of the mighty dollar the leaders and managers are crushing people underfoot. There are no one-on-one conversations around how the team is doing in general, no empathic or supportive conversations when a person is struggling. The key thing is that if you have not hit your numbers over a 3-month period you are out. The pressure on each person is enormous as they live under the threat of losing their job. This kind of stress has implications – people don't think as clearly when their brains are under pressure and the levels of neurotransmitters and glucose don't allow the cognitive brain to fire as well as it needs to.

This can, and has, lead to dubious decisions being made not always in the best interests of the team or organisation. Each person is often so under pressure they are not functioning well; they are not enjoying work; they are experiencing less and less positive emotions; they are more likely to be directive and abrupt with team members; there is very little teamwork and cooperation; no-one will do anything for anyone else as it may affect their ability to hit their numbers and keep their job. All of this has led to a huge turnover rate – in some countries – of nearly 50%. With an estimate of 150% of salary to replace an employee this is placing an enormous cost on the business.

With the above example, this organisation may not choose to exchange the results gained from the culture for a few dollars off the cost base due to reduced turnover. The results may be the ultimate prize. Organisational psychology research shows that organisations need a range of elements in place for individuals and organisations to be successful, and positive relationships are a significant contributor to this.

Toxic emotions and relationships happen all the time in organisations and between individuals and often not intentionally. For example, a behaviour that may have proved successful in the past as an independent contributor becomes destructive when that person changes role – in particular moves into a leadership position.

10.5   Building Positive Relationships Through Individuals

Fowler and Christakis (2009, 2010) found that if a person is happy, the likelihood that a close friend will also be happy is increased by 15%. At two degrees of separation, this likelihood is increased by 10%, and at three degrees of separation, this increase of probability falls to 6% and the effect is still significant. Their 'Three Degrees of Influence' have effects on individual's personal and professional lives.

Reverting to the Gallup item about having a best friend at work, they found this correlated most highly in the most productive workgroups. Gallup also observed that employees who report having a best friend at work were:

- 43% more likely to report having received praise or recognition for their work in the last 7 days
- 37% more likely to report that someone at work encourages their development
- 35% more likely to report co-worker commitment to quality
- 28% more likely to report that in the last 6 months, someone at work has talked to them about their progress
- 27% more likely to report that the mission of their company makes them feel their job is important
- 27% more likely to report that their opinions seem to count at work
- 21% more likely to report that at work, they have the opportunity to do what they do best every day

This last point links to positive psychology research around strengths – ensuring that employees have the opportunity to do what they do best every day.

10.6   Engagement at Work: Using Strengths

Positive relationships may be enhanced at work if institutions encourage people to use their strengths every day – again this links to the third item on the Gallup list.

A standard tool in many organisations is the 360°-feedback tool, where people assess themselves, and then choose managers, direct reports, peers and maybe clients to assess them too, on a range of behaviours or competencies. Interestingly, the first place a recipient of such a report looks at is the page about development opportunities or the Bottom Ten behaviours. Exploring where improvements can be made is important, yet perhaps counterintuitive. If people spend all their time focusing on doing things they are not good at and don't like doing, it will affect morale and motivation and perhaps reduce performance. A strengths-based approach, as explored by the positive psychology research, suggests looking at what employees do well and encouraging this in their day-to-day work. Strengths-based research indicates that people are happier and find more fulfilment when they are playing to their strengths (Linley et al. 2009).

The VIA (Values in Action) Signature Strengths, devised by Chris Peterson and Martin Seligman, focuses on 24 specific strengths classified under six broad virtues. These virtues are considered universal across all cultures – wisdom, courage, humanity, justice, temperance and transcendence. Substantial research into these strengths has resulted in the *Character Strengths and Virtues Handbook*, which provides detailed data into each of the 24 areas, including gender, age, cross-cultural elements and interventions (Peterson and Seligman 2004). Utilising these strengths in the workplace can lead to increased engagement for employees and in turn increased positive relationships if used in a constructive manner to support organisational goals. The VIA can be completed free of charge online and embedded into the workplace.

Case Study

Consider an organisation that asks each member of the team to complete the VIA Signature Strengths test online when they join the organisation. Each employee's top five strengths are posted on their intranet page (including the CEO) and everyone is encouraged to use this information when they are working with each other. The CEO encourages team members to consider his strengths when they are asking for approval of new projects. This aids communication and builds positive relationships.

Individual strengths are also used to create growth targets in addition to standard key performance indicators (KPIs). Each person identifies and agrees one or two growth targets aligned with their strengths and the business goals and at the end of the year they are rewarded if the target is achieved. Camp Quality Sydney, NSW, Australia

Case Study

Consider the leadership team who complete their strengths test regularly throughout the year, and share these as a team when they are offsite discussing the strategy for the future. The team as a whole builds stronger relationships by working to these strengths and encouraging each other to use them every day in the workplace. Langley Group

10.7 Flow

Another element to consider for engagement is the work of Csikszentmihalyi around 'flow' states. Flow is the mental state that occurs when a person is fully immersed in an activity with a feeling of energised focus, full involvement and success in the process of the activity or 'the capacity for full engagement in an activity' (Csikszentmihalyi 2003). Flow is focused intrinsic motivation; it is such absorption in a task that time disappears. It is about being contained yet energised by the task. Flow can be experienced at any time, yet for most people, it will be when they are doing something they do best.

The experience of more positive emotion and perhaps a higher sense of accomplishment can translate to positive business outcomes.

Understanding strengths can help build positive relationships at work in various ways. Often, organisations will ask employees to complete a personality or thinking styles profile in order to improve team understanding, which may not be as beneficial as strengths and are often used as an excuse for behaviour. The ideal use is to understand and appreciate everyone's individual strengths and use the knowledge to communicate more effectively. Whether an organisation is exploring personality strengths, learned skills or signature strengths, using these in the workplace can help build stronger relationships and higher performance.

When strong engagement is felt in a workgroup, employees believe that their co-workers will help them during times of stress and challenge. In this day of rapid-fire change, reorganisation, mergers and acquisitions, having best friends at work may be the true key to effective change integration and adaptation. When compared to those who don't, employees who have best friends at work identify significantly higher levels of healthy stress management, even though they experience the same levels of stress (Gallup 2008).

10.8 Meaning at Work

Providing meaning at work can enhance positive relationships – whether a leader is providing the purpose behind a task or linking it to a bigger vision, or an individual gains understanding of how their work makes a difference. Research has found successful organisations over time are clear on their purpose, vision and values and embed that into the culture of the business (Collins and Porras 1994). Research also suggests individuals who have a greater sense of meaning have more flourishing lives.

> Our positive emotions evoke thought-action tendencies in humans that broaden human attachment to others and to community service. From thence comes meaning and purpose (Vaillant 2008).

Research on meaning at work by Wrzesniewski (1997) found that people who see their job as a calling as opposed to a job find more meaning in their work and are more likely to be using their strengths (Bunderson and Thompson 2009). Wrzesniewski's work on jobs, careers and callings provides insight into how people find meaning in what they do and how this contributes to the overall sense of well-being and satisfaction (Wrzesniewski and Dutton 2001).

Wrzesniewski defines the meaning of work in the following ways:

- A job has a focus on financial rewards and necessity rather than pleasure or fulfilment; not a major positive part of life
- A career has a focus on advancement
- A calling has a focus on enjoyment of fulfiling, socially useful work

Her work explores the psychological and social processes through which these work meanings develop. An organisation that can tap into the sense of meaning that can develop for their employees will often find that this enhances workplace relationships (Wrzesniewski et al. 1997). Helping employees find meaning through connecting their role to something bigger than themselves is important here.

From a young age, a child often asks 'why' – longing to learn and know and understand. As adults, often the same principle applies in the workplace; creating a sense of meaning through purpose, values, efficacy and self-worth is important.

10.9 The Neuroscience of Relationships

Social neuroscience also provides insights into building positive relationships in the workplace. One theory is that the human brain has evolved to the size and complexity it has in order to deal with our social networks (Dunbar 1998). When people experience social pain, such as being excluded from a project or the promised promotion doesn't happen, it activates the same area of the brain as physical pain.

Equally, brains respond to fairness – the brain's reward centre activates when fairness and cooperation is experienced. This has implications for the workplace with respect to fairness between colleagues, fairness in the allocation of work or rewards and cooperation during meetings (Tabibnia and Lieberman 2007).

Human relationships also impact key areas of our brains. People are more likely to connect with another person if they perceive there are similarities between them. With similarity comes the ability to better infer mental states. If a person is able to find something similar in a new team member, he and she are more likely to empathise and connect with them, which in turn is going to ensure that they converse and build a relationship, leading to more cooperation and teamwork. If a person feels they are significantly different to a new team member, it may be harder to find common ground; the person may be less likely to make an effort to get to know them. This information provides insight into how we handle diversity in organisations.

Diversity is encouraged and embraced in organisations for many more valid reasons than covered in this chapter; however, a key element is that in order to build positive relationships, people need to find something in common – that could be race, gender, background, history, experience or even just the project, favourite colour, sport, etc. These elements that create similarity allow for more positive emotions and therefore more positive relationships to develop (Mitchell et al. 2006).

> When I am facilitating or working with a group in any part of the world, if a participant is from England at some point during the morning tea break or over lunch I can guarantee they will come up to me and ask me what part of England I am from. My accent gives me away and it will be something that another English person can grasp that indicates we are similar. That thought triggers a positive response in the brain, which means we are more likely to connect through conversation and perhaps find other areas of similarity. Sue Langley, ELW, Sydney, Australia.

Creating positive relationships in a team leads to an exploration of mirror neurons in the social neuroscience research. Mirror neurons are particularly important in the workplace as these can influence feelings and actions (Mukamel et al. 2010). To give an example of how mirror neurons work, imagine you are walking down the street and someone smiles at you. The natural reaction is to smile back.

Imagine this same situation in the workplace. There is a subset of mirror neurons whose job it is to detect these smiles and prompt the same response, and a person in a team who can trigger these responses tends to be able to bond a team, which in turns leads to higher performance (Goleman and Boyatzis 2008). A person experiencing positive emotions triggers the mirror neurons of those around him or her; however, so does a person experiencing negative emotions. Mirror neurons mean people are constantly influenced in the workplace by others – those with the ability to create positive relationships and those with the ability to create negative relationships.

10.10 Positive Relationships and the Impact of Effective Communication

Communication at work has a big influence on creating or destroying positive relationships. Research has found that providing negative feedback in a positive way (such as nods and smiles) left people feeling better than if they were given positive feedback in a negative way (Goleman and Boyatzis 2008). Often in the workplace, positive feedback can be given flippantly in a generic way, such as 'great job today' or 'well done, that was good'. This may be nice yet becomes meaningless to a team member if not done in a genuine, connected manner. It is far more important to connect with the person and ensure they know exactly what was good or bad and why, such as: 'Great job with the report today Jim, I loved how you put the summary figures on the front, so they were easy for the project team to see at a glance, thank you so much for doing it', (with a smile and a nod) is more beneficial for both parties.

Communication in the workplace can make or break a relationship or a team. Consider the following scenario:

The team are in a sales meeting discussing new ideas to lift sales and perhaps branch into new niche markets. Peter has an idea.

He's thought about focusing on small to medium enterprises (SMEs) with their new product line as it could really help business owners organise their database and customer relationship more effectively.

He hasn't fully formulated the idea yet so in the meeting he says, "What about SMEs?" Jane immediately replies, "That won't work because they don't have enough funds and we'll spend all our time running around for small contracts." Meilin adds, "Yeah, I'm sure we tried that a few years ago, let's focus on our core corporate markets."

Peter's idea is shot down and the team move on getting bogged down on the usual challenges with growing their corporate sales. Peter still thinks it is a huge untapped market and is now feeling de-motivated and disillusioned – "this always happens, they never listen to new ideas, they didn't even let me finish."

This may be common in meetings – one person has an idea and another person suggests why it won't work. The idea may not work; yet dismissing the idea contracts the conversation and may make the person less likely to share other ideas in the future. The team does not explore the new idea, and relationships and neural connections are reduced (Fredrickson and Losada 2005).

Gottman first explored the positive/negative ratio with his work on marital relationships (Gottman et al. 1998), and this has continued in the positive psychology field around individuals and teams. Fredrickson and Losada (2005) explore a 3:1 positivity ratio for individual experience of positive emotions in relation to negative, and Losada and Heaphy (2004) found that high-performing teams worked at a ratio of 5:1 – meaning that they had five positive interactions to each negative. This does not mean people can only say nice things.

The language used in communicating to others in the workplace can either contract or expand relationships and conversation. In the example above, Jane's response immediately contracted the conversation and Peter's idea was crushed. Does it mean that Peter's idea was great and would have worked? Not necessarily. It may well have been a ridiculous idea, yet the way it was dismissed contracts the workplace relationship between each person. How could Jane and Meilin have created a more positive outcome?

Consider an alternative with a more positive team response:

> The team are in a sales meeting discussing new ideas to lift sales and perhaps branch into new niche markets. Peter has an idea.
>
> He's thought about focusing on small to medium businesses with their new product line as it could really help business owners organise their database and customer relationship more effectively.
>
> He hasn't fully formulated the idea yet so in the meeting he says, "What about SMEs?" Jane immediately replies, "Tell us what you had in mind?" Meilin adds, "Yeah, we did think about that a year ago. I am not sure we ever really explored it. How do you see it working, Peter?"
>
> Peter expands on his idea and as he does a few others in the meeting are able to add some elements that means it may be viable. They agreed to draft an outline of how it could work and review at the next meeting. Corporate sales are higher revenue, yet SMEs could be something new. Peter is happy with the outcome of the meeting. He doesn't really know if it will work, he is just happy he has been heard and getting input from the rest of the team really made him feel like he belonged at last.

The final outcome of this may mean that Peter realised all by himself that the idea is not viable, in which case it is still a better outcome for the relationships in the group and his own levels of positive emotion. By expanding the conversation also, Peter was able to feel heard and connected to the others in the team and the others were able to contribute to what may turn out to be a viable option.

This method of active constructive responding (Gable et al. 2004) is much more powerful in workplace relationships, as it preserves a positive dynamic between two people and expands the communication.

Consider the team member who can use that style of communication to connect with internal clients and encourage cooperation between groups. Consider how this works across borders or with virtual teams. It can really expand and explore the topic whilst at the same time building the relationships.

10.11   Positive Relationships and Social Capital

Positive relationships build social capital, which facilitates co-operation and mutually supportive relations. This may be applicable between two people in an organisation as well as in communities and nations as a means of combating some of the social disorders in modern society (Putnam 1995). This building of social capital could be reciprocity between two people in an organisation, and it may be specific – 'I do something for you and you do something for me' – or general – 'I do something for you and maybe you will do something for someone else' – and so on. This reciprocity is more likely to occur when people are in a positive mood as people are generally more helpful and altruistic when feeling positive (Post 2005).

Dutton (Dutton and Ragins 2007) is a key researcher in social capital and identifies it as 'the resources that inhere in and flow through networks of relationships' – they could include knowledge, advice, information, goodwill, help and emotional support, as well as material goods and services. Whilst social capital can be negative, this chapter focuses on the positive elements.

When people experience high-quality connections at work, research has found that physiological functioning increases, learning and engagement increases, attachment and commitment increases, as well as cooperation and collaboration and individual performance (Baker and Dutton 2007).

High-quality connections are defined as 'short-term, dyadic, interactions that are positive in terms of the subjective experience of the connected individuals and the structural features of the connection'.

These high-quality connections have an impact on individual and organisational outcomes, and one of the keys is positive relationships and link heavily to respect. The five key areas are:

- Conveying presence, which is about being psychologically available to someone
- Being genuine, which is about authenticity
- Communicating affirmation, which is about finding the good in people and sharing it
- Effective listening
- Supportive communication, which links to the active constructive responding elements from Gable's work (Stephens et al. 2011)

Maintaining positive self-regard and being able to make positive contributions is critical for individual flourishing in the workplace (Ramarajan et al. 2007). This links to motivation and the Gallup questions around 'doing quality work', 'my opinions count', and 'doing what I am good at'. People like to feel they are contributing to something bigger than themselves. This is prevalent in the meaning research and also contributes to enhancing positive emotions.

If organisations want to build flourishing workplaces, they need to provide the means to allow each person to build their own positive self-regard, to build their self-confidence and levels of positive emotion. Many people don't know how to do this every day. They have had past experiences and past relationships that have led them to some unproductive workplace behaviours. These behaviours may get results in the short term. Providing training around emotional intelligence and positive psychology can allow individuals to learn how to handle their own emotions, build resilience, manage themselves more effectively, and therefore consider the impact they are having on others and adjust their behaviour accordingly.

People's subjective experience of their social interactions with others has 'immediate, enduring and consequential effects on their bodies' (Heaphy and Dutton 2008). One way organisations can encourage flourishing relationships is to be aware of the impact these social interactions have on employees and encourage these. The current way of working is to use email and virtual conferencing for all interactions – every day people will send an email to a person that sits beside them at work. Social media and internal networks reduce personal interactions. In the workplace, perhaps we need to strive to keep social interaction alive, for the sake of our bodies as well as our minds?

This sense of appreciation is key to generating powerful neurotransmitters and positive emotions in both people. Appreciation has several meanings – it means thank you, and it means growth (Thompson 1995). Appreciation is often about thanking a person, and when this is done well, the level of positive emotion increases. Appreciation is a win-win situation – when one person appreciates another, both people are likely to experience positive responses.

10.12 Making Things Practical: How to Increase Positive Relationships

What positive psychology tools can help people build better relationships and enhance performance?

10.12.1 Positive Psychology Training

Teaching all individuals how to build their own levels of positive emotions – simple techniques, such as three blessings (Seligman et al. 2005), resilience training (Reivich and Shatte 2002), reappraisal and labelling (Lieberman 2007).

10.12.2 Emotional Intelligence Training

Teaching individuals emotional intelligence techniques to manage negative emotions more effectively: emotional intelligence training helps build skills in emotional awareness of self and others, as well as emotional management. Building resilience through emotional management includes the four As – awareness, acceptance, adjustment and action.

There are various models of emotional intelligence (Palmer et al. 2007); the model itself is only powerful when it is translated into tangible tools and techniques that can be built into individual and team behaviour (Vella-Brodrick and Page 2009: 117).

Resilience in the workplace helps individuals bounce back from setbacks and challenges. People who are more resilient are likely to be more successful (Reivich and Shatte 2002).

10.12.3 Social Neuroscience Learning

Building similarity across diversity – encourages teams to find elements of similarity whether across functional borders or country borders; find the common ground.

Teaching people more about how the human brain works and encouraging individuals and leaders to practise what is known about social neuroscience and allow for the desire for status, certainty, autonomy, relatedness and fairness where possible (Rock 2009).

10.12.4 Developing Communication

Improving communication between individuals and in meetings by increased understanding of active constructive responding and the positive negative ratio helps build relationships. Providing tools and techniques to manage this allows individuals to be more aware of how their communication is impacting their relationships at work.

Helping individual create high-quality connections through their daily communication habits and interactions (Heaphy and Dutton 2008).

10.12.5 Developing Strengths

Building strengths into the framework of the business so each person can use their strengths each day in what they do. The VIA Strength Survey is a well-researched tool, and many interventions exist exploring how to develop each strength.

10.12.6 Create Meaning and Contribution

Ensuring that there is a framework of meaning through purpose, vision and values so each person knows where they fit into the bigger picture and how what they do every day makes a difference.

Providing a sense of meaning through leadership as well as allowing people more control over what they do and where it fits to the bigger picture.

10.13   Conclusion

An organisation comprises the people who work there. It is individual performances and the relationships between people that impact on how effective and successful the organisation is in meeting its goals.

There are many elements that contribute to positive relationships in the work-place, including job roles, leadership role models, pay scales, culture and environment, competition and markets. Above that, making changes to an organisation needs to happen through the people who are employed there. People matter and it is people who make a difference. If each individual does one thing slightly better, or is slightly more positive, or has a few more self-management tools under his or her belt, this person will create a dynamic impact on the whole.

Positive psychology has a lot to offer in helping organisations improve flourishing in the workplace and increasing the opportunity for positive relationships to occur. Focusing on the key areas of positive emotion, engagement and meaning can help increase positive relationships, which in turn create positive institutions.

References

ABC (Australian Broadcasting Corporation). (2009). *All in the mind: Dialogue with the Dalai Lama Part 3*. Transcript Accessed January 3, 2011 from http://www.abc.net.au/rn/allinthemind/stories/2009/2766891.htm

Baker, W., & Dutton, J. E. (2007). Enabling positive social capital in organisations. In J. E. Dutton & B. R. Ragins (Eds.), *Exploring positive relationships at work: Building a theoretical and research foundation*. Mahwah: Lawrence Erlbaum Associates.

Barsade, S. G., & Gibson, D. E. (2007). Why does affect matter in organisations? *Academy of Management Perspectives, 21*(1), 36–59.

Barsade, S. G., Ward, A. J., Turner, J. D. F., & Sonnenfeld, J. A. (2000). To your heart's content: A model of affective diversity in top management teams. *Administrative Science Quarterly, 45*, 802–836.

Bernstein, S. D. (2003). Positive organisational scholarship: Meet the movement. *Journal of Management Inquiry, 12*(1), 1–6.

Buckingham, M., & Coffman, C. (1999). *First, break all the rules: What the world's greatest managers do differently*. New York: Simon and Schuster.

Bunderson, J. S., & Thompson, J. A. (2009). The call of the wild: Zookeepers, callings, and the dual edges of deeply meaningful work. *Administrative Science Quarterly, 54*, 32–57.

Caruso, D., & Salovey, P. (2004). *The emotionally intelligent manager*. San Francisco: Jossey-Bass.

Carver, C. S., Scheier, M. F., & Segerstrom, S. C. (2010). Optimism. *Clinical Psychology Review, 30*(7), 879–889.

Collins, J., & Porras, J. I. (1994). *Built to last: Successful habits of visionary companies*. New York: Harper Collins.

Csikszentmihalyi, M. (2003). *Good business: Leadership, flow and the making of meaning*. London: Hodder and Stoughton.

Diener, E., & Kahneman, D. (2009). The Easterlin paradox revisited, revised and perhaps resolved. *Social Indicators Network News, 100*, 1–3.

Dunbar, R. I. M. (1998). The social brain hypothesis. *Evolutionary Anthropology, 6*(5), 178–190.

Dutton, J. E., & Ragins, B. R. (Eds.). (2007). *Exploring positive relationships at work: Building a theoretical and research foundation*. Mahwah: Lawrence Erlbaum Associates.

Ekman, P. (1999). Basic emotions. In T. Dalgleish & M. Power (Eds.), *Handbook of cognition and emotion*. Chichester: Wiley.

Fowler, J. H., & Christakis, N. A. (2009). *Connected: The surprising power of our social networks and how they shape our lives*. New York: Little Brown and Company.

Fowler, J. H., & Christakis, N. A. (2010). Cooperative behavior cascades in human social networks. *Proceedings of the National Academy of Sciences of the United States of America, 107*(12), 5334–5338.

Fredrickson, B. L. (2001). The role of positive emotions in positive psychology: The broaden-and-build theory of positive emotions. *American Psychologist, 56*(3), 218–226.

Fredrickson, B. L., & Dutton, J. E. (2008). Unpacking positive organizing: Organisation as sites of individual and group flourishing. *The Journal of Positive Psychology, 3*(1), 1–3.

Fredrickson, B. L., & Losada, M. (2005). Positive affect and the complex dynamics of human flourishing. *American Psychologist, 60*, 678–686.

Gable, S. L., Reis, H. T., Impett, E. A., & Asher, A. R. (2004). What do you do when things go right? The intrapersonal and interpersonal benefits of sharing positive events. *Journal of Personality and Social Psychology, 87*(2), 228–245.

Gallup. (2008). *Employee engagement: What's your engagement ratio?* Washington, DC: Gallup Consulting.

Goleman, D., & Boyatzis, R. (2008). Social intelligence and the biology of leadership. *Harvard Business Review, 86*(9), 74–81.

Gottman, J. M., Coan, J., Carrere, S., & Swanson, C. (1998). Predicting marital happiness and stability from newlywed interactions. *Journal of Marriage and Family, 60*(Feb), 5–22.

Heaphy, E. D., & Dutton, J. E. (2008). Positive social interactions and the human body at work: Linking organisation and physiology. *Academy of Management Review, 33*(1), 137–162.

Kahneman, D., & Deaton, A. (2010). High income improves evaluation of life but not emotional well-being. *Proceedings of the National Academy of Sciences of the United States of America, 107*(38), 16489–16493.

Lemonick, M. D. (2005). The biology of joy: Scientists know plenty about depression. Now they are starting to understand the roots of positive emotion. *Time, 165*(3), 12.

Lieberman, M. D. (2007). Social cognitive neuroscience: A review of core processes. *Annual Review of Psychology, 58*, 259–289.

Linley, P. A., Harrington, S., & Garcea, N. (2009). *Oxford handbook of positive psychology and work*. Oxford: Oxford University Press.

Losada, M., & Heaphy, E. (2004). The role of positivity and connectivity in the performance of business teams: A nonlinear dynamics model. *American Behavioural Scientist, 47*, 740–765.

Maslow, A. H. (1943). A theory of human motivation. *Psychological Review, 50*, 370–396.

Mitchell, J. P., Macrae, C. N., & Banaji, M. R. (2006). Dissociable medial prefrontal contributions to judgments of similar and dissimilar others. *Neuron, 50*, 655–663.

Mukamel, R., Ekstrom, A. D., Kaplan, J., Iacoboni, M., & Fried, I. (2010). Single-neuron responses in humans during execution and observation of actions. *Current Biology, 20*, 750–756.

Palmer, B. R., Gignac, G., Ekermans, G., & Stough, C. (2007). A comprehensive framework for emotional intelligence. In R. J. Emmerling & V. K. Shanwal (Eds.), *Emotional intelligence: Theoretical and cultural*. New York: Nova Science Publishers, Inc.

Peterson, C., & Seligman, M. E. P. (2004). *Character strengths and virtues: A handbook and classification*. New York: Oxford University Press.

Pink, D. H. (2009). *Drive: The surprising truth about what motivates us*. New York: Riverhead Books.

Post, S. (2005). Altruism, happiness, and health: It's good to be good. *International Journal of Behavioural Medicine, 12*(2), 66–77.

Putnam, R. D. (1995). Bowling along: America's declining social capital. *Journal of Democracy, 6*(1), 65–78.

Ramarajan, L., Barsade, S. G., & Burack, O. R. (2007). The influence of organizational respect on emotional exhaustion in the human services. *The Journal of Positive Psychology, 3*(1), 4–18.

Reivich, K., & Shatte, A. (2002). *The resilience factor: 7 keys to finding your inner strength and overcoming life's hurdles.* New York: Broadway Books.

Rock, D. (2009). *Your brain at work: Strategies for overcoming distraction, regaining focus, and working smarter all day long.* New York: Harper Collins.

Seligman, M. E. P., Steen, T. A., Park, N., & Peterson, C. (2005). Positive psychology progress: Empirical validation of interventions. *American Psychologist, 60*(5), 410–421.

Stephens, J., Heaphy, E. D., & Dutton, J. E. (2011). High-quality connections. In K. Cameron & G. Spreitzer (Eds.), *Handbook of positive organizational scholarship.* New York: Oxford University Press.

Tabibnia, G., & Lieberman, M. D. (2007). Fairness and cooperation are rewarding: Evidence from social cognitive neuroscience. *Annals of the New York Academy of Sciences, 1118*, 90–101.

Thompson, D. (Ed.). (1995). *The concise oxford dictionary.* Oxford: Oxford University Press.

Vaillant, G. (2008). *Spiritual evolution.* New York: Broadway Books.

Vella-Brodrick, D. A., & Page, K. M. (2009). Positive leadership: Accentuating and cultivating human resources. In J. C. Sarros (Ed.), *Contemporary perspectives on leadership: Focus and meaning for ambiguous times.* Prahran: Tilde University Press.

Wrzesniewski, A., & Dutton, J. E. (2001). Crafting a job: Revisioning employees as active crafters of their work. *Academy of Management Review, 26*(2), 79–201.

Wrzesniewski, A., McCauley, C., Rozin, P., & Schwartz, B. (1997). Jobs, careers, and callings: People's relations to their work. *Journal of Research in Personality, 31*(1), 21–33.

Sue Langley is Director of the Langley Group Pty Ltd. Her consultancy company is focused on human development within organisations, using emotional intelligence and positive psychology interventions. Sue has worked in many different industries across the world and is a regular speaker at positive psychology conferences. Contact: sue@langleygroup.com.au

Chapter 11
Positive Professional Relationships

Elizabeth Gillies

11.1 Introduction

We live in a world of relationships: from birth to death, we are part of social groups in our families, with friends, at work, in school and in our local communities. In this social world, we will, at many times, look to others for help and support for different reasons or problems. This chapter is about the role of the effective helper in a professional relationship, when someone buys in assistance, whether this is of a practical or professional nature. This role brings with it responsibilities and expectations that impact the nature of this work and hence the outcome. Positive professional relationships contribute to the quality and progression of that work and have an impact on life when the work is over.

In recent years, there has been a move in many helping professions away from the traditional expert model with passive client to a collaborative empowering partnership. This new relationship calls on professionals to view clients as experts in their own right, owning their own strengths and skills, working alongside them to achieve their goals and paying attention to the factors that enhance the relationship.

This chapter will initially address broad issues about helping and the positive approach, then go on to examine how elements from current research from the field of psychological help can be useful to a wide range of professional relationships.

E. Gillies (✉)
Educational Psychologist, International Mental Health Professionals, Tokyo, Japan
e-mail: elizabeth_gillies@mac.com

S. Roffey (ed.), *Positive Relationships: Evidence Based Practice across the World*,
DOI 10.1007/978-94-007-2147-0_11, © Springer Science+Business Media B.V. 2012

11.2 Positive Professional Relationships Matter

A friend recently hired a construction company to renovate their house. Their experience was a highly positive one for several reasons:

The clients knew what they wanted to achieve and the builders provided expertise about how best to realize their goal. Options with the pros and cons were presented and discussed. Decisions always remained with the clients.

There was good communication by both parties: there was honesty about delays, issues were clarified and information flowed. When the clients didn't understand something, it was explained - often through demonstration.

The builders valued the open communication and provided this feedback to the clients.

At a time of potential conflict the workers and client were courteous, willing to negotiate and arrived at a compromise. The positive relationships already established facilitated this process.

There were conversations about life beyond the project, which enabled each side to see they were more than clients and builders.

The builders were unfailingly polite, did what they said they were going to do, were reliable, conscientious and worked long days towards the end of the project to fulfill their time commitment. The clients expressed their appreciation.

The above illustrates a collaborative process where respect, trust, knowledge and expertise from both sides were valued, solutions worked through and reflection about how the project was progressing took place. Importantly, they discussed how they were working together. Though the ongoing work and the eventual outcome were important, it was the process that enabled this to occur that made the difference to the satisfactory completion of the project. This comprised the relational qualities between the workers and clients that created a positive environment. Though the 'clients' in this example were the people who paid for the time and skills of the builders, they also felt a sense of inclusion, of this being a project where their full involvement was welcomed.

The case study highlights critical aspects in making professional relationships work well; they are about the nature of knowledge, how it is valued and who has power to make decisions. According to Dutton and Heaphy (2003), the features of 'high quality connections' are where a wide range of emotions are part of the dialogue, flexibility exists to withstand difficulties and there is creativity and openness to new sources of ideas. Here both parties recognised the value of creating and fostering their collaborative relationship.

11.3 The Positive Force

As humans, we are drawn into action when we feel challenged and react with our fight/flight response. When things are going well or are just ticking over, our attention is less. Noticing the details when things are working well requires a different stance. Positive psychology has encouraged us to focus on what we need to do to thrive and flourish. This is a different lens with which to interpret the world (Seligman and Csikszentmihalyi 2000). In many fields, there is growing interest in examining excellence and how it is attained and developed. In *Good to Great*, Collins (2001) researched the important factors of excellence in industry; Robinson and Aronica (2009) write about how individuals find their passion and excel; and Miller et al. (2007) report on how 'Supershrinks' contribute to successful outcomes in therapy. The move in positive working relationships is away from discussing 'corrosive connections' to 'high quality connections' (Dutton and Heaphy 2003). Adopting curiosity about examining and then using what actually works in creating effective professional relationships is an important part of the 'positive' focus.

The positive approach places relationships as central toward attaining quality experiences, actions and outcomes; creating mutually beneficial win-win partnerships where everybody profits in some way needs to focus on the 'how' of creating effective relationships (Covey 1989).

The *positive* contribution in this chapter focuses on the details of successful models and approaches rather than on investigating the problems and difficulties in professional relationships.

11.4 What Is Different About a Professional Relationship?

There are issues and elements that set professional relationships apart from other kinds of relationships.

- The client seeks some expert help, skills and/or support. They have choice in this selection.
- The professional gets paid for their help: it's what they do for a living.
- A contract usually exists outlining practical ways that will enable the work to progress smoothly and professionally: e.g. costs, timing of meetings, a start and end point.
- 'Being a "helper" of some kind is not as simple as it may at first seem'. (Maidment 2006). Work takes place in an environment of increased litigation and where there are favoured best practice models that can often direct and dictate professional action. Competition exists between professionals. There is demand for quality and satisfaction amongst clients.
- Professionals usually belong to organisations or associations where core values, principles and standards are set to uphold professional practice and offer protection to the public in their selection and work with professionals. With membership comes agreement to work in ethical ways: e.g. being competent to carry out specific professional roles, continuing professional development, knowing the limits of your professional skills, etc.
- Within such relationships, there are guidelines that recommend rules in the relationship or boundaries in order to ensure professionalism and safety in the interaction.

11.5   How Professionals Go About Helping

Professional relationships can be varied and range from seemingly simple tasks to complex situations: e.g. hiring a plumber to repair a leaking tap, going to a doctor or consulting a psychologist. Within these different partnerships are ways of relating that bring quality to the relationship: ways that make or break the common goal, ways that create stress or provide comfort, ways that empower or deskill. It is clear when we have a positive experience, as in the case study above, and is painfully obvious when we don't.

For the professional then, there are important factors that impact on their practice in order to provide a skilled service.

- In *The Customer Revolution*, Seybold et al. (2001) suggest customers have greater control in how they choose and use services. With greater choice come higher demands and expectations. The relationship with clients and their experience matters more than it used to.
- Professionals need to be aware of the changing experiences and expectations of people, especially younger people. Saxton (2004) writes of the 'driving forces of participation' in society that demand greater involvement. With increasing levels of education, people expect to be involved in many levels in society from voting to making health care decisions. The rise of technology has increased searching and sharing information in a highly participatory way with people around the world.
- Clients have access to many sources of information, especially the Internet, and may come into the professional relationship with a level of knowledge and information that was previously less available to them. For example, in the medical world, many patients are 'active consumers of health information', and this can affect how doctors relate with their patients (McMullan 2006).
- We live in a changing diverse society and need to work with people in ways that are culturally sensitive. Professional relationships are culturally dependent; levels of respect and interaction between professionals and clients are related to values and norms in society (Macklin 1999).
- Rights and views of consumers are important and are often protected by law and by professional standards of accreditation.
- Professionals have expertise. It is important for them to understand how to use their knowledge skillfully and successfully to arrive at a positive outcome for the client. It is also valuable for them to understand the positive gains for themselves in helping and how this affects their work.

11.6   A Change of Direction in Helping

The transition from traditional expert role, where experts have the power and knowledge and where clients are silent recipients, to a more collaborative approach is evident in many helping professional fields. In the literature, there is increasing use of terms and discourse that places the client or relationship at the centre of the work and focuses on a working partnership. There is evidence of many positive outcomes of employing such an approach.

In an increasingly global and diverse world, where working and managing from a distance are common, employers want staff to be able to work cooperatively both within their own company and with their partner companies. In their 'Portrait of an ideal helper', Corey and Corey (2006) suggest that knowing your own strengths and weaknesses and understanding who you are as a person are your most important resources in effective helping. With the move toward more collaboration in the workplace, inter- and intrapersonal skills become highly valued (Goleman 2000).

More collaborative approaches are increasingly popular in the medical field and appear frequently in journal articles. Notions of patient-centred care and relationship-centred medicine highlight a change in thinking 'beyond diagnosis to include the person being treated and improving the quality of connection between physician and patient' (Goleman 2006). Elywn et al. (2009) state 'shared decision making' as an important goal for clinical practice. Preference for terms such as 'adherence' to medical treatment is viewed to be more appropriate than 'compliance', suggesting a more collaborative approach between doctors and their patients (Osterberg and Blaschke 2005). Research evidence indicates that a positive doctor/patient relationship leads to higher satisfaction with medical treatment (Fuertes et al. 2009).

Restorative justice practices are used successfully in many countries to deliver a fair and just process to wrongdoing. The aim is to work toward repairing harm and restoring relationships through collaborative processes with the involved parties and a trained facilitator. Sherman and Strang (2007), in a review of research in the UK and abroad, cite positive and powerful outcomes for crime victims and offenders.

In social work too, over the last 20 years, there has been a growing emphasis on engagement with and learning from their clients. 'Partnership with parents has become a central feature of child care policy and practice' (Sheppard 2001). Asking users and carers of their experience of services should be an 'integral part of strategic commissioning' (Schehrer and Sexton 2010).

11.7   Consultation with Schools: Collaboration in Action

Two heads are better than one.

The following example highlights the difference between a more traditional interaction and relationship between client and professional and one in which collaboration becomes centre stage.

In the UK, consultation is a popular and common form of service delivery operating between Educational Psychologists (EPs) who are employed in Local Education Authorities (LEAs) and work in schools with students, teachers, parents and other professionals at an individual, group and system level. This provides an alternative to assessing and counselling individual students as the main way of working.

In consultation, there is often a 'triadic relationship' involving the psychologist and the key adult/s in consultation about a student or an issue (Dougherty 1995). EPs are not employed to work full time in a single school but have an agreed time allocation of hours or visits on an annual basis. They are therefore external consultants with a committed relationship to a patch of schools.

Case Study

An example of systemic consultation is where an educational psychologist regularly met with a group of teachers from different schools who all had children with Down's Syndrome in their class. The group got together after school once a term to share knowledge, approaches and work out new ways forward. The group was both reactive in discussing problems and preventative in sharing information that might be used by other members in the future. Not only was this a more effective use of time for the EP, but also facilitated group support.

Caplan's work in the 1970s influenced consultation being taken into schools in the USA. Different models of consultation are described and discussed in the US literature with evidence that this way of working is popular with psychologists and schools. Over the last 15 years, consultation in the UK has been shaped by Wagner (1995, 2000) who has developed a consultation model in her own LEA and with other services across the country (Watkins 2000). Her model is partly based on Mental Health Consultation but with greater emphasis on social psychological approaches as they 'match the complexity of the social systems with which we work and promote a reflexive stance for the EP' (Wagner 1995). In particular, systems thinking, personal construct psychology, social constructionism and symbolic interactionism are mentioned as helpful. EPs also use solution-focused thinking/approach with their work in schools (Ajmal and Rees 2001). These approaches inform the structure and language of the consultation.

Consultation is defined by several assumptions (Wagner 2008; Brown et al. 2010):

1. It is a voluntary indirect process to resolve issues. The EP works initially or solely with the key adults rather than students.
2. The subject of the consultation can be an individual, group, or organisation.
3. There are two expected outcomes of the consultation: the first is about helping the person consulted to be more skilled in their area of concern; the second outcome is related to improving services for a third party, e.g. differentiated support for a student.

In writing about 'active consultation', Kanter (1994) highlights the need for developing 'mechanisms - structures, processes and skills in order to achieve real value from the partnership'.

In structure, a typical consultation might look like this:

A teacher has a concern about a student in their class. They request a consultation with the EP who works in their school. The teacher would prepare for the consultation by thinking about or writing questions that will set the scene for the consultation and provide thinking time prior to meeting. Typically, this is presented as a Consultation Request Form. The questions asked encourage an interactionist perspective and place value on the teacher's knowledge and skills (Wagner and Gillies 2001).

What do you hope to get from the consultation?
What strategies have you already tried?
What effects have you noted?
When does the behaviour you want happen?

In the face-to-face meeting, the EP will give an outline about what will take place in the consultation. A script, a dialogue using set words and phrases that emphasise role and relationship, is used to provide a consistent approach that guides both EP and teacher through the consultation (Kerslake and Roller 2000).

The consultation continues with reflection about what the teacher wants from the meeting by gathering and processing the information presented by the teacher. The underlying psychology informs the questions asked and demonstrates interest in particular aspects, widening the view of the situation and opening up new possible solutions.

What sense does the student make of the situation?
How might other people be influencing what is happening?
When everything is working well, what helps this happen?

Planning what needs to happen next follows with input from both professionals, the teacher and the EP, in a way that meets the needs of the situation and ensures the collaborative process. Sometimes it will be clear to the teacher about what they can implement to make changes; at other times, the intervention will need more input from the EP, further meetings, or direct contact with the student. Plans are recorded with a follow-up meeting arranged.

Reviewing how the consultation met the needs stated at the beginning of the consultation and confidence levels of the teacher in carrying out the intervention close the consultation.

At the end of the school year, the EP writes a summary of the joint work in school. This would then form a basis of reflection on the work together and planning for the year ahead.

The outline above provides a brief overview of the structure of consultation, and of course it is much more than this. Relationship-making skills will be covered in the section on significant factors in a therapeutic relationship.

11.8   Outcomes from Consultation

For many EP services, consultation provided the solution to move from a crisis-referral-based system of individual work with students to an interactive process where psychological conversations and shared responsibility take place. For the LEA where I worked, our impetus for change was to add greater value and

consistency in the psychological contribution to schools and improve client satisfaction with our professional service. Positive outcomes found were:

- Enhanced ratings by schools and parents of our service
- Increase in time allocated to schools
- Increase in joint working and in team project among EPs
- Discussion with other agencies and managers about consultation.
  (From Developing Consultation. A workshop for Educational Psychologists.
  Institute of Education 1998)

The outcomes included greater satisfaction and understanding about consultation from clients with increased opportunities for collaborative work among EPs.

In the UK, discussion and research continue to grow about how EPs use consultation in schools (Kennedy et al. 2008; Leadbetter 2006). The research has mainly
focused on what psychologists say in the consultation though there is evidence
about the benefits for teachers and students of the joint nature of the collaboration
(Timmins et al. 2006).

Overall, consultation has offered a way of asking what help people want and
working alongside them in a professional way to achieve it. Both the specialist skills
and knowledge of the teacher and psychologist are harnessed to make a difference
for teachers and students. It is a good example of high quality connection.

11.9 Significant Factors in a Positive Therapeutic Relationship

Therapy is commonly viewed as a relational activity. 'Relationships are the forum
for change to take place' (Kottler and Shepard 2008). Though the relationship is
valued as a highly influencing aspect by most mental health professionals, it has
only recently been a major focus of attention. A shift has taken place from looking
at what therapies are effective to what therapists do to contribute to effect change
with their clients.

Lambert's (1992) common factor research highlighted the importance of relational aspects in therapeutic work. From analysis of thousands of sessions between
client and practitioner, four sets of factors were seen to contribute to successful
outcome:

- 40% of successful change was attributed to the factors that clients bring with
  them into therapy. These included the clients' own strengths and skills, their
  readiness for change and the other resources available.
- 30% of successful change was attributed to the positive relationship between
  practitioner and client. Skills such as 'empathy, warmth, acceptance, encouragement of risk taking' were seen to be important.
- 15% was attributed to hopes, expectations and placebo factors.
- 15% was attributed to the model or technique that was used.

Client factors and the alliance between the client and therapist were therefore found to have greater influence over techniques and models. Though initially conceptualised as separate factors, it is now recognised that there is an interplay among all these aspects. Research and debate continue about the nature of how things work together to create change, though the relationship between client and professional is viewed to be key. The one constant 'variable' is the 'relationship, co-created and sustained by client and therapist' (Orlinsky 2010).

From extensive research, Norcross (2010) highlights evidence from both sides of the relationship that contribute to effectiveness. First are elements of effective practice of the therapist, then secondly, feedback from clients about their experience of the work together. These do not happen in isolation but work in concert together.

Many therapeutic professionals will recognise the elements of good practice, detailed below. It is not just therapists having and using the skill; it is the client's perceptions of these in the relationship that is important to outcome. This is especially important in relation to empathy and positive regard. Even though this is known to be an important characteristic, levels of low empathy are sometimes found in professional helpers (Reynolds 2008). Professionals are not always able to accurately ascertain or predict others peoples' experience.

The following are desired elements of a therapist in a helping relationship:

- The role of the empathetic helper, in being sensitive and open to understanding life from the clients' point of view, initially highlighted by Carl Rogers (Rogers 1980).
- Building an alliance by creating a positive working partnership, especially in the early stages of work; having a clear idea about how to build relationships especially in complex circumstances; using positive communication skills, empathy and openness.
- Collaboration in agreeing goals and a focus for work.
- Positive regard for the client through an accepting, caring and respectful attitude.
- Genuineness and openness shown by the therapist in relating to the client.
- Providing considered positive feedback to clients that adds to the partnership.
- Addressing and repairing difficulties when they arise.
- Infrequent personal disclosures that are significant in the context of the work and that will enhance the relationship.

The following important factors are given in client feedback:

- The fit and the quality of the relationship both matter. The consistent client voice says to 'cultivate and customize the … relationship' (Duncan et al. 2004).
- Pay attention to how the clients experience the work. Good outcomes are related to client feelings of empathy and collaboration.
- Ask for feedback on how the relationship is going while you are working together. This demonstrates collaborative work in action and provides a voice for the client; the feedback can inform how the work proceeds in the future and helps know what is contributing to what is working in this particular case. 'If evaluation only happens at the end, it is too late' (Egan 2002).

'How are we doing?' is a question regularly asked by a colleague during group and individual work. Just asking the question and using word 'we' both emphasize the goal of joint work and is open to receiving a variety of feedback.

- At the end of the work, ask what has helped. Below is an example of seeking the client's view:

I like to follow-up with people when our work is over, to ask a few questions about what was helpful in our time together.
This primarily helps me improve my work with others.
So, if you were to say 3 things that you thought helped, what would they be?

In my experience, clients have definite ideas about what has helped them. Often it is about the positive thinking space that leads to different ways of viewing their issues and subsequently new possibilities for action.

The rise of relational factors has led to closer examination of what successful therapists or 'Supershrinks' do in creating positive relationships and change (Miller et al. 2007). Literature about experts from many fields and the distinctive behaviors of skilled professionals were translated into a 'formula for success' for therapists. The elements are both process- and outcome-focused and act as a 'cycle of excellence'.

- Creating a baseline in order to measure effectiveness: knowing where you are starting from in order to gauge success.
- 'Engaging in deliberate practice' happens when there is a focused effort to improve performance. This involves hard work with increased attention on the process as it is happening and on the outcome.
- Asking for feedback and acting on the information to inform/change the process.

There are a variety of tools available to provide feedback on the working relationship and outcome (Lambert 2010; Kelly et al. 2010). Two well-researched scales have been developed by Duncan and colleagues (2003). The scales are completed at the end of each session and are straightforward to complete, taking only a few minutes. There are scales for adult and child feedback, and the questions focus on aspects of the working relationship and on progress.

The Session Rating Scale (SRS) has four scales to be completed by the client about the current session in the following areas:

- The relationship – being heard, understood and respected.
- The goals and topics – was the work appropriately focused on what the client wanted to talk about.
- Approach – the goodness of fit of the therapist method.
- Overall – how the session worked.

The Outcome Rating Scale (ORS) again asks for four sets of feedback, focusing on client movement toward their goal in the following areas:

- Personal wellbeing
- Relationships with family and friends
- Work relationships
- General sense of wellbeing

Benefits of asking for feedback have been found to increase positive outcomes and client retention (Miller et al. 2005). The process covers many of the desired elements of effective therapists highlighted by Norcross (2010) earlier in the chapter and provides a space for the client voice.

> When using the SRS in a recent piece of work with a 9 year old student, his rating for the overall way the session worked was much less than I anticipated. When asked about this, he replied he liked to learn through games and wanted to know if I had games that might help him learn some new ways of doing things. This proved to be very useful feedback that helped me change my approach and helped him towards his goal.

Current therapeutic research highlights the factors that make helping more effective: the focus is on skillfully creating a collaborative working relationship while understanding the needs, impact and experience of the other person in the process. Using models that include these elements as central is important. Such frameworks inform the wider scope of professional relationships and are highly desirable.

11.10   How Solution-Focused Thinking (SFT) Builds Positive and Effective Relationships

Brief Therapy is an effective model that is used with a wide range of clients. It is a collaborative, strength-based approach based in a positive psychology paradigm. A wellness belief exists about clients who are viewed to have skills and resources. Through examining what is already working and adopting a future orientation, clients are helped to uncover their own solutions. Solution-focused thinking (SFT) has developed from Brief Therapy, using the principles and techniques in areas other than in therapy. A wide range of successful applications is found, for example, in education (Durrant 1995; Parsons 2009), social work (de Jong and Berg 2001), coaching/management (Greene and Grant 2006) and nursing (McAllister 2010).

In adopting the assumptions below, the techniques and questions provide practical tools that are used in a deliberate way to create an expectation of change and improve the situation:

- Every client/situation is unique.
- Strengths and resources within the client/situation exist and can be used to create solutions.
- An emphasis on the past and details of the problem are not necessary for the development of solutions.
- Knowing the client goal will focus where and what is wanted.
- Change is constant. There are always exceptions to problems; it is not an all-or-nothing situation.
- In trying to bring about change, begin by starting small.

Walter and Peller (1992) suggest a three-part 'pathway to constructing solutions':

11.10.1 Find Out the Client's Goal

Constructing goals together is a respectful approach that brings clarity to what needs to happen and acts as a guide to navigate through the work.

> In presenting at a conference in the UK in 2000, John Murphy described his job as similar to a travel agent. The client knowing or working out together the desired destination helps them on their journey as briefly and directly as possible (Murphy 2000).

Iveson (2005) talks about the 'Power Handover' when writing about solution-focused therapists who ask the not-knowing question of 'How can I help you?' He recognises that this is a question asked by many professionals in determining a work contract. The focus centres on what the customer wants, and the therapist joins with them in a 'common project' (Korman 2004).

11.10.2 Look for Positives in the Current Situation and Build on These Strengths

This involves exploring details of what is already working well or is something positive that already exists in the situation.

Scaling questions emphasise the notion of change and can act as a way to measure progress, compare situations, or gain feedback. The client is an active participant in monitoring differences and change.

> In relation to your goal, where are you now on a scale of 0–10 with 10 achieving your goal?
> If you were one point higher on the scale, what would be happening?
> What has been your highest point on the scale?
> On the 0–10 scale, how would you rate the helpfulness of this work?

Exception questions can help unpick the dynamics of the positives and build on what is already going well:

> When things are going well, what is different?
> What do you do that is different?
> Who else in involved or notices?

Uncovering client skills, then enquiring how they can use them in the problem scenario, makes use of what the client resources and encourages new thinking.

> A young client who wanted to be an actor when he grew up decided he could use his talents in acting like the student that all the teachers wanted.

11.10.3   Find Out What Needs to Happen Next and Do Something Different

Bill O'Hanlon (1999) quotes a Dakota tribal saying: 'When you discover you are riding a dead horse, the best strategy is to dismount'. This philosophy goes against the grain of 'try, try again' and moves the focus to trying new different things.

Talking about positives and possibilities brings a new view to the situation and provides hope for change. It can be a short step then to ask:

So what needs to happen next?
What will it take for that to happen?

Due to the interest in what is working, oral and written feedback is a common feature, both during the work and at the end of a session.

How are we doing? Tell me if you feel I'm going at a snail's pace with my questions? I can change gear! (Rees 2001).

Commonly toward the end of the session, there is a short break in the meeting. This time for reflection can be used by both therapist and client to actively review and then plan what happens next (Sharry et al. 2001).

Feedback letters aim to 'capture the essence of the conversation' and remind the client of their strengths and the changes they have made (Stephenson and Smith 2001).

SFT offers many different professionals hopeful assumptions and tools to use flexibly and creatively. It places collaboration with the client at the centre. Clear strategies attend to and use the positives that already exist in the situation. Giving and gaining feedback is important to the process.

11.11   Implications for Developing Positive Relationships

Relationships are a core component of helping. They matter on a number of levels and need to be cultivated and reviewed. Professional training brings a level of expertise and knowledge. Clients also have expertise, and many are knowledgeable about their situation. Adopting a collaborative solution-focused approach where the professional is attentive to the process, asks for ongoing feedback, and is open to change will go a long way to create a positive working relationship.

The example at the beginning illustrates many of the points made in the chapter. The workers in this situation may not have had formal training on how to create positive working relationships, yet they were able to put many aspects into practice. It might just be that along the way, they attended to what has worked well for them and their clients and that they know how to continue to maintain high quality connections.

They know the benefits of evidence gained as they are involved in their day-to-day work. For others, we can look to the research literature and implement findings into our practice that will promote our working relationships.

References

Ajmal, Y., & Rees, I. (Eds.). (2001). *Solutions in schools*. London: BT Press.

Brown, D., Pryzwansky, W. B., & Schulte, A. C. (2010). *Psychological consultation and collaboration: Introduction to theory and practice* (7th ed.). New York: Merrill.

Collins, J. (2001). *Good to great: Why some companies make the leap … and others Don't*. New York: Harper Business.

Corey, M. S., & Corey, G. (2006). *Becoming a helper* (5th ed.). Belmont: Brooks Cole.

Covey, S. (1989). *The seven habits of highly effective people*. New York: Simon and Schuster.

de Jong, P., & Berg, I. K. (2001). Co-constructing with mandated clients. *Social Work, 46*(4), 361–375.

Dougherty, A. M. (1995). *Consultation: Practice and perspectives in school and community settings* (2nd ed.). Pacific Gove: Brooks/Cole.

Duncan, B. L., Miller, S. D., Sparks, J. A., Claud, D. A., Reynolds, L. R., Brown, J., & Johnson, L. D. (2003). The session rating scale: Preliminary psychometric properties of a 'working' alliance measure. *Journal of Brief Therapy, 3*(1), 3–12.

Duncan, B. L., Miller, S. D., & Sparks, J. A. (2004). *The heroic client: A revolutionary way to improve effectiveness through client-directed, outcome-informed therapy*. San Francisco: Jossey-Bass.

Durrant, M. (1995). *Creative strategies for school problems*. New York: Norton.

Dutton, J. E., & Heaphy, E. (2003). The power of high-quality connections. In K. S. Cameron, J. E. Dutton, & R. E. Quinn (Eds.), *Positive organizational scholarship: High quality connections 27 foundations of a new discipline* (pp. 263–278). San Francisco: Berrett-Koehler.

Egan, G. (2002). *The skilled helper*. Belmont: Brooks/Cole.

Elwyn, G., Edwards, A., Eccles, M., & Rovner, D. (2009). Decision analysis in patient care. *The Lancet, 358*(9281), 571–574.

Fuertes, J. N., Boylan, L. S., & Fontanella, J. A. (2009). Behavioral indices in medical care outcome: The working alliance, adherence, and related factors. *Journal of General Internal Medicine, 21*(1), 80–85.

Goleman, D. (2000). *Working with emotional intelligence*. New York: Bantam.

Goleman, D. (2006). *Social intelligence. The new science of human relationships*. New York: Bantam.

Greene, J., & Grant, A. M. (2006). *Solution focused coaching: Managing people in a complex world*. Harlow: Pearson Education.

Institute of Education. (1998). *Developing consultation*. A workshop for Educational Psychologists organised by EP Consultation Group from various LEAs.

Iveson, C. (2005). Teaching the difficult craft of not knowing. *Solution News. Bulletin of the United Kingdom Association for Solution Focused Practice, 1*(3), 3–5.

Kanter, R. M. (1994, July –August). Collaborative advantage: The art of alliances. *Harvard Business Review, 72*, 96–108.

Kelly, S. D., Bickman, L., & Norwood, E. (2010). Evidence-based treatments and common factors in youth psychotherapy. In B. L. Duncan, S. D. Miller, B. E. Wampold, & M. A. Hubble (Eds.), *The heart and soul of change. Delivering what works in therapy* (2nd ed.). Washington, DC: American Psychological Association.

Kennedy, K., Frederickson, N., & Monsen, J. (2008). Do educational psychologists 'walk the talk' when consulting? *Educational Psychology in Practice, 24*(3), 169–187.

Kerslake, H., & Roller, J. (2000). The development of 'scripts' in the practice of consultation. *Educational Psychology in Practice, 16*(1), 25–30.

Korman H. (2004). *The common project.* Accessed November 29, 2010, from http://www.sikt.nu/Articl_and_book/Creating%20a%20common%20project.PDF

Kottler, J. A., & Shepard, D. S. (2008). *Introduction to counseling. Voices from the field* (6th ed.). Belmont: Brooks/Cole.

Lambert, M. J. (1992). Implications of outcome research for psychotherapy integration. In J. C. Norcross & M. R. Goldfried (Eds.), *Handbook of psychotherapy integration.* New York: Basic Books.

Lambert, M. J. (2010). Yes it is time for clinicians to routinely monitor treatment outcome. In B. L. Duncan, S. D. Miller, B. E. Wampold, & M. A. Hubble (Eds.), *The heart and soul of change. Delivering what works in therapy* (2nd ed.). Washington, DC: American Psychological Association.

Leadbetter, J. (2006). Investigating and conceptualizing the notion of consultation to facilitate multi-agency work. *Educational Psychology in Practice, 22*(1), 19–31.

Macklin, R. (1999). *Against relativism: Cultural diversity and the search for ethics.* Oxford: Oxford University Press.

Maidment, J. (2006, January–March). The quiet remedy: A dialogue on reshaping professional relationships. *Families in Society, 87*, 1.

McAllister, M. (Ed.). (2010). *Solution focused nursing: Rethinking practice.* Basingstoke: Palgrave Macmillan.

McMullan, M. (2006). Patients using the internet to obtain health information: How this affects the patient-health professional relationship. *Patient Education and Counseling, 63*(1), 24–28.

Miller, S. D., Duncan, B. L., Sorrell, R., & Brown, G. S. (2005). The partners for change outcome management system. *Journal of Clinical Psychology: In Session, 61*, 199–208.

Miller, S. D., Hubble, M., & Duncan, B. (2007, November/December). Supershrinks. Who are they? What can we learn from them? *Supershrinks. Psychotherapy Networker, 31*(6), 26–35, 56.

Murphy, J. (2000, September 14–15). *Solution focused intervention for school problems.* Cardiff Conference

Norcross, J. C. (2010). The therapeutic relationship. In B. L. Duncan, S. D. Miller, B. E. Wampold, & M. A. Hubble (Eds.), *The heart and soul of change. Delivering what works in therapy* (2nd ed.). Washington, DC: American Psychological Association.

O'Hanlon, B. (1999). *Do one thing different.* New York: William Morrow and Company.

Orlinsky, D. E. (2010). Foreword. In B. L. Duncan, S. D. Miller, B. E. Wampold, & M. A. Hubble (Eds.), *The heart and soul of change. Delivering what works in therapy* (2nd ed.). Washington, DC: American Psychological Association.

Osterberg, L., & Blaschke, T. (2005). Adherence to medication. *The New England Journal of Medicine, 2005*(353), 487–497.

Parsons, R. D. (2009). *Thinking and acting like a solution-focused school counselor.* Thousand Oaks: Corwin.

Rees, I. (2001). Solution world. In Y. Ajmal & I. Rees (Eds.), *Solutions in schools.* London: BT Press.

Reynolds, W. J. (2008). Do nurses and other professional helpers normally display much empathy? *Journal of Advanced Nursing, 31*(1), 226–234.

Robinson, K., & Aronica, L. (2009). *The element: How finding your passion changes everything.* New York: Viking Penguin.

Rogers, C. (1980). *A way of being.* Boston: Houghton Mifflin.

Saxton, G. D. (2004). The rise of participatory society: Challenges for public administration. *PA Times, 27*(11), 4–5.

Schehrer, S., & Sexton, S. (2010). *Involving users in commissioning local services.* York: Joseph Rowntree Foundation.

Seligman, M. E. P., & Csikszentmihalyi, M. (2000). Positive psychology: An introduction. *American Psychologist, 55*(1), 5–14.

Seybold, P. B., Marshak, R. T., & Lewis, J. M. (2001). *The customer revolution*. New York: Crown Business.

Sharry, J., Madden, B., Darmody, M., & Miller, S. D. (2001). Giving our clients the break. Applications of client-directed, outcome-informed clinical work. *Journal of Systemic Therapies, 20*(3), 68–76.

Sheppard, M. (2001). The design and development of an instrument for assessing the quality of partnership between mother and social worker in child and family care. *Child and Family Social Work, 6*(1), 31–46.

Sherman, L. W., & Strang, H. (2007). *Restorative justice: The evidence*. London: Esmee Fairbank Foundation, The Smith Institute.

Stephenson, M., & Johal-Smith, H. (2001). Discovering the expert. In Y. Ajmal & I. Rees (Eds.), *Solutions in schools*. London: BT Press.

Timmins, P., Bham, M. S., McFadyen, J., & Ward, J. J. A. (2006). Teachers and consultation: Applying research and development in organizations. *Educational Psychology in Practice, 22*(4), 305–320. doi:10.1080/02667360600999419.

Wagner, P. (1995). *School consultation: A handbook for practicing educational psychologists*. London: Kensington and Chelsea EPCS.

Wagner, P. (2000). Consultation: Developing a comprehensive approach to service delivery. *Educational Psychology in Practice, 16*(1), 9–18.

Wagner, P. (2008). Consultation as a framework for practice. In B. Kelly, L. Woolfson, & J. Boyle (Eds.), *Frameworks for practice in educational psychology: A textbook for trainees and practitioners (chapter 7)*. London: Jessica Kingsley Publishers.

Wagner, P., & Gillies, E. (2001). Consultation: A solution-focused approach. In Y. Ajmal & I. Rees (Eds.), *Solutions in schools*. London: BT Press.

Walter, J. L., & Peller, J. E. (1992). *Becoming solution focused in brief therapy*. Levittown: Brunner/Mazel.

Watkins, C. (2000). Introduction to the articles on consultation. *Educational Psychology in Practice, 16*(1).

Elizabeth Gillies is a UK Educational Psychologist who has lived and worked in the UK, America, Japan and Australia. She currently has a private practice in Tokyo, working in international schools and as a consultant for an Employee Assistance Programme. She is the Vice President of International Mental Health Professionals in Japan.

Contact: elizabeth_gillies@mac.com

Chapter 12
Positive Mentoring Relationships: Nurturing Potential

Ann M. Brewer

12.1 Introduction

In today's fast-developing world, whatever one's age, and whether one is working or studying, raising a family or volunteering, it is important to learn and go on learning throughout life. All relationships involve learning, but in mentoring this is especially so and both formal and informal mentoring continues to be popular. Mentoring has its roots in ancient times with Homer in *The Odyssey* telling the story of Telemachus, the son of Odysseus, and his coming of age under the tutelage of a mentor while his father was absent at war. It has endured throughout the ages to the present day and is used, for example, with children in primary school who are paired with older students, early career professionals with more-experienced counterparts, youth workers working with young people, women seeking directorships on boards and young people using reverse mentoring with the less technologically savvy.

Mentoring is a relationship built on trust, with two people conversing together and one giving guidance, support and encouragement to the other (Hartley 2004). It occurs in a range of contexts: personal, professional and organisational. A typical mentoring relationship involves the mentor: a more experienced person, a trusted counsellor and the mentee: the recipient of the mentoring relationship referred to here as a protégé. Protege has been selected as 'Mentee' is simply a descriptor referring to a person who has a mentor, whereas a protégé conveys potential and untapped talent and therefore active learning. Influence in this relationship is never unidirectional, with one party being shaped and dominated by the other. The 'equality' of the partnership, however, depends upon the more experienced person doing what they can to neutralise any power imbalance. While mentorship is

A.M. Brewer (✉)
Office of Vice Chancellor Strategic Management,
University of Sydney, Sydney, Australia
e-mail: ann.brewer@sydney.edu.au

S. Roffey (ed.), *Positive Relationships: Evidence Based Practice across the World*,
DOI 10.1007/978-94-007-2147-0_12, © Springer Science+Business Media B.V. 2012

characterised as dyadic, with differential experience between the mentor and protégé, this is not always the case. For learning to occur, the social exchange between the mentor and protégé involves mutual influence, as will be demonstrated throughout this chapter.

The focus here is on understanding mentoring and the reasons for its endurance. Several questions will be addressed: What do we understand by mentoring? What is it about the mentoring relationship that allows a person's potential to emerge, be shaped or flourish? What are the types of mentoring available? How is the mentoring relationship qualitatively different from other types of relationships? What are the benefits for mentors and which ways of mentoring are more effective than others? Does it make a difference the way this relationship comes about? What about training for mentors?

Case Study

Mitchell helped Diana rethink her start-up business, which, although making a small margin, had an ad hoc approach. One thing Mitchell revealed was that he does not always follow his own advice but varies it depending on business context. Mitchell was a reluctant mentor at first but took this assignment on because he was asked by a mutual friend. One of the first tasks he got Diana to think about was what success would look like in, say, 2 years time and to write it down. That helped her work with a more structured business plan than she currently had, and over the course of the next 6 months, he assisted her:

- *Improve her negotiating skills with suppliers*
- *Refuse potential clients seeking free advice*
- *Develop relationships with new networks of clients*
- *Develop and align her marketing plan to her newly formulated business plan*
- *Select an accountant to improve her budgeting and capital planning*
- *Price her services to improve her margin*
- *Better manage her time between home and work*

At the end of the 6 months assignment, Mitchell reported that Diana had renewed confidence in herself and this allowed her to make better business decisions. This chapter attempts to show how this successful mentorship was achieved.

12.2 What Do We Understand by Mentoring?

Mentoring forms the backbone of most learning relationships including coaching, consulting, person-centred counselling and the shadowing of more-experienced people that occurs in professional and organisational learning contexts. The focus of both parties together is on the potential goals, performance, relationships, leadership capability and motivation of the protégé. A mentor intervenes in the learning process through facilitation, listening, counselling, challenging and providing overall support to assist the protégé in identifying and examining the above and to see whether these are aligned to actions and plans. A formal mentoring conversation usually includes preparation, dialogue, commitment and closure to each meeting. It also involves agreement about goals around the process, accountability of each party to the relationship and a plan. Following up and identifying outcomes, opportunities for further development or advancement, assessing progress towards goals and using feedback are important in producing the desired learning. Mentors need to assess their own capability for assisting the protégé, either through self-assessment or peer review by a colleague or friend.

Mentors do not try to persuade or coerce, but rather encourage and challenge their protégés. Mentorship ensures accountability of both parties and abides by the professional standards and ethics of the participants relevant to the context (school, organisation or profession). For example, if a teacher is acting as a mentor with a younger person, then the professional and ethical standards apply, as does the relevant sphere of accountability.

A positive mentoring relationship develops gradually over time as the key ingredients, mutual trust and respect, take time to develop. It allows the protégé to connect personally at a deeper level with a significant other, usually but not always a more experienced person. This personal connection is important for mirroring other types of critical relationships for the protégé, such as teacher, parent, supervisor, client or peer, depending on the type of mentorship. More importantly, such relationships expedite learning in a way that may otherwise not occur or take longer if the mentorship did not exist. For example, the mentor may offer insights or opinions that may not have been shared except within this exclusive relationship. *Trust* is vital in this situation as privileged insights, knowledge and information are often private and both parties are relying on the other to respect confidentiality. The protégé may describe a situation, for example, where they are feeling oppressed or bullied, and ask the mentor whether this situation is familiar to them, and if so, how would they deal with it. Intervention by the mentor is not requested as this can lead to a conflict of interest or an ethical concern for the mentor. They may have the authority to act on this but cannot do so due to the privileged nature of the communication. An example of this is where a junior medico is being 'bullied' by a more senior colleague.

Underpinning mutual trust between the mentor and protégé are shared values and perspectives, vital particularly in youth mentoring where the adult needs to work within the 'headspace' of the protégé. Both parties to the mentoring relationship need to agree to participate, with the mentor taking responsibility for supporting the protégé. Essentially success is dependent upon the meeting of two minds to achieve a certain shared 'relaxed space' that will progress reflection and learning. When mutual trust and respect lead to positive outcomes, this helps develop a rhythm and synchronicity to the pair's cooperation. The notion of 'mentis', the Latin word for mind, is core to mentorship. Protégés are often encouraged to build a different *mindset*, sometimes actively countermanding a prevailing one. The new mindset is a catalyst for new learning and critical to the process of development.

Central also to mentoring is the use of *narrative* (Britzman and Gilbert 2004). This is where two people come together and tell stories to each other about both big and small things such as past achievements and failures, present and future aspirations. Unsolicited advice does not have a place in these conversations, as this is likely to be ignored unless something occurs to trigger it being replayed in the protégé's mind.

12.3 What Is It About the Mentoring Relationship That Allows a Person's Potential to Emerge, Be Shaped or Flourish?

Learning is frequently accidental, whether planned or not. Mentoring facilitates the protégé in progressing from inadvertent learning towards active learning, self-knowledge and building personal capability to deal with the ups and downs of life. The unfolding narrative facilitates meaning between the participants about what is going on in their situation and what meaning it has for them. What can they learn from this? A lack of self-focus can be valuable in getting the protégé to see themselves as others see them. There is a paradox here, as the protégé also becomes the *centre of attention* in the relationship to assist their own internal locus of evaluation, a catalyst for transformational learning.

What does a mentor offer another person and how does this influence them throughout the relationship and beyond? In many situations, public and private, people learn from each other informally through observation, modelling or shadowing, and also through conversations and conflicts. How many times does one hear the expression 'if only I'd thought of that at the time' indicating that people reflect on past conversations after the event and learn from the further contemplation about the experience. Mentoring facilitates further contemplation which is where real learning occurs.

Whilst mentoring varies from situation to situation, it requires the following three dimensions: learning, transforming and ultimately a capacity to rebuild. Take the example of a young person working with an adult where the mentor is attempting to steer the protégé in a new or life-changing direction. Both have to believe in each other and that any change of direction is based on the mentor's belief that this is in the protégé's best interest. The protégé has to assume that the mentor is acting in good faith. Trust is crucial for 'unpicking' the current action and formulating new goals. Building new personal capacity requires expanding networks of relationships, and this also takes time. Often in mentoring, the protégé has to step back rather than forward, a process that is never easy for young people who are keen to progress rapidly. Helping them to take a step back and rebuild to fortify personal capability can be crucial for their development.

12.3.1 The Role of Influence in Mentoring

Mentoring is about influencing rather than 'telling' or 'advising', and each party to the relationship is subjected to the other's energy, control and resistance. Although the mentor influences the protégé, this is never a one-way exchange. The challenge for each is to accept or counter the other's influence depending on the nature of the persuasion and the purpose being addressed. The protégé should never be dominated by the mentor, who may be revered for their achievement or status (seniority), as this would defeat the purpose of mentoring. The protégé does, however, need to be accepting of the mentor's influence and consider alternative directions if they are to learn. This requires both belief in each other and an evaluation of the learning that occurs. One of the outcomes of mentoring is to improve one's capability to influence others and not be dominated by them, particularly where one's own ideas are being subjugated. Mentoring reveals the role that power and influence play in every relationship and how to act vigorously to participate in this process and not stand on the sidelines. Selecting an appropriate mentor is important in balancing the power within this relationship. Mentors need to be well connected so that they can use a range of resources, although ideally these should not include the protégés' supervisor as the capacity to be open may be thwarted by the possibility of gaining incentives or receiving sanctions. Having said this, supervisors frequently use mentoring to develop skills in those reporting to them, and this can work effectively.

An unsuccessful mentoring relationship makes people reluctant to participate in another similar relationship. 'A negative relationship can affect morale, stress levels and even turnover rates. Those who have a bad experience with mentoring are often reluctant to take part in another relationship' (Cranwell-Ward et al. 2004: 209). Empowering participants rather than incapacitating them is the key to exerting positive influence. The quality of the mentoring relationship is therefore critical both for the present and the future.

12.3.2 What Makes a Successful Mentoring Relationship?

In the first instance, protégés themselves need to have a commitment to act on their new learning. This includes making decisions about how to modify what they do, how they think and their approach to others. Mentoring encourages self-reflections, evaluation and a commitment to change. It facilitates change and development in mindsets. It is a form of learning where the protégé has to be 'present' and cannot be 'absent', unlike in other learning situations, such as the classroom or in a clinical therapeutic situation where the 'learner' does not necessarily 'buy into' the process. If they become preoccupied, the mentor needs to be attuned to this and bring them back into the moment.

Secondly, mentoring takes time – although the amount of time will vary depending on its nature and the roles and experience of the people involved. Some pairs will meet regularly and frequently while others will agree to get together as needed. The former is suited where young and less experienced protégés are involved, and the latter, where it involves professional equivalents or differently experienced people of similar status. Whatever the circumstance, successful mentorship requires frequent meetings in the beginning of the relationship to establish a good foundation for moving forward. Meetings do not always require personal contact and could be achieved through Skype, email or phone. Peer mentoring can be done in a similar way and through electronic discussion fora too.

Thirdly, sponsorship may be a significant feature of the mentoring relationship whereby the mentor can draw their influence and networks to gain some advantage for the protégé. This advantage may be in the form of additional resources, career opportunities and the like. For example, in Australia and other western countries, women aspiring to become board members of listed companies are seeking out formal mentors with the expectation that this will give them a real opportunity to gain a seat on boards (Korporaal 2010).

12.3.3 Outcomes of Mentoring

A core benefit of mentoring for both parties is multidimensional learning. Feedback on how to make decisions, how to impact on others and how to align individual goals with actions, resources and plans may take place simultaneously. Mentors offer valuable knowledge and skill development based on their own experiences of finding pathways out of life's cul-de-sacs. Protégés can offer valuable resources to the mentor to reciprocate their support (Mezias and Scandura 2005). Mentoring provides for both, individually and together, feedback about their assumptions and roles (Hall 1996) and is an effective way for both to broaden their vision on career development (Liu et al. 2009).

Other benefits from a positive mentoring relationship are within the affective domain. This includes feeling more self-aware and self-confident, more closely connected to the organisation and finding work more satisfying and meaningful. For example, some of the positive outcomes of mentoring for law students, who were paired up with lawyers acting as volunteer mentors through a university alumni programme, include:

> "I enjoy the one to one contact with my mentor; it helped reduce the gap between teacher and student and its helped me with my career decisions too".
> "I am much more interested in law as a career now than I was before I started this program".
> "I have an increased awareness of my professional responsibilities now".

Mentoring increases knowledge and connections extending to others outside the mentoring relationship, including throughout an organisation. 'It helps people build new relationships and strengthen existing ones; people become more collaborative in their performance and learning, and individuals feel more prepared to offer themselves as mentors to others' (Zachary 2005: 9). This is important given the labyrinthine career paths that people, especially women, find themselves having to navigate. Some comments from women include:

> "I've been inspired to push myself beyond my limits and that has resulted in my promotion – thank you".
> "I felt so frustrated about my opportunities but my mentor helped me open the door to new ones that I hadn't even seen".

12.4   How Is the Mentoring Relationship Different?

Mentoring covers the full gamut of learning relationships and can be beneficial from the novice to the highly experienced. It can also include elements of counselling, coaching and team building. Although the learning outcomes are critical, the process itself is also an important source of modelling, transforming and education. Learning occurs at any stage of this spectrum if the mentor is someone that the protégé admires. This process entails unpacking the thinking and feelings of the protégé, reflecting on the degree of coherence between emotions and reasoning, intentions and aspirations, implementation and follow up. The effectiveness of mentoring is dependent on the degree of engagement and the nature of the interpersonal communication between the mentor and protégé. This builds a store of information including sensitivity to contextual meanings, perceptions and interpretations as well as being able to tease out the distinctions between these. Effective mentoring is primary a *conversation* where protégés feel 'protected' by the mentors and that they are 'there' for them. This is particularly important for Generation Y workers who respond well to management when they are provided prompt feedback and credit for results achieved (Martin 2005; Southard and Lewis 2004).

This personal, intimate conversation transmits shared meaning and is responsive, deeply satisfying, trusting and influential (Nezlek 2001). All of these characteristics make life more fulfilling. Intimacy inherent in mentoring is impossible in situations where there are more than two people present, such as group training sessions, apprenticeships or on-the-job training. A one-on-one mentoring relationship can therefore become highly significant and worthwhile. While mentoring does *occur within, overlap* and *parallel* other forms of collaborative, learning relationships, these rarely contain the particular ingredients and benefits that mentoring affords its participants, both for the mentor and the protégé (Tenner, 2004).

12.5   Types of Mentoring

Mentoring relationships are established through different ways.

12.5.1   Traditional One-on-One Mentoring

Traditional one-on-on mentoring is a type of apprenticeship whereby the more junior protégé learns from a more experienced mentor. Its aim is to prime the protégé for their next step, focusing on values, decisions and performance. This is often formalised, although rarely compulsory, and the mentor and protégé are often selected and matched. It is used in schools and other organisations for supporting people to develop or learn new skills. Mentoring can, however, also be informal where one party seeks out the other. Whether formal or not, traditional mentoring may vary in its philosophy in regard to whether the mentor's viewpoint is that the protégé's thinking needs to be 'aligned' to that of, say, an organisation (dubbed 'alignment mentoring') or allows the protégé to come to their own position through reflection and reflective practice, more akin to professional mentoring.

12.5.2 Professional Mentoring for Practitioners

This is similar to traditional one-on-one mentoring and primarily focuses on reflective inquiry into how the junior professional is improving the quality of their decisions and actions as a practitioner, for example, a medical practitioner, lawyer, teacher, social/youth worker, counsellor or nurse. Professional mentoring is often mandatory, such as peer supervision for psychologists, coaches and the like. It provides a standards and ethical base that enables the practitioner to evaluate their own approach, analyse their dilemmas and work through problems to resolution.

12.5.3 Mentoring and Sponsoring

Sponsoring is a form of mentoring with one difference: 'Sponsors go beyond giving feedback and advice; they advocate for their mentees and help them gain visibility in the company' (Ibarra et al. 2010: 83).

12.5.4 Cross-Cultural Mentoring

Cross-cultural mentoring encourages and assists the protégé to probe into their underlying assumptions, values that impact on their perceptions and actions in the host culture. It is mentoring between people of different cultures such as in 'expat' situations. It works through an approach whereby the protégé is required to walk along two paths. A good example of this would be integrating an indigenous approach within mainstream culture especially where the protégé has to deal with people from the former cultural background. Napier has explored the cross-cultural exchanges between foreign 'experts' who work as mentors in developing countries and local 'learners' who possess a great deal of locally relevant knowledge that the foreigner needs and lacks (Napier 2006). The dialogue, learning, teaching and support across cultural differences are a vital component of cross-cultural mentoring relationship. The interaction between the two parties happens within the institutional context, and the decision to engage in those actions is influenced not only by the individual but also by the institution's culture, staff expectations, mission and history.

12.5.5 Peer Mentoring

Mentoring between peers of similar status such as school or university students is beneficial in sharing information, problem solving and support for each other. It overlaps with informal mentoring and is probably the most common and, therefore, invisible form of mentoring. The key factor here is that peer mentoring includes personal approaches that are not always dealt with in formal programmes. Some examples of feedback from two different peer mentoring experiences between lecturers and students conducted as part of a course include:

> A wonderful experience, which definitely contributed to my experience as a teacher. It encouraged me to be more reflexive regarding my own teaching practices – something we don't often take the opportunity to think about. (Lecturer group)
>
> It allowed us leadership opportunities and also encouraged us to be more innovative in our approach to our learning. (Student group)

12.5.6 Reverse Mentoring

The protégé stereotype is usually that of a young or 'junior' status person paired with a more experienced, older person (Wanberg et al. 2003). Effective mentors could, however, just as easily have less experience and still provide a basis for new learning for others. The notion of Generation Y approaching work with different expectations compared to previous generations may be oversimplified. Over the ages, humans have wanted similar things from their working life regardless of whether it is a short or long career, continuous or temporary. They desire security, satisfaction, a sense of belonging, acknowledgement and growth. Many motivational theorists and research attest to this (Watson et al. 2003; Montana and Lenaghan 1999; Macky et al. 2008; Cennamo and Gardner 2008). The stereotypes applied to Gen Y could therefore just as easily be applied to the over 50s. If one thinks about the baby boomer generation, the amount of change and innovation that has occurred in their lifetime has far outstripped that of Gen X or Gen Y. They were the first teenagers, the first hippies, some transmogrified into 'yuppies' and more recently, 'sea-changers' and 'tree-changers'.

While structured mentoring schemes are well established for senior mentors and junior protégés, reverse mentoring schemes are relatively new (Greengard 2002). The over 50s generation are paired with a Gen Y, for example, with a specific purpose in mind. There is widespread recognition, however, that reverse mentoring is more common than is acknowledged, if only because it happens informally and goes unnoticed. Reverse mentoring originates in the trend away from concepts of knowledge and power that parallel traditional mentoring to a more equal relationship, whereby all participants, regardless of age, have something of value to contribute (Darwin 2000; Tempest 2003).

Trust is also essential in reverse mentoring especially where one member acts as a sounding board or takes on the role of the questioning partner: 'Why are you doing that? What are you trying to achieve? Wouldn't you be better doing it this way?' and so on. (Welch and Welch 2006). This approach benefits younger people, giving them a leadership voice and enabling them to feel more confident and valued by others (Cotugna and Vickery 1998; Leh 2005; Morgan and Streb 2001). This may be of particular value to Generation Y, whom some authors claim to be more interested than earlier generations in the moral, civic and social value that their work provides (Allen 2004; Cone 2006; Crampton and Hodge 2009; Glass 2007; Pekala 2001). The benefits of reverse mentoring also open up networking and other benefits for young people (Leh 2005; Wong et al. 2008; Zanni 2009).

An example of how trust came about is exemplified in the following quote from a Gen Y participant working with a much older staff member:

> Bob was so gracious in letting me guide him through the process that, although I was showing him the technical side of things, when I think back on it, I was actually learning from him about how to let others take the lead.

Rather than relying on staff to approach their supervisors when they had a problem, this programme reverses the accountability and puts the control back on to the younger staff, allowing them to help older workers and, in doing so, have a conversation with them where they discover other 'pearls of wisdom' in the process. Learning occurs both ways and helps to break down the generation gap.

12.5.7 Group or Situational Mentoring

Although it is often thought that learning is best served through a traditional one-on-one mentoring experience, sometimes it works better when people interact with multiple learners (group mentoring) or with multiple experts (situational mentoring). Different learning situations are important (Emelo 2010), and various approaches may need to be trialled and used. Some employers have experimented with forms of peer coaching for cultural change and personal transformation. Others have established mentoring circles for the purpose of facilitating development. An example of this is where a senior leader, trained in managing group dynamics, meets with a small circle of people regularly to discuss particular issues that may be shared among them and uses the group's skills and knowledge to learn.

12.6 Gender Differences in Mentoring

Mentoring plays different roles in men's and women's professional development. Professional women might experience more mentoring than professional men. In a 2008 Catalyst survey of more than 4,000 full-time professional men and women,

83% of women and 76% of men say that they had one or even more mentors at certain time in their career. However, more mentoring does not necessarily lead to career advancement. A 2010 follow-up survey showed that men received 15% more promotions than women. One of the main reasons that mentoring failed women in terms of promotion is the difference between having a mentor and a sponsor. Women tend to have mentors and men have sponsors (Ibarra et al. 2010). Compared with men who are more ready and willing to both offer and seek a mentor, women mentors need to be encouraged and sought out (Laff 2009). And they will provide more psychosocial functions since they are more relationship-oriented (Okurame 2007).

Women's mentors usually possess less organisational power due to their position in the hierarchy. In the 2008 survey, 78% of men versus only 69% of women were actively mentored by a CEO or other senior executive. This is a real disadvantage, as a mentor's position in organisations is closely related to their protégé's career advancement. Both men and women find mentors themselves instead of relying on formal programmes. However, the different mentoring (formal or informal) does make a difference to promotional prospects. In the 2010 follow-up survey, women with mentors through formal programmes received more promotions than women who found mentors by themselves (by a ratio of nearly 3 to 2) (Ibarra et al. 2010).

12.7   The Benefits for Mentors

Sometimes a mentor is viewed as the one giving all or even making sacrifices for the other; however, this is rarely the case. The benefits to each participant will vary according to the quality of the relationship that is generated between them. Mentors can learn from their protégés how to become more constructive and/or appreciate the need to extend their own professional or social networks. The interaction can heighten mentors' performance and acknowledgement for this work especially where outcomes are substantiated (Ragins and Scandura 1994; Russell and Adams 1997). This in turn can afford them enhanced career satisfaction, renewed effort and interest from collaborating with others (Johnson 2002: 87).

Being a mentor inevitably fosters one's understanding about how other people think, feel and act including in relation to others. The mentoring relationship is a microcosm of the protégé's behaviour. As a result, mentors not only assist protégés and provide them with feedback on their interpersonal dynamics but also find that they learn to communicate more effectively themselves regardless of whether it is a traditional or reverse mentoring relationship. Seeing life through the eyes of others is an important learning source for mentors (Eby and Lockwood 2005; Wanberg et al. 2006) and one that is often overlooked. Different perspectives such as these broaden the mentors' understanding and allow them to address some of the challenges they face in their own lives. Through self-reflection activated during the mentoring process, mentors learn by appreciating how they themselves (or their roles) impact others and how this leads them to modify their approach as well as enhance their communication with people who have different values and backgrounds.

12.8 Different Ways of Mentoring Are More Effective Than Others

Mentoring, formal or informal, is more effective when it is voluntary by both parties, and both respect each other and believe that they are achieving some value from it. Voluntary mentoring relationships have better chance to succeed because of the self-motivation inherent in the voluntariness. Take the Lawyers Encouraging and Assisting Promising Students (LEAPS) project for example; this is 'a workplace learning program in which young people are each provided with a mentor from a law firm. The mentors work through lessons on study skills, ethics and career planning with the students' (Australian Youth Mentoring Network 2010).

12.9 Does It Make a Difference the Way the Mentoring Relationship Comes About?

The manner in which mentoring programmes are established leads to different outcomes. Formal and informal mentorships vary in the ways they are established and acknowledged. One should not replace the other. Often informal mentorships are established by selection of participants based on mutual appeal and convenience, which may not be officially endorsed by management.

On the other hand, the institutional orchestration of formal mentorship means that formal mentors may not view the protégé as worthy of special attention and support; protégés may be seen as undeserving of the benefits of mentorship or the special attention it affords them. Such 'assigned' relationships may lack compatibility, interpersonal ease, as well as the longevity required to develop trust and the provision of psychosocial dynamics so critical to achieve the best outcomes (Chao et al. 1992). Mentors in formal programmes may be more visible and therefore less able to sponsor and promote their protégés because these actions may be construed as favouritism by co-workers (Ragins and Cotton 1999). DeLong et al. (2008) see a disadvantage. They claim that mentoring often relies on the selection of 'A-grade performers', that is, the top 10% of the internal workforce, and does not include the 'B- or C-grade performers', that is, the bulk of the internal workforce who are good, albeit invisible, workers who get more than the lion's share of the work done, especially the burdensome work, and often remain loyal to the organisation for longer periods. However, much of the value of those exclusive, one-on-one, power-dependent mentoring relationships depends on context-specific knowledge, which is less and less relevant to sustaining career learning especially as career mobility increases (Darwin 2000).

12.10   Training for Mentors

Potential mentors and protégés need to be identified in all institutions, whether staff, students or leaders. A path can be planned for each depending on how their knowledge and experience is to be developed and utilised. The new recruit, student or staff, in the organisation can be assigned a mentor, and their progress tracked. Similarly, a training pathway for the mentor can be designed and planned. This approach can suit one-on-one mentoring or a circle of peer mentors. Performance feedback training for mentors will be of value in terms of their effectiveness as a mentor as well as their retention in the organisation.

Leaders need to be responsible for seeking out 'ways to help people foster their own developmental networks that include relationships providing various types and amounts of support' (Chandler et al. 2010: 49). They could then ascertain information about, for example:

What is it like to join this organisation as a newcomer?
What does it feel like to be promoted or not promoted here?
How are people treated when faced with leaving?
What do we learn when we take on a new management or leadership role?
What is it like to change career focus?

Answers to these questions are vital for designing mentoring programmes.

12.11   Handling Conflict in the Mentoring Relationship

Good mentors understand that conflict is all-pervading. No matter how productive conflict can be between two people, it is challenging. Influence, conflict and negotiation are important parts of mentoring especially for the protégé to learn and test their skills and reactions to conflict. Mentorships will sometimes produce disagreement, strain relationships and even be distressful for individuals (Johnson et al. 2000; Johnson and Nelson 1999; Levinson et al. 1978; O'Neil and Wrightsman 2001). Learning to cope with conflict and examining both sides of an argument, while suspending judgment, are critical for everyone to learn. As conflict and change are inevitable in relationships, conflict handling is a vital skill for effective mentoring.

12.11.1   Communication

Communication training boosts confidence and credibility with the protégé and strengthens the mentor relationship. Mentors need to listen well so as to give those frequently not heard a voice in what sometimes can be described as 'silent culture' in organisation, where difficult issues are not voiced and avoided. In learning how to voice issues, protégés gain a sense of being a more powerful unique self.

12.11.2   Team Building

Training in team development is critical to mentoring. It permits diverse perspectives to be shared so as to facilitate a common outlook on issues, which in turn is more likely to engender trust and transparency amongst team members and leaders (Jones et al. 2007; Reilly and Lojeski 2009). In spite of best efforts and attention, some people will be poorly suited to mentoring.

12.11.3   Boundary Setting

All human relationships have boundaries or 'rules' about what is or isn't allowed in the relationship. Boundaries are expectations of what can be achieved and are essential for framing a mentoring relationship and distinguishing it from other relationships. Mentors need to think in advance about setting appropriate boundaries, expectations and accountability with their protégés, and discuss these to reach an agreement about them from the outset.

For example, respect is an important boundary in any relationship. Respect is relevant in informal mentoring and peer mentoring, where personal issues are more likely to be dealt with. Personal issues are explored in other mentoring situations when they might interfere with the protégé's positive feeling about themselves in the school, workplace or organisations. Confidentiality is an essential element here too. Mentors need to establish rules of confidentiality in the relationship and discuss it with the protégé at the outset.

12.12   Choosing Mentors

In formal mentoring programmes, individuals who are deemed desirable (a teacher, a good student, a good citizen, a good manager) are usually invited to become mentors. However what is more important in selecting mentors is ensuring they can form positive relationships and have the resources and capability to contribute positively to the growth of the protégé. As one protege told me: 'He helped me define what I thought were impossible goals, and then I went on to achieve them'. As a consequence of this, the protégé felt 'freer', which gave her permission to test out other ideas that she had.

Mentors do not always require the technical expertise to be successful. In many circumstances, the personal qualities of a mentor make a big difference: a good listener, capable of encouraging and creating opportunities to realise hidden talents and wanting to help people develop and succeed.

Allowing potential protégés to have a say in the choice and selection is important. Using social media is one way of achieving this. Establishing mentoring groups, according to special interests, is one way. Facilitating people to link with a group with common needs through a website is a good way to achieve this. Support for informal group creation, either by the mentoring programme administrator or the participants themselves, including searches of mentor and protégé profiles to facilitate group formation, is advisable. A SharePoint with designated areas for group discussions, question and answer sessions, group event notices, project postings and document uploads encourages interaction and collaboration among group participants. Group administration and moderation is essential to assure programme monitoring, evaluation and safety.

12.13   More than a Fleeting Connection

Mentorship, if effective, can become the mainstay of a significant learning relationship for both mentors and protégés and may even develop into a friendship that extends beyond the initial need. Durable mentoring is valuable for young people in particular. In order to maximise mentoring, it is recommended that mentoring programmes are planned and designed according to the principles outlined in this chapter, assuring quality and consistency. This prepares potential mentors and protégés from the time they enter their organisation whether this be as a student, employee, client or citizen. Mentoring requires strong support from within institutions and the community to encourage as many people as possible to volunteer and participate. Mentors are never paid extra for this work as this would impinge on the relationship.

This chapter has shown how mentoring can occur and how it contributes to life learning, enhanced perspectives of thinking and values as well as outcomes. Economic and social changes have somewhat transformed us and the communities in which we reside and the institutions in which we study and work, and mentoring connects both mentor and protégé to these changes. Increasingly, people are engaged in small- to medium-sized organisations with flatter hierarchies, with people working alongside their 'bosses' or collaborating with their teachers or lecturers. Although there is increasing ageism, it is not the inter-generational issues that are the points of difference between different experience levels in mentoring. What distinguishes people today are their views about the environment, education, the economy, refugees and our national resources. People, young and old, expect social justice and 'fair play' in all aspects of their lives, and they believe that our leaders have an obligation to deliver this through procedural fairness. People want better lives, and given that work and study is a fair chunk of this, they want leaders and followers to work together on common challenges and endeavours. Mentorship is an important micro-relationship to assure that this happens at the macro-level.

The challenges for us are to integrate the view of all layers of society into a defining vision and reflect this in laws, regulations, opportunities and educational programmes. By reconciling the financial imperative with social justice and innovation, mentoring harnesses the power of relationships to develop resolution to numerous social and economic issues. Through mentoring, we have the opportunity to 'invent' the culture in which we want to work and thrive.

References

Allen, P. (2004). Welcoming Y. *Benefits Canada, 28*(9), 53.

Australian Youth Mentoring Network. (2010). *LEAPS*. Accessed November 22, 2010, from http://www.youthmentoring.org.au/program_details.php?id=220

Britzman, D., & Gilbert, J. (2004). What will have been said about gayness in teacher education. *Teaching Education, 15*(1), 81–96.

Cennamo, L., & Gardner, D. (2008). Generational differences in work values, outcomes and person-organisation values fit. *Journal of Managerial Psychology, 23*(8), 891–906.

Chandler, D. E., Hall, D. T., & Kram, K. E. (2010). A developmental network and relational savvy approach to talent development: A low-cost alternative. *Organisational Dynamics, 39*(1), 48–53.

Chao, G. T., Walz, P. M., & Gardner, P. D. (1992). Formal and information mentorships: A comparison on mentoring functions and contrast with nonmentored counterparts. *Personnel Psychology, 45*, 619–636.

Cone, Inc. (2006). *The 2006 Cone Millennial cause study*. Boston: Cone, Inc.

Cotugna, N., & Vickery, C. E. (1998). Reverse mentoring: A twist to teaching technology. *Journal of the American Dietetic Association, 98*(10), 1166–1168.

Crampton, S. M., & Hodge, J. W. (2009). Generation Y: Unchartered territory. *Journal of Business and Economics Research, 7*(4), 3.

Cranwell-Ward, J., Bossons, P., & Gover, S. (2004). *Mentoring: A Henley review of best practice*. New York: Palgrave Macmillan.

Darwin, A. (2000). Critical reflections on mentoring in work settings. *Adult Education Quarterly, 50*(3), 197–211.

DeLong, T. J., Gabarro, J. J., & Lees, R. J. (2008). Why mentoring matters in a hypercompetitive world. *Harvard Business Review, 86*(1), 115–121.

Eby, L. T., & Lockwood, A. (2005). Protégés and mentors' reactions to participating in formal mentoring programs: A qualitative investigation. *Journal of Vocational Behaviour, 67*, 441–458.

Emelo, R. (2010). Increasing productivity with social learning. *Industrial and Commercial Training, 42*(4), 208.

Glass, A. (2007). Understanding generational differences for competitive success. *Industrial and Commercial Training, 39*(2), 102.

Greengard, S. (2002). Moving forward with reverse mentoring. *Workforce, 81*(3), 15.

Hall, D. T. (1996). Long live the career—a relational approach. In D. T. Hall (Ed.), *The career is dead—long live the career: A relational approach to careers* (pp. 1–12). San Francisco: Jossey-Bass.

Hartley, R. (2004). *Young people and mentoring: Towards a national strategy, Big Brothers Big Sisters Australia*. Dussledorp skills forum and the Smith family. Accessed November 16, 2010, from http://www.thesmithfamily.com.au/webdata/resources/files/tsf_Mentor_May04.pdf

Ibarra, H., Carter, N. M., & Silva, C. (2010). Why men still get more promotions than women. *Harvard Business Review, 88*(9), 80–85.

Johnson, W. B. (2002). The intentional mentor: Strategies and guidelines for the practice of mentoring. *Professional Psychology: Research and Practice, 33*(1), 87.

Johnson, W. B., & Nelson, N. (1999). Mentoring relationships in graduate education: Some ethical concerns. *Ethics and Behavior, 9*, 189–210.

Johnson, W. B., Huwe, J. M., & Lucas, J. L. (2000). Rational mentoring. *Journal of Rational-Emotive and Cognitive-Behavior Therapy, 18*, 39–54.

Jones, K. W., Hardcastle, V., & Agnich, L. (2007). *A guide to mentoring*. Lexington: University of Kentucky.

Korporaal, G. (2010, August 11). Women make mark on boards. *The Australian*. http://www.perthnow.com.au/business/business-old/women-make-mark-on-boards/story-e6frg2qu-1225903781801

Laff, M. (2009). The guiding hand: Mentoring women. *T + D, 63*(9), 32–35.

Leh, A. S. C. (2005). Lessons learned from service learning and reverse mentoring in faculty development: A case study in technology training. *Journal of Technology and Teacher Education, 13*(1), 25–41.

Levinson, D. J., Darrow, C. N., Klein, E. B., Levinson, M. H., & McKee, B. (1978). *The seasons of a man's life*. New York: Ballentine.

Liu, D., Liu, J., Kwan, H. K., & Mao, Y. (2009). What can I gain as a mentor? The effect of mentoring on the job performance and social status of mentors in China. *Journal of Occupational and Organisational Psychology, 82*(4), 874–876.

Macky, K., Gardner, D., & Forsyth, S. (2008). Generational differences at work: Introduction and overview. *Journal of Managerial Psychology, 23*(8), 857–861.

Martin, C. A. (2005). From high maintenance to high productivity: What managers need to know about Generation Y. *Industrial and Commercial Training, 37*(1), 39–44.

Mezias, J. M., & Scandura, T. A. (2005). A needs-driven approach to expatriate adjustment and career development: A multiple mentoring perspective. *Journal of International Business Studies, 36*, 519–538.

Montana, P. J., & Lenaghan, J. A. (1999). What motivates and matters most to Generations X and Y? *Journal of Career Planning and Employment, 59*(4), 27–30.

Morgan, W., & Streb, M. (2001). Building citizenship: How student voice in service learning develops civic values. *Social Science Quarterly, 82*(1), 156–169.

Napier, N. K. (2006). Cross cultural learning and the role of reverse knowledge flows in Vietnam. *International Journal of Cross Cultural Management, 6*(1), 57–74.

Nezlek, J. B. (2001). Causal relationships between perceived social skills and day-to-day social interaction: Extending the sociometer hypothesis. *Journal of Social and Personal Relationships, 18*, 386–403.

O'Neil, J. M., & Wrightsman, L. S. (2001). The mentoring relationship in psychology training programs. In S. Walfish & A. Hess (Eds.), *Succeeding in graduate school: The complete career guide for the psychology student* (pp. 113–129). Hillsdale: Erlbaum.

Okurame, D. E. (2007). Perceived mentoring functions: Does mentor's gender matter? *Women in Management Review, 22*(5), 418–427.

Pekala, N. (2001). Conquering the generational divide. *Journal of Property Management, 66*(6), 30–38.

Ragins, B. R., & Cotton, J. L. (1999). Mentor functions and outcomes: A comparison of men and women in formal and informal mentoring relationships. *Journal of Applied Psychology, 84*(4), 529–550.

Ragins, B. R., & Scandura, T. A. (1994). Gender differences in expected outcomes of mentoring relationships. *Academy of Management Journal, 37*, 957–971.

Reilly, R., & Lojeski, K. S. (2009). Leading the dispersed workforce. *Mechanical Engineering, 131*(11), 30–34.

Russell, J. E. A., & Adams, D. M. (1997). The changing nature of mentoring in organisations: An introduction to the special issues on mentoring and organisations. *Journal of Vocational Behaviour, 51*, 1–14.

Southard, G., & Lewis, J. (2004). Building a workplace that recognises generational diversity. *Public Management, 86*(3), 8–12.

Tempest, S. (2003). Intergenerational learning: A reciprocal knowledge development process that challenges the language of learning. *Management Learning, 34*(2), 181–200.

Tenner, E. (2004). The pitfalls of academic mentorships. *The Chronicle of Higher Education, 50*(49), B7–B10.

Wanberg, C. R., Welsh, E. T., & Hezlett, S. A. (2003). Mentoring research: A review and dynamic process model. In J. J. Martocchio & G. R. Ferris (Eds.), *Research in personnel and human resources management 22* (pp. 39–124). Oxford: JAI Press/Elsevier Science.

Wanberg, C. R., Kammeyer-Mueller, J., & Marchese, M. (2006). Mentor and protégé predictors and outcomes of mentoring in a formal mentoring program. *Journal of Vocational Behaviour, 69*, 410–423.

Watson, I., Buchanan, J., Campbell, I., & Briggs, C. (2003). *Fragmented futures: New challenges in working life* (pp. 20–30). Annandale: Federation Press.

Welch, J., & Welch, S. (2006). *Winning, the answers: Confronting 74 of the toughest questions in business today* (pp. 96–98). London: HarperCollins. 187–189.

Wong, M., Gardiner, E., Lang, W., & Coulon, L. (2008). Generational differences in personality and motivation. *Journal of Managerial Psychology, 23*(8), 884–885.

Zachary, L. (2005). *Creating a mentoring culture: The organisation's guide.* San Francisco: Jossey-Bass.

Zanni, G. (2009). Reverse mentoring: An effective strategy for career growth. *The Consultant Pharmacist, 24*(6), 465–467.

Professor Ann M. Brewer is Deputy Vice-Chancellor (Strategic Management) and CEO, Centre for Continuing Education and Sydney Learning Pty. Ltd. at the University of Sydney, Sydney, Australia.

Contact: ann.brewer@sydney.edu.au

Chapter 13
Spirited Leadership: Growing Leaders for the Future

Hilary B. Armstrong

13.1 Spirited Leadership

> There are, and always have been "little sacraments of daily existence", those subtle weavings
> of the heart that move us on a minute to minute basis – the fabric of our existence, which
> we ignore but which are the DNA that binds us together.
>
> (David Malouf, The Great World, 1990)

Currently when organisations and communities seek to develop leadership, there are a number of key activities they use, mainly based on taken-for-granted leadership theories and practices. One of these is a common practice of positive psychology, organisational coaching. What is not clear, though, is why certain interventions are chosen over others and what learning outcomes leadership programmes hope to produce. One consequence of the lack of clarity about leadership is that organisations still promote and reward people based on technical expertise (easier to quantify) and then wonder why their newly appointed CEO fails. In many cases the failure of a new senior recruit is because of his/her lack of 'soft skills' or ability to build positive relationships based on emotional intelligence – and rarely is this considered seriously enough for it to become the driver for successful recruitment. The significance of emotional intelligence is well known but more difficult to quantify. At all levels of leadership, there is a knowing/doing gap partly at least because there is more talk than action and soft skills are (unfortunately) rarely rewarded or valued.

Recently writers drawing on the emerging neuroscience research have added weight to the arguments for 'soft skills', particularly in the area of what is being termed social intelligence. What this is telling us is that leadership at all levels must include social as well as emotional intelligence (Boyatzis and McKee 2005; Sinclair 2007; Hughes et al. 2009). The aim of this chapter is to unpack what is meant by

H.B. Armstrong (✉)
Institute of Executive Coaching, Sydney, Australia
e-mail: hilarya@iecl.com

S. Roffey (ed.), *Positive Relationships: Evidence Based Practice across the World*,
DOI 10.1007/978-94-007-2147-0_13, © Springer Science+Business Media B.V. 2012

positive relationships in the context of leadership by reporting on the experience of people who are identified as 'leaders of the future' in a number of organisations. We employ the results of a piece of research done with aspiring leaders to understand more about the connection between positive workplace relationships and leadership. In particular we propose the notion of a 'spirited' leadership that has as its heart a form of relationality that enables the leader to inspire and innovate (transform). This specific aspect of social intelligence named by respondents is, with the exception of Sinclair, not usually taken into account. Spirited leadership requires a particular form of sensibility – the ability to 'read' others and the social/cultural dynamics present. A spirited leader does this to be constructively subversive – to challenge taken-for-granted practices. A spirited leader needs this to conform, but just enough and not without the critical thinking. But to be spirited – to challenge, stretch and grow people and organisations beyond their perceived limitations – requires positive relationships. This is the new face of leadership, and in the tradition of strength-based or positive psychology approaches, we will explore and elucidate this more in order to grow it.

Initially we critically reflect on the received wisdom about leadership to reposition it as a set of reflective and relational practices that are socially located within an organisational/cultural structure. The evidence we use comes from a piece of research designed to explore the benefits of organisational coaching in leadership development. Our aim here is not to prove or disprove the effectiveness of coaching but to reposition leadership based on what the respondents reported. The 280 people identified as 'leadership talent' who completed the survey work in a broad range of organisations, public and private, not-for-profit and government, and at all levels. There are CEOs, people in high office, leaders in schools and universities, mid range leaders, team leaders and leaders of small not-for-profits. One thing they agreed on, wherever they are positioned, was the vital importance of positive and constructive workplace relationships, a view that is contrary to much of the received wisdom about leadership.

13.2   The 'Heroic' Leader

Stories of heroic leadership are firmly embedded in the cultural psyche, and although books on leadership multiply yearly, they mostly, implicitly or explicitly, just add to the 'already said' about leadership. Leadership is seen as an individual endeavour attached to material success, involving extraordinary willpower and even redemption. It is portrayed largely in heroic terms – tales of an individual's transformation of (and in) crisis and difficulty. This ability to transform (hopefully for good) is depicted as being due to intrinsic (hence psychological) heroic attributes that are mostly innate, even if enhanced through discipline, ambition and focused learning.

The ideology of the leader as hero, like any dogma, is interesting not only for what it inspires in us but also for what it ignores or represses. When we hear of acts of heroism, we feel excitement, enjoyment and perhaps some relief at being (simply) voyeurs; we are moved and frightened and simultaneously given hope that our 'ordinary' struggles will finally be transcended. But there is another side, an implicit and competing aspect of this dogma. Leadership is something a person can get right, or horribly wrong. It is paradoxical. We see this most in political and historical arenas. Leadership is both our possible salvation (Ghandi or Obama) and our shadow (Hitler, or Stalin). It is regarded as the answer to the current woes of the world as well as something that has the power to enslave and ultimately destroy us. The possibility of finding the 'right' leader/hero fills us with hope and routinely lets us down.

Individualistic assumptions about leadership mislead us in several ways. Firstly, they remove leadership from the essentially social relationship that defines it; a leader does not exist without a follower. Secondly, they propagate a specific structure of social relationship: Heroic acts are performed by mainly men conquering mainly thorny problems. In our prevailing mythology, effective leaders only work for 'good' (although it is their right to make the call about what is 'good'). Thirdly, individualistic assumptions perpetuate the myth that leadership is practised only by 'chosen' people who are born to it ('it's innate') or through ambition, have gained the skills. Finally, these assumptions trap us either into competitive striving for exceptionalness through subliminal messages of deficit ('you haven't got what it takes', 'you're not good enough') or into passive acquiescence and learned helplessness. Of course, there are some people who are wise to this, but unfortunately in organisations, most of us find ourselves pulled around by these assumptions. Gender equality in leadership is still minimal, and immoral leadership still exists. Hierarchical structures still silence people, and many young people in organisations feel under pressure to strive and deliver at the expense of their own and their families' health.

13.3 Leadership Learning Goals

The proposition that I am making is that leadership practices, whether at macro or micro levels, depend on the implicit ethos of positive relationships (the quote at the beginning of the chapter) to be truly transformative. An aspect of this is the health of our inner worlds. But this is not enough. Sensibility to the other, including the outer world and its culture and social dynamics, its power and politics, is also required. And from the research, high potential individuals are increasingly aware that individualistic assumptions about leadership, though still influential, are no longer sufficient. In a pre-work survey undertaken before their leadership development (including coaching), respondents were asked to clarify their learning goals. Table 13.1 shows the goals, including a summary of the meanings attached to them ($n=280$). They fall into five categories.

The first two categories reflect the role of emotional and social intelligence in leadership and the need to understand its social location. What is important here is that participants are asking to be able to develop and learn about these things. The goals they identify reflect qualitative aspects of leadership, including managing relationships with others and the bigger picture as well as self-awareness and self-management. Less important are the more instrumental aspects of leadership: performance, goal setting, results, planning. Although this may not be surprising, it was the degree of importance placed on the top

Table 13.1 Leadership learning goals

Goal	%	Summary
Managing everyday relationships at work	99	Speak openly; give feedback; conduct robust conversations; manage up, down, sideways; manage conflict; empathy; respect for difference; power and politics; political savvy
Team building	95	Delegate, model roles, understand relational dynamics, mentor/support, understand 'bigger picture'
Learning about self in relationship to others and work	81	Awareness of personal values, self talk, strengths/challenges, personal history and psychology
Reduction of stress	65	Improve work–life balance, wellbeing; learn to manage stress at work
Improve workplace organisation and planning	62	Improved task performance, setting goals, planning of work, prioritising, achieving results

three categories that interested us, and because we regard them as aspects of a spirited leadership, we will address in more detail.

The first aspect is an obvious one. In the first three categories, respondents are asking to learn about managing relationships and self-in-relationship at work. This indicates that they consider leadership to be relational rather than individualistic. This is confirmed by the world stage. Leaders at any level are deemed successful (or not) because of their ability to mobilise and inspire others. And the opposite is also true: without a network of relationships, leadership cannot emerge. Our attention might be diverted to the wonder of a heroic act attributed to a single human being at a particular time. But where leadership really waits is not in the spotlight but in the shadows, emerging out of the nexus of events that materialise in communities of people weaving their lives together in invisible and unspoken ways. What happens is that thousands of acts of relationality come together and are expressed as ongoing guidance, support, sharing of experience and inspiration of one another. These are the everyday interactions and humane acts that build communal relationality and connectedness, producing new possibilities for the ways we live our lives – and a leader emerges. This is again most visible on the world stage, when a leader like Barack Obama appears 'out of nowhere' at a particular point of history in a particular location.

Leading at its best then is a relationship of mutual influence that dwells in our connection with others as we mobilise them through our responsiveness, mindfulness and curiosity, political savvy, group dynamics, modelling robust conversations, respecting difference and influencing. When one reads these characteristics of leading, it becomes obvious it is not a one-way street, i.e. it involves both parties, and the quality of relationality happens through mutual influence (for example, being mindful of our intentions as well as monitoring how they are landing on another). As Goleman and Boyatzis (2008) report, from neuroscience research: '... the leader-follower dynamic is not a case of two (or more) independent brains reacting consciously or unconsciously to each other. Rather, the individual minds become, in a sense, fused into a single system... great leaders are those whose behaviour powerfully leverages this system of brain interconnectedness'.

13.4 'Outsight', Voice and Mindfulness

At the basis of political savvy, group dynamics and managing diversity is 'outsight' – as opposed to insight (Armstrong 2009). Many leadership learning interventions (including coaching) are directed at interior/individual change alone – something unexpected when the majority of theories that are drawn upon emerge from individualistic theories and pedagogies drawn from mainstream psychology and developmental theories, new age concepts, positive psychology, the human potential movement and motivation and goal-setting processes (Grant and Cavanagh 2004). From these perspectives, 'outsight' is regarded as a product of increased self-awareness rather than also a likely producer of it and the goal becomes one of changing/eliminating 'distortions of perception' that get in the way of the 'natural' potential of individuals. However, in our study the goals that respondents identify indicate that leading also includes awareness of social dynamics. Distortions of perception are not necessarily only subjective and individual. In fact people in organisations will usually acknowledge that judgements about validity ('true' or 'just a perception') are more likely to be based on where the speaker (as well as the listener) is located in the social dynamics (including organisational hierarchy).

Another aspect is the issue of voice: speaking openly, robust conversations, feedback conversations, managing conflict, indicating the correlation between positive relationships and conversation. To achieve results, a leader is engaged in countless conversations in a day or a week. How these conversations are conducted will shape the relationship. As Buber (1923) said: 'The inmost growth of the self does not take place through our relationship to ourselves but through being made present by the other and knowing that we are made present by him'. Or, more simply put, the conversation is the relationship (Scott 2004). Spirited leadership recognises that quality conversations are the basis of success. If a conversation is shallow or leads to misunderstandings, the relationship becomes shallow and full of misunderstandings. If a conversation is lively, respectful and productive, then the relationship is positive and leads to mutually productive outcomes.

And, conversations are complex. They can never be separated from the milieu in which they occur, making them both personal and social. For example, a senior leader when asking for input or feedback should take into account that his/her position and/or perceived power may affect peoples' decisions on how/whether to speak. In these situations, a leader requires 'outsight'. One respondent managing in a cross-cultural context reported: 'Through the conversations [in coaching] I realised that I was expecting too much of my leadership team. It's a cultural thing as well as a positional thing. In their culture they would not speak up in the group. But after the meeting I would spend all morning with them, one at a time, in my office, telling me what they really thought. It was me who had to change'. In this case, awareness of the social and cultural dynamics produced the learning and the leader introduced changes that reflected this and shifted the group towards more positive and therefore productive relationships (Armstrong 2009).

At the heart of leadership in all its relational complexity is mindfulness, the reflective capacity to self-regulate and adapt in the moment in ways that build and maintain relationship. Being mindful means reflecting and accepting the stories that have shaped one's life, as well as awareness of others and their stories and using this awareness to self-monitor and adapt in order to build rapport. Awareness of the connection between inner and outer, subjective and objective, echoes what Buber is really saying in the statement quoted above – that the gap between inner and outer collapses as both parties mutually shape the relational space. Therefore, self-awareness practices to enhance mindfulness are central to spirited leadership. Heifetz (1999) called this the ability to be 'on the balcony and in the dance' simultaneously. As he suggested, this ability, which we all can learn, enables us to notice, to be with another, to recognise the effect of the environment and to adapt and change in order to maintain a strong relationship.

Finally, spirited leadership, or leadership grounded in positive relationships, necessarily incorporates a positive psychology, or more precisely in the present context, a strength-based approach to learning and leadership. One participant gave an example: 'It was not until I was asked about how I had got where I was that I realised I had faced my problem before in another context. It was then I realised I could get through this time and I had all the skills to do it'. The assumption underlying this approach is that a problem focus tends to grow the problem, while a focus on resourcefulness grows peoples' strengths. There are several strength-based approaches that build positive relationships – some grouped around a psychological framework (Seligman 1990; Greene and Grant 2003) which regards strengths as based on inner resources and psychological processes. Others are grouped around a social epistemology (de Shazer 1993; White and Epston 1990; Armstrong 1999), and they emphasise the weaving of outer as well as inner resources and strengths through language and meaning. The latter places the focus on the nexus of the relationship between people rather than the individual. How this looks in practice is that achievements, strengths and personal resources are identified and 'talked up' in the conversation, including where they are employed and the effects this deployment has on others. The focus and 'talking up' of personal strengths validates them, and this reflective and iterative process of recognition, acknowledgement and confidence generates application of existing resources and strengths in new areas of major challenge. This practice is not new. It expands the foundations of the experiential and 'whole person' learning traditions (Kolb 1985; Boud et al. 1993) which are grounded in the idea that learning is a social process based in, and building upon, peoples', existing resources. Recently, with the popularity of positive psychology, this idea, which can be seen as countercultural, has gained popularity, and there is excellent evidence that a 'gold-miner's' mentality (that the other has the gold within) will grow and enhance positive relationships (Seligman 1990) and transform leadership.

13.5   Benefits from Leadership Coaching

I have described these aspects of spirited leadership in detail because they are the aspects of leadership described by participants in the study when asked to identify benefits gained from leadership coaching. The survey[1] lists 32 benefit items which participants are asked to rate in two different ways; the extent of benefit (learning) and the significance of that benefit to their work and leadership goals. The benefits, grouped under thematic headings, are listed below in the rank order of importance assigned to them (Table 13.2).

Table 13.2 Benefit groups listed in order of importance

Benefit groups	Summary of items in group
Mindfulness	Awareness of personal values, self talk, strengths/ challenges, personal history and psychology
Voice: communicating of self to other	Speak openly, give feedback, robust conversations, managing up, managing conflict
Listening: responsiveness to others	Understand relational dynamics, empathy, respect for difference, relational power and politics
Leadership and teambuilding	Delegate, role model, group dynamics, mentor/ support, 'bigger picture'
Professional aspirations	Clearer personal vision, deeper appreciation of collective, meaning, confidence
Work organisation and performance	Improved task performance, planning of work, prioritising, solving problems
Wellbeing in work	Job satisfaction, stress level, work/life balance

Although the most important benefit named is mindfulness, taken together, the top four areas of greatest impact are those to do with learning about *self in relation to others*. This confirms leadership as personal *and* social, a shift away from abstract and rational to individualistic notions about leadership to the myriad practices and ways of relating that is leadership – a view given its first major attention through a notion of 'servant leadership' (Greenleaf 1977). However, the transition from an individual focus in leadership to a relational focus was initially not apparent in the results. The benefit groups below are ranked by the average proportion of coachees rating benefits in relation to items in the group from 'considerable' or 'very considerable' with the latter average shown in parentheses (Table 13.3).

---

[1] In 2004 research was initiated to assess the effectiveness of a socially located coaching practice in growing talent and leadership in organisations. Our interest was twofold. One was to ascertain both the benefits that coachees were gaining from coaching and the significance of these benefits on their leadership journey. The second was to ascertain how coaching was working to create these benefits. The research employed several approaches: a before and after online survey with a space for open-ended comments, both qualitative and quantitative methods with responses from coachees and from people (third parties) who worked with them. The coachee respondents all completed six to ten sessions of hourly coaching with a coach accredited in the approach described above. For yearly reports of the results, please refer to www.iecoaching.com

Table 13.3 Average scores of items in each benefit group

Benefit group	Extent of benefit Top 2 (Top 1)%
Self-awareness	67 (36)
Communicating with others	64 (26)
Responsiveness to others	57 (24)
Leadership and teambuilding	56 (30)
Professional and career aspirations	55 (22)
Work organisation and performance	49 (20)
Personal wellbeing in work	43 (18)

The percentage of people who ranked the benefit of individual awareness as considerable or very considerable is greater than for other benefits. This seems to show that it is increased self-awareness that was the clear area of change that respondents experience and value most. However in the survey, respondents were also asked to rate not only the benefits they received from coaching but also the significance that they placed on these benefits when they thought about them in the context of the workplace.

What is interesting in the following table is that although increased self-awareness is the highest ranked in terms of benefit gained, it is not regarded as the most significant (Table 13.4).

Table 13.4 Average scores of items in each benefit group

Benefit group	Extent of benefit Top 2 (Top 1)%	Significance of benefit Top2 (Top 1)%
Self-awareness	67 (36)	69 (38)
Communicating with others	64 (26)	75 (39)
Responsiveness to others	57 (24)	69 (31)
Professional and career aspirations	56 (30)	59 (33)
Leadership and teambuilding	55 (22)	63 (32)
Work organisation and performance	49 (20)	55 (28)
Personal wellbeing in work	43 (18)	50 (25)

The variation or 'gap' between rating of the significance and the rating of extent of benefit is interesting. While gains in self-awareness and professional and career aspirations are rated as very significant, the gap between their significance and the extent of benefit experienced is slight, indicating that participants are achieving the level of gain that they consider desirable. For other dimensions, the significance is rated generally 10% higher than the benefit that is experienced. This gap is most marked in benefit areas concerning positive relationships (communicating self to other and responsiveness), leadership and team building. This suggests that what is most important to this group of respondents is learning to build positive workplace relationships, suggesting that the complexity of everyday relationships in the workplace and their management is the most pressing issue.

When we asked respondents to be more specific, they identified conflictual relationships with especially others who did not report to them (colleagues and those who are more senior) and the difficulty of presenting their ideas, trying out new things, fielding questions, encouraging innovation and creativity and assisting people to feel engaged and part of the workplace.

Finally, a key question this paper asked was: How do leadership interventions produce the benefits? We were particularly interested in organisational coaching, but the coaching approach is basically an extension of best-practice adult learning principles. How learning interventions such as coaching produce learning outcomes is therefore translatable to any adult learning context. More interesting perhaps is that they also translate into spirited leadership, in that the conversational practices that respondents identified as assisting them in their leadership learning are the same practices that help build positive workplace relationships. Table 13.5 reports on these (see also Armstrong 2007).

Table 13.5 Practices and qualities that contribute to achieving benefit

	Mean %	Top 2 %	4 %	3 %	2 %	1 %	n/a %
A person who asked *reflective questions* that got me thinking about things differently	91	60	31	5	1	0	2
A person who *challenged* the assumptions I am making in constructive ways	86	51	35	8	2	1	3
A *safe place* to talk about problems and issues that I can't discuss with anyone else (the politics)	85	56	29	8	3	2	2
A '*sounding board*' where it was safe to express and test ideas	84	51	33	11	2	0	3
A person who was interested and able to *monitor* my learning and development	80	45	35	21	6	2	1
Someone who could join with me in *brainstorming* ideas for my work or professional future	73	35	38	16	8	1	3
Someone who really *understands* my situation and the issues I face	70	31	39	17	8	3	3
Someone I could depend upon to give me *support* while I made significant changes	68	33	35	21	6	3	3
A structured *learning framework* for me to develop new behaviours and work processes	56	24	32	27	10	4	3

These rankings show the extraordinary value of asking reflective questions that stretch and challenge people to think differently and outside the assumptions of their everyday organisational culture and social milieu. When people are given a 'safe' space away from the politics and the confining routines of their everyday work life, they can reflect and be challenged to see themselves and others in new and transformative ways. More 'instrumental' aspects of learning – a structure, monitoring and having subject matter expertise – are less important, again suggesting the significance of building positive relationships in leadership. It is not heroic acts but courageous conversations, small and seemingly insignificant conversational practices, the sacraments of everyday life, that matter.

People seem to also indicate the enjoyment of being challenged and stretched, suggesting another very important aspect of learning and leadership. There is a middle ground between overchallenging someone to the point of distrust and disrespect and underchallenging them through the tyranny of wanting to be liked. This is where courage and everyday heroics enter. The practice of relational risk taking, the dance between sustaining trust and challenging people to go beyond their comfort zone and draw new, previously 'unspeakable' topics into the conversation, is central to both learning and leadership.

Providing a safe place is implicitly gesturing to the politics of organisations and the ethical dilemmas people find themselves in when they work inside organisations. Organisation systems and cultures shape peoples' thoughts and behaviours more strongly than people are able to shape their organisation culture. There are always complex social dynamics; there is always a complex three-way relationship between self/other and the organisation. A 'safe' place meant to respondents awareness of these things – of ethical quandaries that exist with all employees, of transparency, confidentiality and responsibility.

Finally, what we consider to be the most important aspect of any leadership intervention is the modelling of the learning objectives during the learning. Relational risk-taking (Mason 2005) is a delicate dance that cannot be learned from a book, only through modelling and experience. Modelling reflective questioning (the understanding of safety in political environments, the challenging of assumptions, focused listening skills, strength-based practices) is arguably the most powerful form of learning and leadership.

And, if knowledge and new learning is generated in the space, both parties benefit and learn – another reinforcement of the importance of relationality. Spirited leading involves active processes of ongoing attention, action and engagement in order to appropriately introduce reflective questions that challenge and 'disturb' (bring into question) routine assumptions and 'ways of being/acting' in the workplace without doing it in a way that is alienating or judgemental.

These findings confirm that leadership learning should focus on relationality rather just on removing individual distortions of perception. In other words, it is the quality of the conversational practices that enables positive relationships and therefore spirited leadership.

In conclusion, spirited leadership is a form of leadership aimed at creating and sustaining positive relationships in the workplace. This expresses a different view of leadership from the received wisdom that paints leadership as an independent, individualistic role usually held by a male who overcomes adversity on his own. I propose a different expression of leadership; one that is embedded in social and emotional intelligence to weave inner and outer worlds through language and meaning to acknowledge and build peoples' strengths and resources. The practice of spirited leadership requires qualities and skills that are not exceptional (except for their rarity). They require a finely tuned sensibility to 'other' and to the context and to the courage to respond to them.

13.6   Conclusion

Through the study into organisational coaching and its success as a leadership intervention, we were able to provide evidence of spirited leadership as well as unpack what it looks like in practice. What we found was a shift of focus from the individual and their internal processes to the ways people relate in their everyday worlds. The ways people relate are the taken-for-granted relational practices – the 'little sacraments of daily life', including the everyday conversation through which people in organisations achieve their results and goals.

When people can dance between insight (knowing our own story and role) and outsight (how we and the environment are mutually influencing each other), they are more likely to be demonstrating spirited leadership. As the adage goes, it is not who we are, but what we do with who we are. Leaders always depend on others for their success. A significant part of this is emotional intelligence. But we also swim in a sea of language and/or social practices that shape who and what we are. Through social intelligence – the recognition of our interconnectedness – we can change our relationships and influence others, building together new and alternative ways of being and doing that that fosters leadership at all levels of an organisation.

References

Armstrong, H. B. (1999). *Dead certainties and local knowledge, post structuralism, narrative and conflict in experiential learning.* Unpublished Thesis, UWS, Sydney.

Armstrong, H. B. (2007). Hestia and coaching: Speaking to the 'hearth' of the matter. *The International Journal of Evidence Based Coaching and Mentoring* Special Edition, 70–81.

Armstrong, H. B. (2009). Integral coaching: Cultivating a cultural sensibility through executive coaching. In M. Moral & G. Abbot (Eds.), *The Routledge Companion to international business coaching.* Oxford/New York: Routledge.

Boud, D., Cohen, R., & Walker, D. (Eds.). (1993). *Using experience for learning.* Buckingham: SRHE and Open University Press.

Boyatzis, R., & McKee, A. (2005). *Resonant leadership: Renewing yourself and connecting with others through mindfulness, hope, and compassion.* Cambridge: Harvard Business School Press.

Buber, M. (1923). *I and Thou* (R. G. Smith, Trans., 1958). New York: Charles Scribner's Sons.

de Shazer, S. (1993). Creative misunderstandings. In S. Gilligan & R. Price (Eds.), *Therapeutic conversations* (pp. 59–80). New York: Norton.

Goleman, D., & Boyatzis, R. (2008). Social intelligence and the biology of leadership. *Harvard Business Review*, September Edition, 1–8. www.hbr.org

Grant, A., & Cavanagh, M. (2004). Towards a profession of coaching: Sixty-five years of progress and challenges for the future. *International Journal of Evidence Based Coaching and Mentoring., 2*(1), 1–16.

Greene, J., & Grant, A. (2003). *Solution focused coaching*. London: Pearson Education Ltd.
Greenleaf, R. (1977). *Servant leadership: A journey into the legitimate nature of power and greatness*. New York: Paulist Press.
Heifetz, R. (1999). *Leadership without easy answers*. Cambridge/London: The Belknap Press of Harvard University Press.
Hughes, M., Thompson, H. L., & Terrell, J. B. (2009). *Handbook for developing emotional and social intelligence, best practice, case studies and strategies*. San Francisco: Jossey Bass Wiley.
Kolb, D. (1985). *Experiential learning*. New York: Prentice Hall.
Malouf, D. (1990). *The great world*. UK: Random House.
Mason, B. (2005). Relational risk taking and the therapeutic relationship. In C. Flaksas, B. Mason, & A. Perlesz (Eds.), *The space between: Experience, context and process in the therapeutic relationship* (pp. 157–171). London: Karnac Books.
Scott, S. (2004). *Fierce conversations: Achieving success at work and in life one conversation at a time*. New York: Berkley Publishing Group.
Seligman, M. E. P. (1990). *Learned optimism*. New York: Knopf.
Sinclair, A. (2007). *Leadership for the disillusioned: Moving beyond myths and heroes to leading that liberates*. Sydney: Allen and Unwin.
White, M., & Epston, D. (1990). *Narrative means to therapeutic ends*. New York: Norton.

Hilary B. Armstrong is the Director of Education at the Institute of Executive Coaching and a Master Coach. Hilary holds a PhD in critical social sciences with a speciality in critical and narrative psychology and was an academic at the University of Western Sydney, Sydney, Australia, holding senior academic positions for a number of years. She is on the advisory panel of the International Coaching Psychology Review and a professional associate of the St James Ethics Centre, Sydney. Contact: hilarya@iecl.com

Chapter 14
Positive Community Relations: Border Crossings and Repositioning the 'Other'

Florence E. McCarthy and Margaret H. Vickers*

14.1 Introduction

The word 'community' has a range of connotations. It can refer to those who share a geographical location, who belong to a school or a neighbourhood or who share common knowledge, understandings and values. This chapter shows how active respect among communities that differ but live in the same locality, can break down barriers and construct more positive community relationships. This chapter provides an example of how this might be put into practice and the factors and processes that can contribute to positive outcomes.

Positive psychology has an extensive literature focusing on promoting the strengths of people, groups and institutions (Aspinwall and Staudinger 2002; Seligman 2002). Ingram and Snyder (2006) note the extensive forays of the positive psychology approach in areas of life, including schools (Baker et al. 2003), sports (Curry and Snyder 2000), multicultural relations (Sandage et al. 2003) and other disciplines (Held 2004). Rather than focusing on the negative aspects of individual mental health or group or institutional dysfunction, the aim is to establish knowledge about what people do well, the knowledge they have and the resilience and strength they exhibit (Seligman and Csekszentmihalyi 2000; Held 2004;

*The views expressed in this article reflect those of the authors and do not reflect the views of the Australian Literacy and Numeracy Foundation, the Papulu Apparr-kari Aboriginal Corporation or the University of Western Sydney.

F.E. McCarthy
Centre for Educational Research, University of Western Sydney, Rydalmere, NSW, Australia
e-mail: ide@iinet.net.au

M.H. Vickers (✉)
School of Education, University of Western Sydney, Rydalmere, NSW, Australia
e-mail: mhv@uws.edu.au

S. Roffey (ed.), *Positive Relationships: Evidence Based Practice across the World*,
DOI 10.1007/978-94-007-2147-0_14, © Springer Science+Business Media B.V. 2012

Murray 2004. See also chapters in this volume). These benchmarks are then used to establish concrete ways of responding to individual needs. This approach has led to studies of wellbeing (Noble et al. 2008), resilience (Frederickson and Tugade 2004; Masten 2001) and persistence. By shifting the focus on the 'subject' from a concern with negative aspects to more positive ones, different approaches are being constructed to work with people so as to position them as participants rather than as marginal others (Dooley 2009; Pate 2008; Bond 2009). As Gable and Haidt (2005) argue, much of conventional social psychology has focused on prejudice and conflict and on deficit models of others. However, following their lead, this chapter explores the conditions that lead to trust, acceptance and compromise rather than conflict and division among disparate inhabitants within one local community.

14.2 Power Relations Within Communities

Most communities embody well-established patterns of exclusion and segmentation, where the dynamics of power and factors of race, gender, socio-economic status, poverty and ethnic and cultural differences tend to set people apart. These factors are often well entrenched and function to sustain institutional and individual borders that can be difficult to cross. Typically these divisions involve dominant and subordinate groups, with the dominant positioning the subordinate as the 'other'. These 'others' are characterised as deficient, inferior and in need of direction, but rarely consulted or heard (Armstrong 2000). Situations such as these raise a significant challenge for positive psychology, namely, to address the age-old question of how innovative programmes can destabilise both the discourses and patterns of community divisiveness. To the extent that positive psychology includes an emphasis on general wellbeing, strength and resilience and recognition that people and their experiences are embedded in social contexts (Seligman and Csekszentmihalyi 2000), it is well positioned to respond to this challenge. However, as Held (2004) reminds us, positive psychology is not without its negative aspects, particularly the negativity that arises from its dominant separatist message (Held 2004:10).

It is recognised that of the 'three pillars' of positive psychology identified by Seligman (2002), that of positive institutions and communities is the least well developed (Gable and Haidt 2005). Beginning with this recognition, our goal in this chapter is to explore ways in which community relations can be improved through 'border crossing' strategies that are created and sustained by both resident/local and visiting/outsider participants supporting some common goals. These strategies will be illustrated though the development of a case study based on Tennant Creek, a remote rural community in the Northern Territory of Australia.

14.3   Indigenous Australians: History, Politics and the Tennant Creek Context

Indigenous history in Australia provides a bleak record of maltreatment, injustice and destruction through the interaction of White settlers with the original inhabitants. Nothing exemplifies this history more than the construction of the new continent as a 'terra nullius' (empty land) upon the arrival of the British who disregarded the presence of roughly 500,000 Indigenous people and over 300 different languages and cultures. As Reynolds (1992) argued, 'discovery' was deemed to give Europeans automatic sovereignty over the land, eliminating recognition of native title. Government policies that dominated the twentieth century were based on the premise that Indigenous Australians would become extinct and their children should be assimilated into White society. An example of these policies was the forcible removal of Indigenous children from their families, placing them in government homes and mission schools (Hollinsworth 2003). From 1900 to 1970, between one tenth and one third of all Indigenous children were removed from their parents. Despite such policies, Indigenous Australians have survived and wherever possible focus on sustaining and reviving their languages and traditions that uphold the distinctive features of their own countries and communities.

This case study illustrates the possibilities that can be created when historical antagonists are involved in new undertakings that reposition them in relation to each other and provide spaces for alternative relationships to develop. Prilleltensky and Prilleltensky (2006) write about the distinguishing characteristics of transformative interventions in community change. They argue that when values of self-determination, participation, social justice and respect are valued and people work together in partnership – doing things 'with' rather than 'to' or 'for' each other – transformative and sustainable change can take place.

The partners in this project include Indigenous Elders ('the Ladies'), Indigenous high-school and primary school students, teachers of the Tennant Creek primary and high schools, pre-service University Secondary Masters of Teaching students from the University of Western Sydney and staff of the Australian Literacy and Numeracy Foundation (ALNF). The role of this outside agency was to act as a catalyst in stimulating new possibilities for all community stakeholders.

14.3.1   The Recent and Relevant History of the Community

It is important to contextualise the relational nexus existing in Tennant Creek. A central feature of this case study revolves around the struggle to sustain first-language learning in the context of schooling and the relations between Whites and

Indigenous people in a small isolated town in the Northern Territory of Australia. The main focus is the development of a language preservation and acquisition programme (Community Action Support programme) for young Indigenous primary school students, together with the transformations that occurred in the relational nexus bringing major stakeholders of the community and outside institutions together as participants in this programme. By creating new spaces for cooperation, participants were able to envision possible new roles for themselves and alter pre-existing notions of 'others' (Armstrong 2000).

Tennant Creek is the fifth largest town in the Northern Territory (NT), founded in 1934 in response to the discovery of gold in the area. The town is located in country traditionally held by the Warumungu people, but even from the 1880s, large portions of this land were designated as pastoral leases, forcing Warumungu and other Indigenous people off their own land to work as stockmen or domestic servants on the cattle stations or move to reserves established for them. Tennant Creek was officially off limits to Indigenous people until the 1960s, and their attempts to move into the township in the 1970s met with opposition from officials and Anglo-European town people. In response to this opposition, Indigenous people began to form their own organisations focused on gaining representation, infrastructure and services for their community (Aboriginal Child Language Acquisition project (ACLA) 2008). Along with a health service, an office of the Central Land Council (the regional representative body for Indigenous people) and the Barkly Regional Language Centre (Papulu Apparr-kari Aboriginal Corporation), the Julali-kari Aboriginal Council Corporation was formed. It originally concerned itself with Indigenous housing but has expanded its focus over time. Within the town, Indigenous people live either in one of the eight residential town camps or at 'street addresses' on residential streets. These 'place of residence' divisions signify borders of segregation and exclusion.

After a 10-year legal battle, Indigenous people of the region now have rights to the country surrounding the town. This means the return of the traditional Warumungu lands to their control and jurisdiction. While some mining and mineral exploration still continue in the area, the main gold mines have largely closed down, reducing the town from a population of roughly 9,000 people in 2001 to a current estimate of 3,185, of which 1,176 are Indigenous (ABS Census 2001). The town is located about 1,000 km south of Darwin and about 500 km north of Alice Springs and is situated at the crossroads of the two major roads in the Territory, the Stuart and Barkly highways. Being extremely isolated, it is difficult to obtain permanent teachers for its one primary and one secondary school or doctors or nurses for the small, local hospital. The mine closures saw the exodus of permanent mine managers and employees, leaving the reduced non-Indigenous population in control of the local council and other positions of consequence in the town. Because Tennant Creek is a regional centre of the Barkly Division, it has Commonwealth government offices, various civic and non-profit organisations, as well as branches of the Charles Darwin University and Bachelor University, which is an Indigenous higher education institution.

14.3.2   Bilingual Education

It is widely accepted that children whose mother tongue is not English learn more easily if they first achieve literacy in their mother tongue (Collins 1999). Indigenous children who speak one or more languages other than English will require explicit instruction in English as a second language (ESL) in order to adequately learn English (Simpson et al. 2009). These issues are critically important for many Indigenous children in the Northern Territory as they may come from families where Aboriginal English or Indigenous languages are spoken as first languages. Aboriginal English is a non-standard form of English that has its own grammatical rules and follows many constructions found in Indigenous languages (Turpin 2008). It is a form of Creole that arises when adults speak many different languages. Many Indigenous children speak more than one Indigenous language, and the formal Standard Australian English taught in public schools is not necessarily familiar to them. In Central Australia, where Tennant Creek is located, the main language families are Arandic, Ngarrkicc and Western Desert, in addition to Warumungu. Each language family has numerous dialects, but 'overlapping dialects/languages share common vocabulary and grammatical features' and are mutually intelligible (Turpin 2008:1). An example of the complexity of languages is found around Tennant Creek where groups speak Wakaya, Alyawarre, Warlpiri or Warlmanpa, Julalikari or Kaytetye, in addition to Warumungu (ACLA 2008).

Bilingual education began in the Northern Territory in the 1970s; though strongly supported then, it has since become a major area of political disagreement. During the time that bilingual education was supported by the Commonwealth government, 22 two-way schools were created in remote rural settlements where both first-language and ESL instruction were provided to children (Turpin 2008). These schools were staffed with a teacher-linguist and were supported by a Literacy Production Centre that created bilingual texts and useful instructional materials.

With the attainment of self-government in 1978, the new Northern Territory government withdrew support from bilingual education, closed 11 of the 22 two-way schools and by 2008, virtually closed all bilingual education by instituting a policy under which the first 4 years of schooling for all children must be only in English. This decision bode ill for many of the endangered Indigenous languages in the Territory; it ignored the language rights of Indigenous people and also ignored the considerable research which indicates that learning outcomes for children for whom English is not their first language are significantly enhanced when bilingual and ESL instruction is employed (Simpson et al. 2009).

14.3.3   The Main Players in Education in Tennant Creek

In communities such as Tennant Creek, where social disadvantage is well established and seemingly intractable, schools are the main institutions that bring different, disparate groups together. All children are required to attend school, and while attendance and interest in schooling may vary greatly within different groups, the required presence of children in schools offers an opportunity to reach out to parents and their communities. Most parents would like their children to receive a useful education and be treated fairly and with respect in the classroom. They desire schools that are welcoming and inclusive of their concerns (Pate 2008). When this does not happen, disparities continue to exist among and within schools and their communities. The disadvantage in communities finds its way into schools and class-rooms and is often mirrored in playground interactions together with the treatment of students by teachers.

Given that schools do not operate in a vacuum, any reform activities need to include a range of groups that represent the diverse communities served by the school. The involvement of groups who are marginalised is especially important. Each group will have specific definitions of its traditionally defined functions and purposes. The mean-ings attached to these roles will often incorporate well-established constructions about others in the community. The combination of traditional roles and ascribed construc-tions of others creates symbolic and behavioural boundaries that reinforce the segre-gation existing in the town. Below is a brief description of the main players in education in Tennant Creek that have contributed to creating and running the Community Action Support programme (CAS).

14.3.4 Tennant Creek High School (TCHS)

In 2008, there were 265 students enrolled in the Tennant Creek High School (TCHS) in Years 7 to 12 (NT Govt 2008a). Currently, approximately 80% of all students are from Indigenous families; some are from settlements and small communities even more remote than Tennant Creek. Twenty years ago, there were almost no Indigenous students, the majority being Anglo-Australians. Estimates of student attendance vary from 74% to 79%. The teaching staff is composed almost entirely of Anglo-Australian teachers, several of whom have been at the school for a long time. There is only one Indigenous teacher born in Tennant Creek. She has returned to teach English in high school. There is also an Indigenous student liaison officer who pro-vides support services, such as driving a school bus to transport Indigenous students to and from school.

In 2008, there were no bilingual classes in high school as the school administra-tion felt that there were 'too many Indigenous languages and a lack of qualified language teachers'. In addition, there was no English as a Second Language (ESL) teacher. Attempts to acquaint Anglo-Australian students with aspects of Indigenous culture are found in a 'culture and language' programme being run by an Indigenous woman appointed as an assistant teacher. Students in each Year group do different field trips involving camping and hunting, with the 'Ladies' from the Language Centre providing information about local plants and flowers and telling stories from their culture. This programme was called a 'two-way' programme, providing Anglo-Australian students with some idea about Indigenous life.

14.3.5   Tennant Creek Primary School (TCPS)

The primary school, including a preschool in the same grounds, has a current enrolment of 378 students (NT Govt. 2008b). The primary school engages in various programmes, such as a government-sponsored healthy eating programme where Indigenous women are contracted to provide breakfast, recess snacks and lunch to primary school students. Other programmes feature environmental concerns, including having students design, plant and care for school gardens, featuring desert plants, or develop signboards highlighting the history of the region, featuring the cattle stations, mining and Indigenous culture. Although exact figures are unavailable, it is safe to assume that the majority of students in the primary school are of Indigenous origin. In 2008, there were no bilingual education classes in the school.

14.3.6   Segmentation and Community Relations

This brief description of Tennant Creek and its schools highlights the segmentation of different groups within the boundaries of the town. Anglo-Australians carry the memories of a more affluent time when they constituted the majority living in the town. Those who continue to reside there now assume and exercise the power attendant in dominant social relations and organisations, holding powerful positions in local government and maintaining separate social clubs. However, maintaining these advantages sometimes assumes a defensive posture as many Anglo-Australians are aware of the significant number of Indigenous people in the town. Many businesses rely on Indigenous people as part-time workers or customers. Relationships across the Anglo-Indigenous divide tend to be remote and uneasy, and each segment of the community has largely stereotypic views of the other. There are few venues or cultural events where Anglos and Indigenous people mingle.

The two schools reflect this separation, as the curriculum of the school features basically Anglo-Australian history, values and subjects deemed important by the Department of Education. Efforts to promote Indigenous culture or provide meaningful language instruction as a key to improving Indigenous student achievement are tokenistic or largely missing. Changing the overall relational nexus of the town is unlikely to occur naturally. Although small beginnings can be created in the one place where Anglos and Indigenous people meet, altering the well-established patterns of behaviour and structure of the schools is also difficult. Often, what is needed to destabilise the existing situation is the intervention of an outside agency willing to work collaboratively in creating new possibilities beyond what might naturally occur, given the existing circumstances and players. Creating positive community relations is like looking at a puzzle and putting it together in new ways. This is the role that the ALNF assumed by working with members and staff of the Language Centre at the Papulu Apparr-kari Aboriginal Corporation.

14.3.7 Papulu Apparr-kari Aboriginal Corporation

One of the most important activities of the Papulu Apparr-kari (PAK) Aboriginal Corporation is the management of the Regional Indigenous Language Centre for the Barkly Division. It was founded to preserve, maintain and revive the 16 Indigenous languages of the region (www.papak.com.au, accessed 28/04/2010). The Language Centre runs a variety of programmes. Among them are cultural awareness/cross-cultural courses for businesses and corporations, interpreter services for legal matters, liaison/mediation services between Indigenous peoples and government and corporate entities, and translation services to help promote communication between Indigenous groups and businesses or government offices. Papulu Apparr-kari has also created business ventures to make it independent of outside funding, foster technical skills among Indigenous workers to improve their employment opportunities and serve as role models for other Indigenous people. The media centre, originally designed to support the main work of the Language Centre has expanded to include a range of commercial services.

Many of these activities were funded through the Commonwealth's Community Development Employment Program (CDEP). With this funding, a group of Indigenous Elders, 'the Ladies', has developed considerable skills related to local languages. They have provided a reliable source of information, knowledge and translation of Indigenous languages for linguists, businesses and government organisations for many years. These Ladies are also essential to the new CAS programme with the schools. With the Commonwealth Intervention in 2007 in the Northern Territory, the CDEP was closed, greatly influencing the work of the Centre. Many of the programmes, such as the Media Centre and welding were phased out, and only the translation work of the Ladies was continued.

There was a perception among Indigenous people that their initiatives to exercise independence were not always appreciated by the White community. For example, feelings among some of the PAK administrative staff indicated that: 'Anglos in the town think Indigenous people can't do food' (referring to the efforts of PAK to make groceries available at affordable prices to Indigenous people). Another comment was that: 'Opposition is from Whites who resent Aboriginals doing for themselves and cutting down on Anglo profits'. In regard to earlier attempts by the Ladies to work in the schools, one teacher associated with PAK said that: 'the program stopped because the ladies wouldn't go any more because of behaviour problems from students'. We later learned that these problems arose because the classroom teacher left the room when the Ladies came to present their lessons.

14.3.8 Training Centre, Charles Darwin University (CDU)

The CDU training centre coordinates Vocational Education and Training (VET) and Technical and Further Education (TAFE) equivalent certificate courses. There are three full-time staff: two teach in the adult Language, Literacy and Numeracy

Programme (LLNP). The third person also functions as the coordinator. When other lecturers are needed, instructors are brought from the main campus of Charles Darwin University in Alice Springs. The training centre works closely with Bachelor University, the Language Centre and, in some cases, the high school to provide certificate classes when there is adequate demand. An opinion expressed here by one staff member mirrored that of some school administrators: 'there is only a minimal work ethic among Indigenous people; they didn't need to work because they are on CDEP or get support from dividends from the mines'. As can be seen from these comments, the positioning of the other from both sides of the community was entrenched within a long history of mistrust and stereotyping. Movements across these boundaries required changes within both individuals and organisations. The CAS programme with its inherent values of learning and respect, along with the contributions of new participants, provided the catalyst for initiating this repositioning.

14.3.9   Australian Literacy and Numeracy Foundation (ALNF)

The Australian Literacy and Numeracy Foundation (ALNF), founded in 1999, is dedicated to raising language, literacy and numeracy standards for disadvantaged people. As part of its work, it raises funds to develop, implement and sustain innovative projects for individuals, families and communities (www.alnf.org). The project in Tennant Creek began in 2004 when Mary Ruth Mendel, a co-founder of ALNF, began working with Indigenous women elders in the Language Centre to transcribe and analyse the Warumungu language and transform it into forms that could be used for first-language teaching to Warumungu children. In seeking to develop this programme, the authors of this chapter were invited to Tennant Creek to explore what kind of school-based programme could be developed. Drawing in part on existing partnership programmes between the ALNF and the University of Western Sydney, a cross-generational mentoring programme was created. An important element in the beginning success of the Community Action Support programme was the trust and respect that had developed between the Ladies and the ALNF. These are essential elements in the creation of any new community initiative and will be discussed below. Such an endeavour requires time. It cannot be hurried to meet a budget requirement or an agency deadline.

14.3.10   The University of Western Sydney, School of Education

The Master of Teaching Secondary programme in the School of Education requires all pre-service teachers to enrol in a non-traditional, service-learning-based practicum (known as PE3) where they engage with school-age children but in non-classroom settings. PE3 is meant to foster an understanding about students, their lives and cultures that are often not possible to learn in the regular routine of the classroom

(Power 2010; Vickers 2007; Harris et al. 2004). The service-learning approach involves engaging students in new situations where they are invited to participate in the ongoing activities of a community agency or not-for-profit organisation. Students are required to reflect on their experiences through a range of activities in order to generate new understandings of the people, children and circumstances in which they have been participating (Harris et al. 2004). The key to the success of these arrangements is the reciprocal relationships that are fostered and nurtured between all participants in the undertaking (McCarthy et al. 2005).

14.4   The Community Action Support Programme (CAS)

The Community Action Support programme (CAS) is a cross-generational literacy-support programme in which different groups collaborate together to train and prepare Yr 10 Indigenous high-school students to provide reading and writing support for young primary school children. While the immediate objective is to enhance the learning of primary school students in both English and first language, the long-term objective is to involve Yr 10 Indigenous students in meaningful engagement with learning and teaching in anticipation that this may encourage retention and lead to pathways to further education for them. The role of the pre-service UWS university students was to provide curriculum suggestions and assist in the development of lesson plans with the Ladies and high-school student teachers and also mentor the high-school students in their own academic work. The Ladies provided an orientation to the UWS students regarding Indigenous culture(s) and language(s). Programme design and all curriculum support materials were the result of collaboration among the ALNF, the high school, the Ladies and the UWS students. While the main teaching staff of the primary and high schools were not directly involved in the delivery of CAS, their approval and support were essential. Over time, their support became more vocal as in both schools, they began to see different forms of interest and engagement in learning among their Indigenous students. This collaboration provides an innovation in community dynamics through which central players are encouraged to re-evaluate their constructions of each other in the process of engaging in fruitful new joint activities.

It was anticipated that as an outcome of CAS, aspects of the Indigenous community would be strengthened. For example, the Ladies would have renewed status within the PAK Language Centre and the wider Indigenous community for their work in promoting first-language instruction in the primary school. The communities would benefit from the active language learning their children were receiving, and this was likely to change their attitudes toward the primary school. The successful teaching by the Indigenous high-school students of the younger children would contribute to the completion of their own community studies class. Their presence and that of the Ladies in the classroom altered the view of the younger children to these adults in positive ways.

The creation of situations that build on the strengths of individuals established new pathways to learning, to changed perceptions about themselves and others and views of education and the schools. The increased engagement and interest of Indigenous students in learning were apparent to the mainstream teachers in both schools. This challenged many of the negative views held by teachers about Indigenous students and about their learning capacities (Armstrong 2000).

14.5   Reactions to CAS

The response to CAS has been overwhelmingly positive. Among the Yr 10 students, at least two of the five students have made plans for further education: one to become a teacher, the other to join the army (Jepson 2009). Two other students in the class also successfully passed the Community Studies subject. The new high-school principal termed the project 'highly successful': 'It keeps the doors open between older and younger generation and in all cultures that are slipping'. The vice principal and Community Studies teacher thought that through CAS, Indigenous students could begin to envision a more ambitious future for themselves, not just as teaching aides or teaching assistants but as classroom teachers. UWS pre-service teachers working with high-school classroom teachers brought the latest methods and ideas with them, and this stimulated the high-school teachers to reflect on their own teaching methods. The head of the CDU training centre suggested that the CAS experience expanded the restricted view Indigenous students had about what was possible for them to achieve (ALNF 2009a).

UWS pre-service teachers saw the power of Indigenous teachers teaching Indigenous students, and this experience at Tennant Creek transformed their ideas about Indigenous people and about the nature of teaching (Brace 2009). One or two stated that they would consider accepting an assignment to teach in Tennant Creek. The Ladies and Papulu Apparr-kari were thrilled with the enthusiastic response of the younger children to first-language teaching and with the presence of young Indigenous high-school students playing an active role in teaching and assisting in the children's acquisition of first language. Mrs. Nakkamarra Nixon, the leader of the Ladies, says she is 'relieved when others learn from her because the language needs to be spoken to live. But Indigenous children need good English, too. It is half this and half that, it is difficult. They should learn both ways so it can balance the things in their lives' (Jepson 2009). It was rewarding for the Ladies to interact with these young people and to experience the enthusiasm and respect of the children and high-school students to them as Elders. For the high-school students, the impact they had on the younger students became clear as the children greeted them on the streets outside of school or at the football matches (ALNF 2009b). Clearly, being a role model was new to them, and while they may not admit this, they were pleased about this (ALNF 2010).

14.6   The Construction of More Positive Community Relations

To make this project successful requires the unique contributions of all the players. The withdrawal of any one of them would inhibit programme outcomes. All are equally important but each in a different way. The ALNF was the catalyst that provided the stimulus and the means for local people to try something new. The primary school undertook to select groups of students who would be taught by the high-school students and provided the space and time for this to occur. The high school enrolled students in the Community Studies class and contributed a supervising teacher who teaches the class and works with the other partners to prepare the teaching materials and resources needed. This teacher also is responsible for teaching and demonstrating to the Yr 10 students what and how to teach the lessons to the younger students. The Ladies and PAK bring their considerable knowledge and experience of working with Indigenous languages and the preparation of first-language teaching materials; they also provide cultural orientation to the UWS students, who may have never been in the 'outback' before or interacted with Indigenous students. The Yr 10 students contribute their willingness to teach younger students, and they become role models for the younger students.

Having all the players in place is still not enough. An analysis of the nature of the exchanges that occurred is crucial to the understanding the outcomes. Fundamental to the exchange among the Ladies and ALNF is the issue of *respect* and *giving*. The ALNF came to work with the Ladies on something that was important to them: to develop the means so that young Indigenous children could learn to read and write in their first languages. This involved 4 or 5 years of collaboration in relation to Warumungu as a written language. The ALNF *supported* the Ladies to develop the means to teach Warumungu to young children. This was a way to keep the language alive and, at the same time, to realise that these children also needed to learn Standard English. This contributed to an improved sense of empowerment and control by Indigenous people of this important aspect of their lives. The fact that the intervention is occurring in the mainstream primary school with the support of the high school is immensely important in shaping new possible forms of community relations between Anglo-Australians and the Indigenous communities.

Reciprocally, after CAS was established, the Ladies were willing to consider going back into the primary school to try teaching again. They willingly mentored the Yr 10 teachers and helped them develop teaching materials. The Ladies gave their time and energies to orient the six UWS pre-service teachers, which increased the likelihood that these outsiders would have more success in their interactions with Indigenous children and adults. Relationships built on *reciprocity* were established with *trust and respect* inherent in the interaction between the Ladies and the ALNF. As the Director of PAK said: 'That ALNF is a good mob to work with. We particularly like their enthusiasm and interest in our languages'. Another important feature of CAS is the *continuity* it is establishing. Most visitors to Tennant Creek make one visit and are referred to by Indigenous people as 'fly-in-fly-out' types. The continuity of the connection between ALNF and PAK and the

Ladies is in sharp contrast with this. Ongoing and continuous *communication* among all the players is an important characteristic of the dynamics of CAS. All participants agreed to attend meetings when the ALNF staff were in town; none of the major players were left out. All relevant players participated in the development of the lessons for the primary school children and for the high-school students doing the teaching. Rather than having projects done 'to' or done 'for' Indigenous people or for the local Anglo-Australians by outsiders, CAS was done 'with' everyone. Different contributions were noted and appreciated, and there was no questioning anyone's commitment to making the programme work. This initiative was supported by the newly appointed principals in both public schools as a means of improving Indigenous student retention and improving the literacy development of Indigenous primary school students. The CDU training centre added its support by crediting the teaching experiences of Indigenous students in Community Studies as prior experience in qualifying for relevant TAFE (Technical and Further Education) certificates.

The elements identified here as essential in overcoming conflict and creating more positive connections among diverse groups are widely supported in the field of community development. For example, in the protocol for health professionals to work with Indigenous communities in the northern reaches of Australia, these same values are listed as essential for professional outsiders who are seeking to engage with Indigenous people: respect, reciprocity, trust, communication, time and so on (NHMRC 2003). Other efforts to improve the power and capacity of people to represent themselves are also found in community mapping initiatives (Amsden and Van Wynberghe 2005) or in the 'theories of change' approach which focuses on creating forms of evaluation that capture the complexity, diversity and variability of communities (Sullivan et al. 2002). The elements posited by advocates of positive psychology as crucial are essentially similar to approaches drawn from diverse disciplines and world views. Universally, it appears that efforts to improve community relations are essential ingredients in promoting peace and stability.

14.7 Into the Future

While CAS has only been operating for 1 year, indications of improved community relations are already apparent. Partially, this is found in the new ways that local townspeople and Indigenous people are relating to each other, both as groups and as individuals. These changes potentially break down long-held constructions of 'others' and open spaces for new ways of relating. The Ladies' interaction with the Anglo-Australian teachers in the schools is an example. Stemming also from these interactions are transformative experiences for many players who have been involved. Young Indigenous children have enthusiastically responded to learning first languages and English and have flourished by having Indigenous teachers in the classroom. The high-school students have become role models not only in the classroom but also in other arenas; two of them want to continue with advanced education.

Respect for Elders by younger Indigenous generations has been enhanced and is important, as traditional relationships, as well as language, need to survive.

The Papulu Apparr-kari Centre has potentially gained stature in the town as the Ladies have utilised their own work and relationship with the ALNF to make a difference in the operation of the schools, proving the value of an increased presence of Indigenous people in educational practices. This relationship is built on the recognition that Indigenous children benefit from learning both English and their first languages simultaneously; this is why bilingual education is needed. The contributions of UWS pre-service teachers made a difference to many in the community, but equally important, they experienced a transformation in their own constructions of 'others', which will inform their own practice as teachers in classrooms with Indigenous students. Other research (McCarthy and Murakami 2010; Sato et al. 2009; Ferfolja et al. 2009; King 2004) also supports the transformative effect that participating in unfamiliar situations can have on the views people have of others.

14.8   What Have We Learnt?

The improvements in social dynamics described in this case study illustrate key principles of community relations in the field of positive psychology. The emphasis is on building on the strengths and resilience of people through collaborative endeavours. Established traditional boundaries are breached both by new experiences and by openness to learning – about the self and about 'others'. Inherent in this process is the movement of Indigenous people from the margins to the centre of the relational nexus. Within a safe setting facilitated by third parties, marginalised voices were heard and respectful action was taken. The imbalance in power was minimised as partners were dependent on each other to reach their mutual and separate goals. The specific goal of CAS was the preservation and promotion of Indigenous languages, and the key to its success was a carefully constructed programme built as the outgrowth of a long and profitable ongoing relationship among the major parties. The work done by Nakkula et al. (2010) in the US mirrors many of the principles and understandings developed here, including respect for individual identities, gaining trust, building on assets or strengths and being both pro-active and collaborative. They too used mentoring as a tool for development and gave young people structured opportunities for leadership.

The initial success of CAS is impressive, illustrating how opportunities for positive relationships between Indigenous people and Anglo-Australians can occur. This success is, however, only a small beginning in the long process required to bring about further and other forms of reconciliation between Indigenous people and Anglo-Australians across Australia.

CAS will continue in Tennant Creek. It can be anticipated that as CAS grows, problems will arise that will again require resourcefulness and initiative on the part of all participants. What the programme has in its favour is the firm foundations built within the PAK Language Centre, the continuity provided by ALNF and the ongoing commitment of the schools. If this initiative can be sustained, there is a good chance that real change could occur in the social context and relational nexus of Tennant Creek. What can be learned from this for other endeavours is that community wellbeing only grows out of reconstructed relationships. The key objective must be to disrupt the practices of discrimination and marginalisation that establish and maintain boundaries among disparate groups.

References

Aboriginal Child Language Acquisition project. (2008). *Regions: Tennant creek.* Melbourne University, Victoria, 1–8. Accessed April 26, 2010, from http://www.linguistics.unimelb.edu.au/research/projects/ACLA/tennant.html

Amsden, J., & Van Wynberghe, R. (2005). Community mapping as a research tool with youth. *Action Research, 3*(4), 357–381.

Armstrong, H. B. (2000). *Breaching the norm; a practice for reconciliation.* Paper presented at the Critical Psychology conference, Parramatta.

Aspinwall, L. G., & Staudinger, U. M. (2002). *A psychology of human strengths: Fundamental questions and future directions for a positive psychology.* Washington, DC: American Psychological Association.

Australian Bureau of Statistics. (2001). *Census 2001.* Canberra: Commonwealth Government.

Australian Literacy and Numeracy Foundation. (2009a). *Community Action Support (CAS).* 1–5. Accessed April 28, 2010, from http://www.alnf.org/programs/community-action.php

Australian Literacy and Numeracy Foundation. (2009b). *Case study: Community action support. Richelle Watson.* Tennant Creek: Australian Literacy and Numeracy Foundation

Australian Literacy and Numeracy Foundation. (2010). *Draft annual report.* Sydney: ALNF.

Baker, J. A., Dilly, L. J., & Auppwerlee, J. L. (2003). The developmental context of school satisfaction: Schools as psychologically healthy environments. *School Psychology Quarterly, 18,* 206–221.

Bond, S. (2009). *Learning support programs: Education reform beyond the school.* Victoria: Brotherhood of St Laurence.

Brace, E. (2009). *Draft project outline: Community action support* (pp. 1–13). Sydney: Australian Literacy and Numeracy Foundation.

Collins, B. (1999). *Learning lessons: An independent review of Indigenous education in the Northern Territory.* Darwin: NT Department of Education.

Curry, L., & Snyder, C. R. (2000). Hope takes the field: Mind matters in athletic performance. In C. R. Snyder (Ed.), *Handbook of hope: Theory, measures, and applications* (pp. 243–260). San Diego: Academic.

Dooley, K. T. (2009). Re-thinking pedagogy for middle school students with little, no or severely interrupted schooling. *English Teaching: Practice and Critique, 8*(1), 5–22.

Ferfolja, T., McCarthy, F., Naidoo, L., Vickers, M., & Hawker, A. (2009). *Refugee Action Support (RAS) Program. A collaborative initiative between the University of Western Sydney, the Australian Numeracy and Literacy Foundation and the NSW Department Of Education And Training: Final report.* Sydney: University of Western Sydney.

Frederickson, B., & Tugade, M. (2004). Resilient individuals use positive emotions to bounce back from negative emotional experiences. *Journal of Personality and Social Psychology, 86*(2), 320–333.

Gable, S. L., & Haidt, J. (2005). What (and why) is positive psychology? *Review of General Psychology, 9*(2), 103–110.

Govt, N. T. (2008a). *Tennant creek high school. School profile.* Darwin: Northern Territory Government Education and Training Directory.

Govt, N. T. (2008b). *Tennant creek primary. School profile*. Darwin: Northern Territory Government Education and Training Directory School.

Harris, C., Vickers, M. H., & McCarthy, F. E. (2004). University-community engagement: Exploring service-learning options within the practicum. *Asia Pacific Journal of Teacher Education, 32*(2), 129–141.

Held, B. S. (2004). The negative side of positive psychology. *Journal of Humanistic Psychology, 44*(9), 9–46.

Hollinsworth, D. (2003). *They took the children*. Kingswood: Working Title Press.

Ingram, R. E., & Snyder, C. R. (2006). Blending the good with the bad: Integrating positive psychology and cognitive psychotherapy. *Journal of Cognitive Psychotherapy, 20*(2), 117–123.

Jepson, D. (2009). *Teenage teachers learn to share the gift of reading. Sydney Morning Herald*, November 27, 2009. Ref: 60785763.

King, J. T. (2004). Service-learning as a site for critical pedagogy: A case of collaboration, caring and defamiliarization across borders. *Journal of Experiential Education, 26*(3), 121–137.

Masten, A. S. (2001). Ordinary magic: Resilience processes in development. *American Psychologist, 56*(3), 227–238.

McCarthy, F. E., & Murakami, M. (2010). *Crossing borders at home and abroad: Transformative service-learning for Japanese students*. Paper presented at the International Research on Service-Learning and Community Engagement Conference, Indianapolis, IL, October 28–30.

McCarthy, F. E., Damrongmanee, Y., Pushpalatha, M., Chithra, J., & Yamamoto, K. (2005). The practices and possibilities of service learning among colleges and universities in Asia. *Pacific-Asian Education, 17*(2), 59–70.

Murray, J. (2004). Making sense of resilience: A useful step on the road to creating and maintaining resilient students and school communities. *The Australian Guidance and Counselling Journal, 14*(1), 1–15.

Nakkula, M. J., Foster, K. C., & Mannes, M. (2010). *Building healthy communities for positive youth development*. New York/London: Springer.

National Health and Medical Research Council. (2003). *Values and ethics: Guidelines for ethical conduct in Aboriginal and Torres Strait Islander health research*. Canberra: Commonwealth of Australia.

Noble, T., McGrath, H., Roffey, S., & Rowling, L. (2008). *A scoping study on student wellbeing*. Canberra: Department of Education, Employment and Workplace Relations.

Papulu Apparr-Kari Aboriginal Corporation Web-site. Tennant Creek. 1–8. Accessed April 28, 2010, from http://www.papak.com.au

Pate, A. (2008). *Learning support programs – 'A chance to experience success': An evaluation of four Melbourne City mission learning support programs for children and young people*. Melbourne: Melbourne City mission.

Power, A. (2010). Community engagement as authentic learning with reflection. *Issues in Educational Research, 20*(1), 57–63.

Prilleltensky, I., & Prilleltensky, O. (2006). *Promoting well-being: Linking personal, organisational and community change*. Hoboken: Wiley.

Reynolds, H. (1992). *The law of the land*. Victoria: Penguin.

Sandage, S. J., Hill, P. C., & Vang, H. C. (2003). Toward a multicultural positive psychology: Indigenous forgiveness among the Hmong culture. *The Counselling Psychologist, 31*, 564–592.

Sato, Y., McCarthy, F. E., Murakami, M., & Yamamoto, K. (2009). The impact of service-learning: Reflections from service-learning alumni. In *Lessons from service-learning in Asia: Results of collaborative research in higher education* (pp. 137–151). Tokyo: Service Learning Centre, International Christian University.

Seligman, M. E. P. (2002). Positive psychology, positive prevention, and positive therapy. In C. R. Snyder & S. J. Lopez (Eds.), *Handbook of positive psychology* (pp. 3–9). New York: Oxford University Press.

Seligman, M. E. P., & Csekszentmihalyi, M. (2000). Positive psychology: An introduction. *American Psychologist, 65*(1), 5–14.

Simpson, J., Caffery, J., & McConvell, P. (2009). *Gaps in Australia's indigenous language policy: Dismantling bilingual education in the Northern Territory. Australian Institute of Aboriginal and Torres Strait Islander Studies.* Australian Policy Online. Accessed December 1, 2010, from http://www.apo.org.au/node/17566

Sullivan, H., Barnes, M., & Matka, E. (2002). Building collaborative capacity through 'theories of change'. Early lessons from the evaluation of health action zones in England. *Evaluation, 8*(2), 205–226.

Turpin, M. (2008). *Aboriginal languages.* Central Land Council, 1–8. Accessed April 24, 2010, from http://www.clc.org.au/People_Culture/language/language.html

Vickers, M. H. (2007). Reversing the lens: Transforming teacher education through service learning. In S. Billig & S. B. Gelmon (Eds.), *From passion to objectivity: Cross-disciplinary perspectives on service learning research* (pp. 199–216). Charlotte: Information Age Publishing.

Florence E. McCarthy is an Adjunct Associate Professor of the Centre for Educational Research at the University of Western Sydney.
Contact: ide@iinet.net.au

Margaret H. Vickers is Professor of Education in the School of Education at the University of Western Sydney.
Contact: mhv@uws.edu.au

Chapter 15
Positive Relations Between Members of Groups with Divergent Beliefs and Cultures

Zalman Kastel

15.1 Introduction

The deputy principal of a small town school in Australia's Northern Territory had organised with the interfaith Together for Humanity team to run a Leadership Day as part of a two-day seminar with 11–12 year olds. Almost all the students were Indigenous, so we thought it important to make it culturally appropriate. Shortly before starting, the team sat down for a snack outside, so our Indigenous team member, Auntie K., could smoke a cigarette. I asked Auntie how we might make the Leadership Day more culturally appropriate. Her response did not seem to answer our question. I asked the question differently and still did not get what we were looking for. I stopped and asked myself: "Am I really listening? Am I asking the wrong question?" Then I asked if this whole idea of 11-year-old leaders might have no cultural resonance. Auntie confirmed this.

Ok, we said, we won't have a Leadership Day. What we are really trying to do is encourage respect, initiative and contribution. What does your heritage say on that? Ah! Auntie was in her element. She explained the kinship system and how every person has responsibilities and links to a vast network of people, and custodianship of specific plants, animals and places. The students responded enthusiastically with a range of initiatives including plans for planting a vegetable garden to distribute to the needy, and making a welcoming video for new students about their friendly school. A few months later, the deputy principal reported there was still a different feeling in the school.

This chapter does not set out a path for world peace, nor does it address the broad relationships between religions, peoples or nations. In terms of divergent beliefs, the purpose here is not to promote respect for religions in general or any particular religion, but rather to identify ways in which people holding different viewpoints about religion, or politics, ranging from atheism to religious literalism, and conservatism to communism can respond appropriately and ethically to tensions arising from these differences and other cultural expressions that might make some people feel uncomfortable.

Rabbi Z. Kastel (✉)
National Director Together for Humanity Foundation, Sydney, NSW, Australia
e-mail: zalman@togetherforhumanity.org.au

S. Roffey (ed.), *Positive Relationships: Evidence Based Practice across the World*,
DOI 10.1007/978-94-007-2147-0_15, © Springer Science+Business Media B.V. 2012

'I hate the word tolerance'. That's a refrain heard from those who find prejudice deeply offensive and think we can celebrate diversity rather than merely tolerate it. It is a noble sentiment, but one this author rejects on the ground that for some situations, tolerance would be a significant improvement. The definition here of 'positive relationships' includes a spectrum of stances varying according to what is realistic for different individuals and contexts. These range along a continuum from an improved sense of belonging for people from varied backgrounds and strong support for distinctive and interconnected communities, to more modest states of responding constructively to conflict, such as interacting with people from varied backgrounds in respectful and just ways (Paradies et al. 2009), to conflict containment and reduction of hatred and mistrust in the context of an intractable conflict (Biton and Salomon 2006).

As much as evidence gathered by academics, this chapter draws on the experience of practitioners working and grappling with divergent beliefs, narratives, norms and perspectives in a range of settings. The author's own experience involves work carried out between late 2002 and 2010 with a group of people with diverse religious and political beliefs, who set out to educate Australian school children about replacing prejudice with empathy, awareness of common values and our ability to work together. Initially there were three: a Turkish politically active Muslim, a Quaker suspicious of power and the author, a Hasidic Jew employed by a religiously uncompromising, revivalist Synagogue. Over time, others got involved: a Liberian survivor of civil war, Aboriginal people, people of Arabic backgrounds including Palestinians and Lebanese, an Israeli, Christian believers in the literal truth of the Bible, religious progressives and atheists. Their collaboration, now known as Together for Humanity, engaged face-to-face with over 50,000 students in 7 years. This rewarding journey confronted core participants with the sometimes challenging reality of divergent beliefs and cultures.

15.2   Challenges

I grew up in an ethnically mixed part of Sydney, but my son did not experience growing up here in the country. When I went on an aeroplane with him – this was after the Bali bombing – and a Muslim sat next to us, he was really terrified. To be honest, I wasn't too comfortable either. It made me think about how prejudiced I was. (School Principal in regional NSW, Australia, 2010)

This chapter frames challenges to positive inter-group relations under three broad categories: Beliefs, Identity and Grievance (BIG). Unhelpful beliefs include prejudices on the part of people who hold strong views about religion, such as the attitudes of conservatively religious people about non-religious people and people who are differently religious to themselves, as well as stereotypes about religious people held by people who are hostile to or ambivalent about religion (Bouma and Halafoff 2009).

Mirroring arguments against racism which assert we are all the same, some have tried to deal with religion-linked hostility by proclaiming all religions are 'good'; or in the case of Islam, calling it 'the religion of peace'. These platitudes do not stand up to scrutiny because far too much violence has been committed at least in part in the name of religion. There are legitimate concerns relating to religious difference especially as it interacts with other factors, e.g. coercive enforcement of religious standards of modesty, controversy around gay marriage and abortion and the real threat to many religious beliefs, values and practices posed by western 'godless' cultural influences.

Waleed Aly, an Australian Muslim academic, attributes much misunderstanding between Muslims and the so-called West to arrogance, which he sees in the tendency of some to ignore the basic principle that we cannot assume our own solutions will work for other people's problems. Yet many in the West insist on a reformation of Islam simply because in the history of Christian Europe this helped solve problems (Aly 2007). A reality of Islam, not considered by those offering such advice, is that the religious ideas often associated with terrorism are inspired by people like Abdul Wahab (1703–1792) who is seen by at least some of his admirers as an 'outstanding reformer' of Islam (Baz 2010).

Aly is equally critical of Muslims who see the 'West' as uniform and fail to appreciate its diversity and merits. A case in point is the way in which the range of views and practices relating to sexuality in western countries can be interpreted as wholesale promiscuity.

A middle-aged man is clearly annoyed with the remarks of Dr. Syafi Anwar at the 2010 Yogyakarta World Peace Forum, about his counter-radicalisation efforts. "It is not we who are the problem. The President of France (Nicolas Sarkozy), bans women from wearing the veil, he wants them all to be like his wife and walk around with no clothes on. In Switzerland they ban the Minarets. It is the so-called 'Enlightened West' that is the problem!"

Misrepresenting the 'other', and seeing them in a negative light, is used by some as a way of strengthening their own identity and collective self-esteem (Griffiths and Pedersen 2009). Exclusive identities and the development of 'us and them' ways of looking at groups are strongly present in societies in conflict and even in post-conflict societies (Hamber 2004). Interestingly, it also can be developed between members of the same majority groups, as a white high school girl made clear to Together for Humanity facilitators in an Australian country town: 'People in Mudgee say that people in (neighbouring) Gulgong are born with two heads, and if you look closely at their necks you'll see a red scar at the spot where the other head was cut off'. More broadly, identity plays a role in what has been termed the 'new racism' and the negative attitudes to people whose differences are seen to be irreconcilable and a threat to the social values of the majority (Paradies et al. 2009).

The perceived threat need not be violent. To established groups such as 'white Australians', the behaviour of new arrivals with unfamiliar norms and customs such as playing football at the beach can be confronting (Wise 2010). Muslim migration along with other movements of people from diverse cultures and beliefs was supposed to be accommodated by the policy of multiculturalism. For some people it works well; however, as Australian social researcher Hugh Mackay explains, 'Multiculturalism as a word carries some negative baggage for others. It suggests to some people that subcultures will be preserved in a way that slows the process of establishing social harmony' (Mackay 2007:145). Some assessments of the situation in the UK and the Netherlands are blunt: 'Multiculturalism has run its course and it is time to move on'; 'Multiculturalism has led not to integration but to segregation' and 'The outcome has been to encourage exclusion rather than inclusion' (Sniderman and Hagendoorn 2007).

One of the greatest challenges stems from grievances relating to actual, perceived or feared harm by people of other groups. This could be a direct experience with minority group members who exhibit anti-social behaviour when this behaviour is 'essentialised' and understood to be related to the offenders and their group's basic culture or nature, rather than being explained as a response to a situation (Batterham 2001). Similarly, there are attitudes stemming from what has been called 'indirect-experiential function', where information received from the media or friends about objectionable behaviour such as terrorism shapes the perception of the whole group that is seen to be linked to this behaviour (Griffiths and Pedersen 2009). These factors also contribute to the 'new racism', where people justify their attitudes because they are based on 'empirical facts' (McConahay 1986).

In the cases of post-conflict societies, or societies currently engaged with conflict, this challenge seems insurmountable. The experiences of war, systemic discrimination, dispossession and extreme poverty are unimaginable to those who have not endured them. Victims of political violence might have their sense of belonging undermined, be dehumanised and internalise a perspective that legitimises violence, although the impact varies between individuals and contexts (Hamber 2004). Even with people not directly involved in conflict, the vicarious effect can be substantial both in terms of the experiences and feelings of those swept up in conflict and their perception of the quantity and degree of evil of the 'others'.

15.3 Justice

Clearly inter-cultural and international justice is the most significant factor in positive relations between groups. Ongoing unresolved issues of justice, equity, prejudice and contested uses of force or power will contribute to animosity between groups and must be resolved at a political and practical level. In apparently successful peace-building initiated by the Center of Research and Development of the Indonesian Religion, Ministry of Religious Affairs, youth leaders, trained as 'action researchers', worked together with community leaders to resolve local conflicts. One important element was ensuring that commitments to correct grievances were honoured (Mudzhar 2010). Sometimes the substantial issues are beyond the control of those involved; however, just as the macro level influences the local level, the reverse is also true. Starting with ourselves would seem the most logical place to start.

> Liberian Australian Mohamed Dukuly relates: "That morning, in mid-1990 during the civil war in Liberia, we were sitting in the hut, it was the triangle hut, we build it with thatch. We all slept hungry, and planned to eat in the morning. I saw a young man I knew, Mamade, coming toward us, when he got to us he fell to the ground. He was covered with blood and he had been in water, which made it look worse. We asked him, what happened? He told us that he escaped from captivity".
>
> "Then I sat there looking at him and I was thinking, why? Why? I thought this (Mamade) could be me and it became real. Now I wanted to know: why do they hate us? Why do they want to kill us?! This was the beginning of my journey, to start thinking about why people hate us. Now I can begin to give it meaning."

Self-reflection is essential for learning to relate positively to people who seem different to ourselves, and to imagine 'alternative possibilities' to our entrenched way of seeing reality (Hoffman 1996). It is worth reflecting on our responses to injustice and violence against our group. How do we think, feel and talk about the group against whom our group has a grievance? Do we tend to think of 'them' as essentially evil? Or can we see them as human beings who are responding in a way that for us is terrible, but which might make some sense to them, based on their story? This is not to say we cannot stand up for justice as we understand it: It is rather an argument for refusing to dehumanise the other side.

> An employer and his Jewish employee are doing their annual wage negotiation "dance". The employee wants more money to meet his family's needs. The employer is trying to get the best "bang for his buck". They settle on a fraction of the requested raise. The employee feels cornered into accepting, but fails to tell the employer this. After a number of times the employer turns to the employee and says: "You know you are just like the Palestinians. The Israelis reach an agreement with them, but they always want more." "Hmmm," thought the employee, "so that is what it feels like to be Palestinian."

Some negotiations between people or groups are predominantly positional bargaining, where each side moves from their original position to 'meet each other halfway'. However, the agreements produced can fail to meet key interests of one party or both (Fisher et al. 1999). Particularly in Islamic tradition, there is a view that there can be no real peace without justice. This, of course, is about a perception of justice or injustice. Problems are exacerbated when people on both sides of a conflict are convinced that a perception of truth is the objective truth.

15.4 Religious Truth Claims

The issue of truth, as related to religion, might seem bizarre to those for whom religious beliefs are essentially a matter of personal preference. To them, feeling uncomfortable about someone's religion might make as much sense as becoming angry about a preference for one ice-cream flavour over another. It might be useful to think of religion in the way some of us feel about the environment, free speech, trade unions, abortion or respect between the sexes. People who believe in the absolute truth of their religious beliefs could be afraid that standing side by side with people of other faiths implies an endorsement of beliefs contrary to their own (Feinstein 1959).

Some religious authorities advise that, if the focus is on social action, then the meaning of being together is not an endorsement of each other's faiths but a practical collaboration. In addition, it is worth recognising the range of views about religious 'truth', including Exclusivist, Relativist Agnostic/Indifferent, Pluralist and Inclusivist. An inclusivist stance is essentially that objective truth exists, and adherents believe their understanding of this objective truth is essentially correct. However, there is an allowance for people who do not share one's belief as still sharing in the one 'truth', albeit getting at it in their own way (Engebretson 2009). A variation of this is to assert that, 'While I believe strongly that my belief is true, I must be humble enough to recognise the inadequacy of the human mind to grasp the mystery of the divine with certainty, and respect others' sincere attempts to find the truth'. This might not satisfy those who believe the concept of 'truth' itself is the source of conflict, but recognising the options between absolutism and relativism is a pragmatic and effective way to work with some devout believers.

15.5   Realism

We must work with people and groups as they are, rather than how we wish them to be. This principle might seem obvious, but it is not always recognised in practice. An example of this was the desire of some Jews and Muslims to engage only with those members of the other group who were close to their own view on the Arab–Israeli conflict. A Muslim study centre in Sydney engaged a Jewish speaker who was harshly critical of the State of Israel and Jewish community support for it. Some members of the Jewish community wanted to limit their engagement to Muslims who were not 'anti-Israel'. As the slain Israeli Prime Minister Yitzhak Rabin retorted to those who criticised him for shaking the hand of Palestinian leader Yasser Arafat: 'One does not make peace with one's friends; you can only make peace with your enemies'.

15.6   Honesty

There is an either/or way of thinking about other groups that is unhelpful: namely, either political correctness and denial of problems, or 'saying it like it is' and hyperfocusing on problems.

> 30 men and women were sitting in a circle in a community centre in Western Sydney a short time after the infamous 'Cronulla riots' of 2005. The conflict could be summed up as having three waves: reports of anti-social behaviour by Lebanese on the beaches; people who looked 'Middle Eastern' being attacked by mostly drunken whites, some waving Australian flags; revenge attacks by gangs of mostly Lebanese who smashed cars and went on a rampage. In our circle, half the group were white residents from the Cronulla area and the other half were mostly Muslim of Lebanese heritage. A woman in her 50s asserted that the allegation of violent behaviour by young Lebanese males was baseless and untrue. A tall blond suntanned white man in his 20s interjected with his personal experience of being attacked by 20 young Lebanese on a train on his way home.

Resistance to recognising the faults of members of minority groups might have various motives, some well intentioned. However, pretending everything is ok will not work in certain situations, especially instances of prejudice or animosity relating to negative experiences, either first hand or vicarious. Participants must feel 'safe' to speak honestly and frankly, including talking about negative experiences. If people feel under attack and think they will be labelled as racist, they are less likely to listen or engage (Pedersen et al. 2005). This was powerfully brought home to us in a Together for Humanity seminar with student leaders at a rural retreat at Lake Burendong, Australia.

> Students were asked to build something using plastic connector pieces. A group of Indigenous students made a colourful circle. In the middle they placed a box filled with small black rectangles. They said, "The colours represent the rest of Australia, filled with colour; but in the middle are us blackfellas isolated from everyone else. But we don't want to talk about it."
>
> We moved on, respecting their choice not to discuss their disclosure. However, when we returned to the issue of relations between black and white Australians, it was as if the floodgates had opened. There was impassioned discussion for almost an hour. As one student put it with deep feeling and frustration, "We care about Indigenous issues; but whenever we open our mouth, we are told we are racist so we just shut up."

The difficulty people have with differences can take the form of 'positive stereotypes' where the generalisations about a particular minority group are meant to be complimentary, e.g. 'Blacks are good at sports'. These generalisations are likely to be seen quite differently by those on the receiving end of the 'compliment'. People are not given the chance to be seen accurately as themselves but are assumed to possess certain qualities based on their colour or group. This can result in increased inter-group mistrust (Czopp 2008).

> **Reflection**: One of the traps I fell into was that in rejecting my old prejudices and building empathy with new communities I put the 'other' on a pedestal. I thought if all the false beliefs I had about Muslims were proven wrong, then any concerns I had in working with any Muslim must also be wrong. Of course, every group has its share of saints and sinners, every person has their virtues and vices, and every relationship will have its joys and challenges. I had to deny any problems.
>
> Years later I read "Three Cups of Tea", about an American mountain climber who like me is swept off his feet by the beauty and wholesomeness of an Islamic culture (Mortenson and Relin 2006). When I read how he is stunned by a betrayal by a member of this community he has come to love, I found tears running down my face. Years later, I would say in relation to our Indigenous Australians, "Why is it that people see them either as Savages or Noble Savages? Why can't we see every community for what it is, just people?!"

Of course we can and must recognise each community as a collection of unique individuals, capable of both good and evil. Still, in some cases, the prevalence of antisocial behaviour or other problems, often related to extreme social disadvantage, looms so large that if we are brutally honest then, we would actually be quite brutal. In these cases, it is sometimes necessary to see the other not as they appear to us based on a collection of obvious facts but as they can be based on their human potential, and broader positive aspects of their heritage and community. 'Honesty and realism' must be tempered with imagination, compassion, a broader perspective and openness.

15.7   Openness

> A religious leader from the subcontinent related how his wife opened his mail when they first married. He was shocked, and explained these were letters addressed to him! She respected his wishes and privacy and never opened his mail again. She later told the author how she grew up in a large family where everyone rushed to the door when the postman

arrived and whoever got there first opened the mail for the whole family. When her husband
was asked if he reciprocated his wife's flexibility and willingness to adapt to his norms, he
said, "Yes, I don't open her mail either." He was serious.

To learn to appreciate each other, especially in cases of mistrust and conflict, we
need to listen to the 'other's' narratives with real curiosity, which entails willingness to abandon preconceived assumptions. This is harder than it seems. Genuine
openness requires adopting a stance of 'not knowing', that resists the temptation to
fill in the blanks in the other's story with our own experiences, and drills down
further to understand the other's experience through their eyes rather than ours
(Livyatan et al. 2005).

We also need some openness to values that are different to our own, but this must
be negotiated with respect for our need to be true to our own principles and morals.
It is highly problematic for positive relationships if, to maintain them, people need
to compromise their religious or moral beliefs and important cultural practices.

In 2006, the author and a male Muslim member of Together for Humanity flew across
Australia. The Muslim suggested this would be an opportunity to talk about a sensitive issue.
During the trip, he complained about the inclusion of a female Muslim participant who did
not conform to certain religious norms, yet was representing the faith. One of the Christian
members objected strongly to this "fundamentalist male chauvinism" and threatened to quit
if she was forced out. We had to accept that the decision for how their religion would be
represented was properly that of the Muslim community, yet we were reluctant to ask her to
leave. In the end she chose to bow out to avoid associating controversy with the project.

Other conflicts of values were resolved in favour of secular principles, e.g. a Jewish
male member's religious laws against hearing women and girls singing conflicted
with a group of high school girls invited to sing at a public event. In this case, the girls
sang, and the Jewish member slipped out for that time. A Quaker member of the group
objected to use of power structures such as senior bureaucrats in the Department of
Education who might coerce teachers to invite us. The decision was taken to prioritise
opportunities of working with more students by engaging these powerful people.

Often the clash is less about a real conflict of values and more about a need for
openness to other ways, creativity and flexibility.

15.8   Credibility and Guilt by Association

While we must be realistic about how much or how little agreement we can expect
from 'the other side', there can be limits with whom one can work. There are issues
of being co-opted to legitimise or whitewash evil in its various forms. There are also
practical considerations of maintaining integrity and legitimacy so that one's efforts
to establish contact with the other are seen as legitimate and sanctioned by one's
own group (Alport 1954). The tendency to assign generalised guilt in times of conflict can mean massive social pressure on those engaging with 'the enemy'.

Running too far ahead of one's own group in inter-group conflict situations can
create significant tensions for bridge builders which, if left unresolved, could

delegitimatise them to members of their own side to the point where all progress made in influencing members could be reversed or at least discontinued. Yet there is external pressure to stand up for justice as understood by bridge builders from the 'opposing side'. We must ensure that we operate in a way that leaders of the 'other group' can feel able to participate without compromising themselves or being seen to be selling out their community.

> One of the issues I am finding hard to accept is that I have never ever heard, even from the most liberal of Jews, anyone ever come out and unequivocally state that Israel stands condemned for her actions without qualification.
>
> Why is this so? This seems to be a line that the vast overwhelming majority of Jews will not cross. Is there a religious teaching that prohibits any criticism of what Israel does as a nation? If this is so, this is something that I as a Muslim would find very difficult to come to terms with. (Arabic Australian Muslim bridge builder)

The 'Gaza war' or Operation Cast Lead (late 2008–early 2009), following rockets fired at Southern Israel, really shook the foundations under the fragile bridges being built between Australian Jews and Muslims, and presented a serious challenge to bridge builders themselves. There was a view among some Muslims that the test of sincerity for Jews involved in this work would be their willingness to condemn Israel. These people criticised Muslim bridge builders for engaging with Jewish people who seemed not to care about justice.

We worked through it by expressing genuine concern about deaths of civilians, affirming universal principles and insisting there is a difference between being active in killing and being silent about a particular campaign of violence carried out by people with whom one has strong ties of nationality or faith.

> **Reflection**: It would be far easier for people in either Jewish or Arabic Muslim communities to insist on only working with people who agree with their perspective of the conflict. In fact since September 11, if not earlier, Muslims faced the 'condemnation test', which measured the worthiness of a Muslim by their willingness to condemn violence committed by other Muslims. With the 'shoe on the other foot', I began to question the value of using condemnation as such an important criterion for engagement. In a sense, condemnation on the basis of a lack of condemnation would be an endorsement of the idea of collective culpability practised by Bin-Laden and others that is so offensive in the first place.

15.9 Respect

In 1999, the Nuer and Dinka tribes of Southern Sudan had been waging war, killing each other and destroying each others' cattle. An American Christian, Bill Lowery, and others from the New Sudan Council of Churches brought chiefs from the two sides together, at great risk to the chiefs themselves. One of the rituals involved participants spitting into a gourd filled with water. When it came to Bill, he spat into it too. When everyone had spat, they splashed the water on each other. The spittle on the tongue is meant to be the coldest part of a person, and splashing it symbolised cooling off the hot bodies, charged with the 'heat of conflict'. Bill asked the chiefs to tell stories they heard from their fathers' mothers about how conflicts were resolved in the past. They sat opposite each other, divided by a rope representing the Nile, and discovered the wisdom of their respective ancestors was very similar. They told stories about what was done to them, and finally were asked what they 'remembered' for the future of their daughters' sons.

After three days of story telling, they reached the point of decision. Bill warned his team that this was not a time to give advice. In the end the decision was a 'no-brainer'. The logical conclusion was ending the fighting. One of the oldest chiefs told Bill, "I have been to many meetings with the United Nations. Never before has anyone asked me what I think." (Lowery 2010)

It makes sense to value the traditional wisdom of diverse communities that are adaptive and have withstood the tests of time, including the varying positive roles religion plays in the lives of some groups. It is useful to challenge ourselves about whether we are asking the right questions, e.g. instead of asking how pessimistic Asian Americans are, which assumes pessimism is the same for them as it is for the researcher's group, we might want to ask whether pessimism is harmful or useful for this group. We could then discover that while Asian Americans were generally more pessimistic than other groups, their pessimism correlated with better functioning, perhaps better preparing them for difficulties, and helping them cope (Lopez et al. 2005). Putting into practice the respect for diverse ways of knowing and being requires flexibility and preparedness to change the question or approach, if it is to be more than tokenism.

15.10   Strategies for Change

Three significant factors that improve inter-group relations are empathy, inter-group contact and cognitive approaches that appeal to reasonableness (Trang and Wittenberg 2004), dispel false beliefs (Batterham 2001) or provide information (Pedersen et al. 2005).

15.10.1   Empathy

A strong inverse relationship exists between levels of prejudice and empathy that influences people to behave in a more positive way toward others (Batterham 2001). In our experience, working together as people of different faiths and vastly different backgrounds, we saw this dynamic at work both in our changing feelings about each other and in responses from students. An effective method for invoking empathy is hearing the stories of others. This was found to be effective in addressing perceptions of Indigenous people in Bunbury, Western Australia, as being lazy and not wanting to work. A television campaign, featuring 12 interviews with employed Indigenous people, saw a 15.8% improvement in the way Indigenous people were perceived after these stories were told (Donovan and Leivers 1993).

Invoking empathy can take a variety of forms with a range of results. Some attempts at manipulating empathy have shown no result in reducing prejudice (Batterham 2001). Particular caution must be taken with building empathy with the suffering of 'out-groups'. Asking people to imagine how they would feel personally in that situation could evoke distress as well as empathy (Batson et al. 1997). In research undertaken in Germany, descriptions of ongoing suffering of Holocaust survivors and secondary trauma in their descendants resulted in increased anti-Semitism on the part of German participants. They were assumed to be giving their real views because they were led to believe a lie detector would show any dishonesty. Their motivation might have been to protect a positive image of their 'in-group'. An explanation for these findings is that when confronted with the guilt of their own group, people might turn on the 'out-group' even if in other situations it would elicit sympathy (Imhoff and Banse 2009).

While positive themes evoke empathy and reduce prejudice, and negativity might increase it, we must also consider the desire of people who have suffered to have their experience acknowledged and validated. The 2008 apology that Australian Prime Minister Rudd offered to Indigenous people and the Stolen Generations was profoundly meaningful to many Indigenous Australians. It acknowledged the trauma and injustice of taking children away from their families. Yet if the aim is to invoke empathy in the listener rather than catharsis for the speaker, there is a trade-off that needs to be considered. In our experience, this has not meant avoiding any discussion of discrimination, but rather to talk about it in the context of a challenge on which we can work on together. Of course, the development of empathy is more likely to occur as the result of an experience with the 'other' than simply receiving information.

15.10.2   Inter-group Contact

> When I walked out the gates of [my school], I felt a sense of unity. I felt closer and more in touch with other students the same age as myself. I was able to step outside of my bubble and be exposed to one of the many other cultures that contribute to our society. I felt so privileged to be able to take part in such an eye-opening event. It just goes to show how one day can change a person's life forever. It can give one more respect for others. That one day was the first layer of bricks used to build a world of peace and understanding.
>
> Things worked out better than we had expected. Everyone mixed in with each other, making the day informative while enjoyable at the same time. It was such an honour to be able to take part in such an event. If everyone in our world participated in this programme, imagine the effects on society? (Sydney High School students, quoted in Nayler 2009)

This reflection was written by students who had participated in a two-day Together for Humanity program in 2008, involving seven public and private schools. It brought together students from Christian, Jewish, Muslim and other backgrounds. The student feedback indicates the program's major impact on them. This is consistent with research in various contexts which found inter-group contact to have significant benefits in reducing prejudice (Pedersen et al. 2005).

Shifts in attitudes in some cases were also generalised from specific inter-group contact to other contexts. This was seen in the results of contact between Chinese and Australian students over 6 months in a university residence, indicating increased acceptance and knowledge of each other (Nesdale and Todd 1998). For this to happen, it is useful that, in addition to changing the way we see the other, we revise our own 'group identity', so that the way we think about the idea or word 'us' is expanded to include a wider range.

It is important to note that while inter-group contact can result in positive attitude shifts, this is not always the case: It can at times exacerbate tensions. For positive outcome, certain facilitating conditions identified by Alport (1954) must be met. These include equality between participants, avoiding competition, common goals and sanction for the contact from relevant authority figures.

It is important to ensure that inter-group activity is structured in such a way that participants become interdependent in carrying out the tasks set for them. Walker and Crogan (1998) found that if a group was asked to learn material by cooperation with each other, but there was nothing in the structure of the activity that made cooperation necessary, there was exacerbation of pre-existing tension. If the activity was, however, structured using a procedure such as the 'jigsaw' approach in which the material is divided between small groups of students who will then be required to teach what they learned to other small groups, this resulted in improved feelings toward 'out-group' peers.

An example of both the failure to implement this principle and learning from it is the case of Muslim and Jewish schools in Australia which began a four part inter-group contact-based activity which could not be completed. Teachers in both schools blamed the other school for the breakdown. Teachers of the better resourced, middle class school A saw the problem as being due to lack of commitment on the part of teachers in school B, which served a poorer community. School B teachers had another interpretation:

> When the students met and the teachers went into the staff room for some tea, the teachers of their school all congregated together and the teachers from our school were on the other side. No effort was made to bring us together.

As is often the case, the teachers were expected to develop rapport without a directed effort to do so. In 2010, school A again embarked on an inter-school project, but this time, teachers' interaction at their first meeting was structured by being given a task to do with one of their peers from the other school. At the time of writing, the activity is on track.

15.10.3 Cognitive Approaches

While experiential approaches are known to be very potent and there is a need to provide information that refutes false beliefs, there is also a role for cognitive approaches as the idea of 'reasonableness' is a significant factor in why people reject prejudice (Trang and Wittenberg 2004). The educational programs of Together for Humanity in Australia are one example that combines elements of both cognitive and experiential approaches. Nayler (2009) carried out an independent evaluation of this work. She noted the need for longitudinal research but still found evidence of educational effectiveness: 'These comments by students suggest that the (Together for Humanity) Workshop Program was very powerful in achieving its objectives to develop student appreciation for and empathy with people from diverse groups/ beliefs'.

15.11 Conclusion

The social, historical, philosophical and psychological forces that challenge positive inter-group relations are formidable. To maintain positive relations or at least minimise division requires some seemingly contradictory responses. The recognition that one's own way is not 'normal' but is just one way amongst many needs to be combined with tolerance of people who believe that their ways are the one Truth. Humility to counter our assumptions about others must not lessen our courage to challenge our own groups' self-serving narratives or offences. At the same time, this invaluable challenging of our own must not be a pre-condition for outsiders being offered a seat at our dialogue table. Honesty about the problems and fears between groups is to be restrained by compassion and tact. Realism combined with hope.

Not all of it is complicated though. A lot of it comes down to empathy, fostered by interaction, listening and respect.

Auntie B, an Indigenous woman, attended a Together for Humanity orientation session in Darwin. We sat in a circle, including the author, a Christian facilitator, an African Imam, Auntie K and others. The facilitator began with an exercise where each of us told our names and something we liked about our names relating to our heritage. Auntie told us later that week that she dreamed about the session that night. She described it in a way I could only understand as a profound religious experience. She said, "It was healing." Often, she said, she was invited to meetings and always walked away feeling like no-one was interested in her views.

Interaction, in a spirit of empathy, respect and equality, is a powerful factor in fostering positive relations between members of groups with divergent beliefs and cultures.

References

Alport, G. (1954). *The nature of prejudice*. Reading: Addison-Wesley.
Aly, W. (2007). *People like us. How arrogance is dividing Islam and the West*. Melbourne: Picador-Pan Macmillan.
Batson, C. D., Early, S., & Salvarani, G. (1997). Perspective taking: Imagining how another feels versus imagining how you would feel. *Personality and Social Psychology Bulletin, 23*, 751–758.
Batterham, D. (2001). *Modern racism, reconciliation and attributions for disadvantage: A role for empathy and false beliefs?* Paper presented at 2nd Victoria Post Graduates in Psychology Conference, Swinburne University of Technology, Melbourne.
Baz, Sheikh Abdul Aziz Ibn Abdullah Ibn. (2010). Accessed July 7, 2010, from http://www.ahya.org/amm/modules.php?name=Sectionsandop=viewarticleandartid=180

Biton, Y., & Salomon, G. (2006). Peace in the eyes of Israeli and Palestinian youths: Effects of collective narratives and peace education program. *Journal of Peace Education, 43*(2), 167–180.

Bouma, G., & Halafoff, A. (2009). Multifaith education and social inclusion in Australia. *Journal of Religious Education, 57*(3), 17–25.

Czopp, A. M. (2008). When is a compliment not a compliment? Evaluating expressions of positive stereotypes. *Journal of Experimental Social Psychology, 44*(2008), 413–420.

Donovan, R. J., & Leivers, S. (1993). Using paid advertising to modify racial stereotypes beliefs. *Public Opinion Quarterly, 57*, 205–218.

Engebretson, K. (2009). *In your shoes, interfaith education for Australian school and universities.* Ballan: Connor Court Publishing.

Feinstein, M. (1959). *Sefer Igros Moshe* (Yoreh Deah Part 3, 278). New York: self published.

Fisher, R., Ury, W., & Patton, B. (1999). *Getting to yes, negotiating agreement without giving in* (2nd ed.). Sydney: Random House.

Griffiths, B., & Pedersen, A. (2009). Prejudice and the function of attitudes relating to Muslim Australians and Indigenous Australians. *Australian Journal of Psychology, 61*, 228–238. doi:10.1080/00049530902748275.

Hamber, B. (2004). *The impact of trauma: A psychosocial approach.* Address to the A Shared Practice- Victims Work in Action Conference, Limavady, Northern Ireland. Accessed January 14, 2010, from http://www.brandonhamber.com/publication/pap-trauma1.htm

Hoffman, D. (1996). Culture and self in multicultural education: Reflections on discourse, text, and practice. *American Educational Research Journal, 33*(3), 545–569.

Imhoff, R., & Banse, R. (2009). Ongoing victim suffering increases prejudice, the case of secondary anti-semitism. *Psychological Science, 20*(12), 1443–1447.

Livyatan, I., Paran, R., & Shalif, Y. (2005). *Keshev multicultural listening and dialogue creating a protected dialogue on subjects of conflict.* Jerusalem: The State of Israel, Ministry of Education, Pedagogical Administration, Psychological Consultation Service, Division of Programs for Assistance and Prevention.

Lopez, S. J., Prosser, E. C., Edward, L. M., Magyar-Moe, J. L., Neufeld, J. E., & Rasmussen. (2005). Putting positive psychology in a multicultural context. In C. R. Snyder & S. J. Lopez (Eds.), *Handbook of positive psychology.* Oxford/New York: Oxford University Press.

Lowery, W. (2010). *Conversation with the Author.* Third World Peace Forum, Yogyakarta, Indonesia. http://southsudanfriends.org/News/Update991122.html. Accessed June 7, 2010

Mackay, H. (2007). *Advance Australia where?* Sydney: Hachette Australia.

McCohanay, J. B. (1986). *Modern Racism, ambivalence, and the modern racism scale.* In J.F. Dovidio & S. L. Gaertner (Eds.) Prejudice, discrimination and racism, (pp. 35–60). New York: Academic Press.

Mortenson, G., & Relin, D. G. (2006). *Three cups of tea.* London: Viking Penguin.

Mudzhar, M. A. (2010). *Peace education through participatory action research.* Paper presented at Third World Peace Forum, Yogyakarta, Indonesia.

Nayler, J. (2009). *Students together for humanity: Final independent evaluation report* (Together For Humanity Foundation). http://www.togetherforhumanity.org.au/resources/Final_Report_8-Jan-2009.pdf

Nesdale, D., & Todd, P. (1998). Intergroup ratio and the contact hypothesis. *Journal of Applied Social Psychology, 56*, 82–90.

Paradies, Y., Chadrakumar, L., Klocker, N., Frere, M., Webster, K., Burrel, M., & McLean, P. (2009). *Building on our strengths; a framework to reduce race based discrimination and support diversity in Victoria* (p. 26). Melbourne: Victorian Health Promotion.

Pedersen, A., Walker, I., & Wise, M. (2005). Talk does not cook rice: Beyond anti-racism rhetoric to strategies for social action. *Australian Psychologist, 40*, 20–30.

Sniderman, P., & Hagendoorn, L. (2007). *When ways of life collide, multiculturalism and its discontents in the Netherlands.* Princeton: Princeton University Press.

Trang, T., & Wittenberg, R. (2004). *Love thy neighbour, racial tolerance among young Australians.* Melbourne: Royal Melbourne Institute of Technology, for the Australian Multicultural Foundation.

Walker, I., & Crogan, M. (1998). Academic performance, prejudice, and the jigsaw classroom: New pieces to the puzzle. *Journal of Community and Applied Social Psychology, 8*, 381–393.

Wise, A. (2010). *A nation's line in the sand.* Sydney Morning Herald. http://www.smh.com.au/national/a-nations-line-in-the-sand-20100122-mqrc.html. Accessed October 10, 2010.

Rabbi Zalman Kastel was raised and ordained as a Rabbi in the Chasidic Jewish tradition in Brooklyn, New York, before migrating to Australia. Encounters and work with Christians, Muslims and Indigenous Australians have transformed him. He is Director of Together for Humanity Foundation, an inclusive, interfaith diversity education organisation.

Contact: zalman@togetherforhumanity.org.au.

Chapter 16
Conflict and Confrontation

Lois Edmund

16.1 Introduction

Conflict Resolution Studies, also called Peace Studies or Conflict Transformation Studies, is a nascent interdisciplinary field, differentiating since the early 1990s from a felicitous coalition of law, history, psychology, sociology and the human sciences. This field of scholarship claims goals of understanding the deep roots of human conflict and illuminating the dynamics of healthy and destructive conflictual relationships. It aims to extend both personal and professional methods for resolving conflict that lead to individual needs fulfilment and sustainable relationships. Although there is no definitive 'positive psychology of conflict', the developing branches of positive psychology can point toward insights that support our work in this field. In this chapter, we explore the intersection between positive psychology and conflict resolution studies.

A useful positive psychology of conflict would incorporate the following:

- Acknowledgment that no amount of positive thinking will completely eliminate conflict; rather, we need to accept and respect the endemic nature of conflict and expect that insight can assist in shaping conflict into a potentially positive force in relationships.
- Affirmation that people do use the techniques arising out of positive psychology, as well as broader spiritual-religious practices, to enhance their skills and modify their relationships to decrease the frequency, intensity and destructiveness of conflict.
- Recognition that conflict and healthy relationships can and do co-exist; conflict is normal and does not necessarily lead to dysfunctional patterns or personal harm.
- A search for positive feelings and behaviours which can mitigate the unpleasant and undesirable aspects of conflict.

L. Edmund (✉)
Conflict Resolution Studies, Menno Simons College, Winnipeg, MB, Canada
e-mail: l.edmund@uwinnipeg.ca

S. Roffey (ed.), *Positive Relationships: Evidence Based Practice across the World*, DOI 10.1007/978-94-007-2147-0_16, © Springer Science+Business Media B.V. 2012

- The cultivation of positive character traits that reinforce healthy, effective human relationships in which we tolerate or even grow and thrive under conditions of conflict.
- A distinction between healthy conflict where differences are expressed and common understanding discovered, and destructive conflict which is overly critical or hurtful, undermining power or self-esteem.
- An explanation of how healthy conflict can make a positive contribution to healthy human relationships through providing means for negotiating and balancing power and influence.
- The integration of multidisciplinary theory and research evidence which will develop effective personal and professional practices.

16.2   Exploring Conflict

A commonly used, somewhat consensual definition of conflict is proposed by William Wilmot and Joyce Hocker: 'Conflict is an expressed struggle between at least two interdependent parties who perceive incompatible goals, scarce resources, and/or interference from others in achieving personal goals'. (Wilmot and Hocker 2011:11). This definition is pragmatic because it normalizes conflict as 'struggle' which does not inevitably deteriorate into 'fight', emphasizes the interdependent relationships at the heart of conflict (Lewin 1948) and also summarizes three conspicuous causes of conflict. Relational abuse, power abuse and violence are not themselves conflict – these are ineffective ways of reacting to conflict, which perpetuate the very problems they are intended to address.

Although conflict is inherently risky, it can have strong and constructive purposes. In the best of circumstances conflict, even though intense or unpleasant, helps parties to mature, to create new perspectives. Conflict extends and expands skill capacities and, thus, transforms behaviours and relationships. The relationship that has no conflict at all is either idealistic or carelessly indifferent. The daunting tasks for all disputants are to sustain positive tactics and goals, avoiding destructive behaviour even while perturbed.

We can think about the complex roots of conflict as a simplified 'Triple P': People, Problems and Process.

16.3   People Issues

'People issues' arise from the parties themselves. People matter to each other so the relationship is worth fighting over. Issues arise out of differing needs, goals, intentions or expectations, apparent incompatibility or interference, erupting into struggles that matter. Most people find conflict deeply stressful and react with typical stress responses: fight, flight, tending others or befriending allies (Taylor 2006).

'People issues' are multifarious, rooted in intrapersonal dynamics and catalysed by interpersonal interactions. If issues are processed in the context of well meaning intention, friendly communication and reliable trust, conflict is likely to be constructive and the difficult dimensions can be tolerated.

16.3.1 Intent Is Not Effect

One core factor in 'people issues' focuses on the intentions that motivate actions. There is often a stark contrast between the intention behind an action and its results. Even in conflict, intentions can be pro-relationship: the wish to communicate about an issue or solve a problem, the hope to clarify or strengthen a bond, the desire to heal a past hurt, for instance. Intentions usually express the core values that a person has for the relationship, and these organize and motivate behavioural choices.

Positive intentions can go awry, however, and may be badly expressed, misinterpreted or poorly received. Sometimes the consequences of actions are not at all what was desired. Rather, the harmful effects of conflict are unintended: 'That's not what I meant!'; 'I was not aware that I was doing that'. Often the actor and the recipient of the actions have very different interpretations. This is complicated in that both intent and effect are intrapersonal and not usually shared or spoken, whereas actions are overt. The actor is more aware of the intent and goal than of the consequences; the recipient is aware of the sometimes hurtful results of the actions and may be completely unaware of actual positive intentions. In interpreting events and responsibility for them, we are often caught by the fundamental attributional bias (Ross 1977): actors tend to interpret their own actions to be positive and supportive of relationship; recipients, especially when hurt, are likely to interpret the actor's behaviour as intentionally malicious.

In conflict resolution, useful distinctions are between friendly and hostile intent, and between intended and unintended consequences. If actions are amicably and positively motivated, even negative or hurtful effects can be overlooked or forgiven; if actions have a hostile tone, they will escalate conflict, or the relationship may deteriorate. Conflict resolution begins with a willingness to understand actual intentions and often requires acknowledging unintended, but nonetheless hurtful, consequences of actions, even if they were positively motivated.

16.3.2 Positive Communication

Another core issue in both the development and resolution of conflict is communication. Conflicts frequently develop because people miscommunicate, misunderstand each other, communicate ineffectively or with hostility. Conflicts cannot be sustainably resolved without open communication and accurate listening to authentic concerns. On the other hand, in the context of effective speaking and listening, even hostile communication can be tolerated and need not erupt into serious conflict.

Sherod Miller and his colleagues' (1992) analysis of communication styles catalogues this core 'people' issue. Miller notes that communication is layered with shallow Shop Talk and Small Talk on the surface. Conflict is rarely part of this layer because the topic and interchange are dispassionate and usually factual, but impersonal. This surface level is enriched by nonverbal communication and also touches on playful communication, which is helpful in conflict resolution (Gottman 1999; Segal 2008). At the deepest level of intimacy is Straight Talk, a style of communication which is authentic, mutual and, when it occurs, implicitly communicates trust, care and respect. Conflict is rarely a part of this type of deeply personal interaction because of its elemental honesty and interpersonal welcome. The positive psychology virtues of courage, humanity and temperance are foundational to Straight Talk.

In conflict terms, the middle level of communication is most sensitive to misunderstanding. At this level, Control Talk and Search Talk occur. Control Talk is action oriented and its purpose is to lead or direct the recipient. If used with mutual consent, Control Talk can be benign and helpful. If used supportively, with kindness and respect, it does not cause problems or conflict. For example, employers, teachers and parents appropriately use Control Talk to teach skills; consenting employees, students and offspring benefit from the control. However, Control Talk can be potentially provocative if it is used with criticism or without consent. Then it is highly likely to cause conflict, which then spills over into Fight Talk or even Spite Talk. Fight Talk contains harsh, negative or judgmental words. Its purpose is to dominate or control others through anger or animosity, and it, therefore, often provokes conflict. Although unpleasant or intimidating, Fight Talk does accomplish communication. It can possibly lead to conflict resolution if parties are willing to hear each other's concerns and move toward solving problems identified. If the communicative element of Fight Talk is frustrated by an unwillingness to listen or solve problems, it is likely to escalate to Spite Talk, which is all-out interpersonal war. The only goal of Spite Talk is harm and humiliation, to hurt or defeat the opponent. Problems are not solved because parties have lost the point of the conflict and their interactions have deteriorated into wholly negative tactics, interactions and outcomes.

A complementary middle level communication style is Search Talk, characterized by careful exploration of personal perceptions, problems, feelings and memories. This supports knowing and understanding both self and other. It is crucial to healthy relationship and also to effective conflict processing. Its purposes are to clarify what is uncertain or ambiguous, to improve understanding and to reduce the anxieties of all parties. Using searching questions, the parties can identify and clarify issues so that resolution can move forward. When Control Talk deteriorates into Fight Talk, when Fight Talk or Spite Talk has taken over, this searching inquiry can effectively transform the negative dynamic into something that could be creative and constructive. Search Talk supports trust, which improves disclosure, defusing the controlling dynamic and opening the possibility of effective communication. Parties can then move toward deeper mutual understanding by using Straight Talk.

16.3.3 Trust and Trust-Building

A third core issue in interpersonal conflict and its resolution is trust. Trust is founded in confidence in a partner's good will or 'friendliness', shown in mutually positive actions, reliability when it counts, and predictable care and responsiveness. Although to some extent inscrutable, trust building can be a deliberated strategy. When relating with others, trustworthy people accept open disclosure without judgment, listen with warmth and reliable and accurate empathy, communicate support and unconditional acceptance that transcends disagreement or disapproval (Zimbardo et al. 2009). Trust is nourished by transparent disclosure and reciprocated openness, upholding consistent but not rigid standards, values and behaviour, and not making bad faith promises (Lewicki and Tomlinson 2003).

Interpersonal trust is fragile. When trust is slow to develop, or is betrayed, or when expectations are disappointed, conflict is one logical result. The intensity of erupting conflict is directly proportional to the initial trust and closeness (Tavris and Aronson 2007). Conflict may then fuel defensiveness, further reducing the likelihood of effective resolution (Gibb 1961). Distrust presumes hostility or malicious intent and may then be used to justify destructive behaviour (Eidelson and Eidelson 2003).

Repairing broken trust requires bilateral commitment and effort. Considerations of whether to work toward reconciliation depend on such factors as the nature of the original relationship (for example, a working versus a personal relationship), the character resources of the parties (wisdom, strength, courage) or the severity of the conflict events and history. The first step toward repair is the de-escalation of conflict. The complex and perilous process of trust repair then requires the restoration of trustworthiness on the part of a wrongdoer, and a victim's willingness to reframe and reinterpret offensive events or the character of the offender. A constructive base for effective conflict processing then produces a positive, relationship enhancing attitude, effective and friendly communication and a base of trust.

16.3.4 The Dimensions of Conflict and a Rationale for Resolution

Paul Wehr (1979) notes the necessity for effectively resolving issues while, at the same time, preserving a workable, healthy relationship. He points our discussion toward practical questions that privately determine whether people choose to engage with each other to process conflict, to overlook issues or even to end a relationship because of a conflict:

- Is the relationship important to at least one party?
- Is the issue important enough to argue over?
- Is there time pressure or stress?

If these questions are answered 'no', it is likely that the parties will at least postpone or possibly decline the difficult process of working through the conflict – they will give up. If any of the answers are 'yes' – the relationship matters, the issue is important, and/or there is a sense of urgency to resolve the conflict – the parties are more willing to engage in the struggle openly and with positive goals.

16.4 Problem Issues

'Problem issues' have to do with the focal point of a conflict. A conflict revolves around surface problems that can be easily identified as the topic of the argument, often expressed in differing opinions, viewpoints and needs. However, most conflicts are also attempts to renegotiate or resolve deeper problems of relationship history and pattern, or underlying attitudes. An argument might be about money, for example, but simultaneously address unresolved inequities in previous money decisions and also express the parties' foundational values about money.

Problem issues are enlightened by Johan Galtung's (1990) important analysis of three simultaneous and embedded conflict roots (and solutions): behaviour, structures and culture. Conflict behaviours describe the obvious, identifiably problematic issues that are conscious during a struggle: 'He said... she said...'; 'She did... he did...'. When in conflict, we tend to mirror the behaviours of the opponent. Other influences that shape conflict behaviour include high or hot emotions (especially fear and anger), frustration in goal achievement, a need for power or status, or revenge for previously unfinished conflict episodes.

Galtung's two additional layers of conflict are substratal. Structural conflict results from the ways relationships are organized, particularly when order and existing power are preserved to the detriment of those 'at the bottom'. For example, structural conflict may result from parents' over-control of money in a family, excluding teenage children from decision-making and leading to parent–teen arguments. Structural conflict is perpetuated by power and polarization – the parents 'against' the kids. Conflict then disintegrates to a simple goal of victory/power over the opponent. Sometimes, structural conflict results in certain people experiencing freedom and power, while others experience repression and powerlessness, and this inevitably results in ongoing conflict, even if it is latent and suppressed.

Conflict culture expresses attitudes, beliefs and consequent behaviour patterns that pervade a group, becoming the norm and perceived as normal. These are the values that characterize some people or groups as more or less amiable, and the attitudes actuate both conflict behaviours and structures. For example, members of some groups will react with anxiety when experiencing conflict and address conflict only indirectly or not at all; members of other groups value straightforward interaction and will address conflict with a hopeful, positive attitude. This was also referred to by Kurt Lewin (1948) as the discernible 'conflict climate' of a group, and it strongly influences the behaviour of individuals within a group.

Another important influence on group climate is the broader culture in which a group functions. Deborah Tannen's (1999) contribution was to identify Western culture as an 'argument culture'. By overemphasizing mutually exclusive concepts and positions, people tend to artificially structure conversations as contests. This tendency creates false dichotomies and polarities that can hinder thorough exploration of an issue and heighten the probability of overt conflict.

16.5 Process Issues

Process issues are determined by the ways in which the parties engage with each other when in conflict. People often believe that conflict events unfold inexorably. This is one of the 'common sense' fallacies of conflict process. There are many possible choices along the way, and successive choices during conflict can influence both process and outcome.

16.5.1 Conflict Style

It is useful to identify patterns of conflict response or style and to deliberately cultivate healthy and positive process. Individuals tend to respond with one primary style in approximately 50% of conflicts, selecting and utilizing alternative styles according to such factors as situation, the prior relationship, or the needs contributing to the conflict (Adler et al. 2006). Healthy, mature individuals are able to flexibly use all styles to improve the resolution of the issues. Prevailing Western and Eastern cultures are shaped by core values which differently emphasize the styles described below. Western individuals are more likely to rely on conflict behaviours which assert individual rights, whereas Eastern individuals are more likely to value accommodating behaviour which emphasizes group needs and harmony.

Scholarly consensus has coalesced around the articulation of five styles of behaviour that persistently affect the struggle. Although all styles are motivated to 'keep the peace' and are appropriate under specific circumstances, some are more likely to result in constructive conflict resolution. Kilmann and Thomas (1975) were the first researchers to crystallize these styles, but their work has been expanded and refined by others (e.g. Robert 1982; Gilmore and Fraleigh 1985; Rahim and Magner 1995).

Avoidance is arguably the most reactive response to conflict. Most people have experienced conflict that ended badly with unfinished problems, wounded people and damaged relationships. Therefore, many people do whatever they can to simply avoid an argument through silence or flight, often at the expense of their own wellbeing. Avoidance frustrates any possibility of a solution.

People who use **accommodation** relate by adapting their agenda to that of others. When in conflict, accommodators tend to use appeasement, processing conflict by creating harmony through self-suppression or even self-sacrifice. Such behaviours are in themselves positive and supportive of relationships and often depict maturity (Cassady and Eissa 2008). When contentious issues are hidden and never addressed, however, accommodation can block productive issue resolution.

A third style of responding to conflict is to **coerce** resolution; to force the other party or the conflict process or to use power to silence the opponent. People who use this style attend to the topic of contention at the expense of the relationship. Dominating behaviour is vigorous and assertive, but may be perceived by others to be aggressively forceful. It may provoke resistance at least and will often inflame conflict.

One party who dominates is usually a good partner to another party who accommodates. This pair engages in a symbiotic 'dance' that may meet their short-term needs for 'peace', but it is likely to be pseudo-peace. The dance is ineffective because it cannot resolve the issues, and the relationship that is preserved is amiably unhealthy.

Avoidance, accommodation and coercion patterns do quiet or suppress conflict but rarely in effective or constructive ways. Two other styles, compromise and collaboration, are much more likely to lead disputing parties toward resolution that is long lasting and productive.

Compromise is based on dialogic communication, with reciprocal listening, and assertive negotiation of needs and desires. It is, therefore, effective to simultaneously resolve an issue and maintain the relationship. Compromise is best conducted between parties of similar power, else it devolves easily into domination. The peril of compromise is that the needs or goals of each party are only partially satisfied, and each party is required to relinquish something in order to gain something, so the resolution reached may be experienced as only incompletely favourable.

In all cultures, the most effective and satisfactory conflict style uses **collaborative problem-solving**. Although this can be relatively time-consuming, it attends both to the health of the continuing relationship and also to the importance of the contentious issue. The parties who process conflict in this way mutually disclose their needs, opinions and desires and are committed to the wellbeing of the opponent. They communicate until they can identify the issue clearly and come to a common understanding of the problem when they then can consider several solutions. This provides for further processing as the solution unfolds (Walton 1987). Collaborative problem-solving is respectful of conflict parties and of their needs. It takes seriously the issue that kindled the conflict and works sincerely toward sustainable resolution.

16.5.2   Destructive and Constructive Conflict Process

Process issues are the primary factors that distinguish destructive, futile conflict from effective, creative forms. These issues are therefore often central to positive or contentious relationships. Negative, destructive conflict dynamics tend to overlook common needs or the common good, and instead centre on self-interested process and goals. Parties are querulous, tending to compound and polarize issues and people. Tactics of coercion or passive-aggression ensure costly victory. The destructive goal is to defeat the opponent rather than to settle the difficult issue. When this type of dynamic is used, it is likely to ignite reciprocal behaviours in the opponent, and this will often result in an Escalatory Cycle of conflict during which communication and collaboration decrease and strife increases. In some relationships, a heated escalation is too risky, so a commonly occurring alternative is the Chilling Cycle. When confronted, parties protect themselves by withdrawing engagement and communication. Either increased animosity or diminished engagement can be lethal to a relationship, however, because without reasonable avenues for process, the possibilities for resolution plummet. Both the escalatory and the chilling cycles are correlated with conflict futility, because at the end point neither party's needs are satisfied, the issue remains unsettled, and the future of the relationship is jeopardized (Adler et al. 2006).

Harm and damaged relationship are by no means the inevitable outcome of conflict. Constructive conflict dynamics can creatively and positively strengthen a relationship through improved understanding, broadened communication skills and greater confidence. The relationship matters and effort is invested to ensure its continuation. Conflict parties refuse to withdraw or break but do remain engaged with each other until the conflict is satisfactorily addressed. Parties are mindful and protective of the future of the relationship beyond the current struggle. At the same time, the contentious issue is important, and parties are committed to actively seek productive resolution; they are unwilling to simply give in. Conflict processing is therefore focused. Tactics and manners are cooperative; parties remain supportive of each other while asserting their own needs. The overall outcome of these dynamics is the increased possibility of finding positive, long-term resolution of the issues that satisfies everyone's needs. This outcome is sometimes called a Virtuous Cycle, wherein a positive action generates positive emotions and self-esteem that, in turn, lead to further positive actions. This cycle is correlated with effective conflict resolution for three reasons: problem issues are dealt with and resolved, the relationship is preserved, and the parties have learned and improved their skills for addressing potential conflict in the future.

Constructive conflict 'does not come easily or without struggle' (Wylie 2003). Destructive conflict is, in fact, simpler and more easily finished – but at the tragic cost of relationship and, perhaps, of self-respect. 'Pleasure and satisfaction do not come without expenditures of willpower, courage, applied intelligence, and a positive attitude which signals good character' (Wylie 2003:50).

16.5.3 The 'Good' and the 'Bad' Together

We should not assume, though, that escalation of conflict is always a negative or dangerous phenomenon. Richard Walton's research (1969, 1987) describes healthy interpersonal peacemaking as a sequential process with two broad phases of mounting and diminishing tension. Differentiation is the phase when parties lay their differences 'on the table'. This may be experienced as similar to the escalation of conflict but occurs more naturally than does heated escalation and is probably necessary for enduring resolution. During differentiation, issues and emotions proliferate and intensify. The effect of differentiation, even though it may become tense or intense, is a first step toward problem-solving. By opening issues and spending time and energy clarifying them, the parties come to a clearer understanding of the problems and, in the process, take each other more seriously. If the relationship is strong, the parties can tolerate the escalatory behaviours. One risk of differentiation is the endless drift of issues and emotions, so original problems become obscured.

At some point, one person in the conversation will recognize the critical state of tension or the loss of problem-solving momentum and initiate a turning point in the argument by inserting statements that cool emotions and shepherd parties toward negotiation.

The second conflict phase, inaugurated by the turning point, is integration. This occurs as issues and emotions become focused so that they can be sorted into central issues and lower priority ones. During integration, parties are able to decipher what is 'worth fighting for'. They find or generate common ground, explore possible options for everyone's satisfaction and move toward resolution.

Together, differentiation and integration prepare the parties for mutual, collaborative problem-solving. Conflict is dynamic and can transform in the blink of an eye. Constructive conflict therefore contributes to positive character, motivates participants to engage and to move hopefully toward solution and should inspire positive, relationship building behaviour.

16.6   Positive Conflict Behaviour

Specific patterns of conflict behaviour can be identified as healthy, constructive and likely to lead participants to a desirable resolution. All relationships must deal with negative events, differences and tensions, and these differences or conflicts per se are not indicators of health or relational impairment. In the relationships Gottman studied (1999), 69% of conflicts are not, in fact, resolved. It is the manner of engaging in conflict and what follows conflict that distinguishes partners who are able to use conflict episodes to reinforce the positive.

First, proscribed negative tactics, the so-called 'four horses of the apocalypse' inevitably lead to damaged relationships. Partners in healthy relationships tend to avoid these tactics even during conflict, whereas warring people use them frequently. The horses are: (a) criticism, which judges another party's behaviour or even character with disrespectful animosity; (b) defensiveness, which justifies our own interpretations while preventing us from hearing the truth in another person's argument; (c) stonewalling, which blocks communication and frustrates the resolution of problems; and (d) contempt, the most destructive tactic that blames and shames the other party while signalling resignation of hope for positive change.

Gottman also describes contrasting positive tactics, which move parties toward creative solutions. Healthy, stable partners tend to couch critique within the positive – they use a ratio of as many as 20 positive affirmations to one negative, or as few as five positive to one negative. Unstable, jeopardized relationship partners (Gottman calls them 'Masters of Disaster') favour negative feedback by a ratio of one positive to five negative.

What follows the end of a conflict episode is crucial. Partners who are able to use conflict constructively are those who offer and accept relational repairs after the conflict is over. These overtures reach out to the other party with care that overrides discord, using tactics such as apology, humour, empathy and overt expressions of affection.

Other research adds to this finding, using the concept of emotional contagion. Emotional contagion seems to parallel disease contagion: feelings spread from one individual to another, so that the recipients begin to feel emotions that are not truly their own. Gustave LeBon (1896) suggested that the emotions which are particularly susceptible to contagion are those based in survival: fear and self-protective anger. These emotions are pointedly generative of conflict. There is a positive dimension of contagion, however, which can create a 'Cooperative Cycle', a positive counterpart to the escalatory and chilling cycles discussed above. Rooted in interpersonal empathy or even sympathy, positive behaviours such as cooperation and kindness also spread. 'Cooperative behaviour is contagious and spreads from person to person to person' (Fowler and Christakis 2010). When a person receives a significant kindness such as a relational repair, they are more likely to be generous and offer others kindness. The next person then does the same thing, and the positive momentum of kindness spreads. So, because of emotional contagion, when the parties to a conflict use negative tactics such as the 'four horses', this can unnecessarily escalate a conflict. When the parties are able to offer amicable interactions, relational repairs or kindness, this is likely to be reciprocated with positive, constructive responses that can contribute to positive feelings toward the opponent, even during conflict.

16.7 Complimentary Continua of Conflict and Peace

When does struggle become conflict? At what point does conflict become fight or lead to interpersonal war? Alternatively, how can conflict or contention be transformed into something positive and creative? As we explore the dynamic elements of conflict, we are reminded that conflict actually occurs on a continuum of intensity and valence. Some conflict such as that motivated by rage or hatred is extreme, out of control and very dangerous to all participants. Some conflict is based on differences in participants' points of view or personal factors such as gender or culture and, if occurring in a context of respect and appreciation, can actually enrich the parties. This type of conflict can be intriguing and positive. In fact, relationships that exhibit a neutralized absence of conflict are likely to be apathetic and unmotivating.

The goal of all conflict is authentic, appreciative peace. Johan Galtung's (1990) discussion of 'negative peace' and 'positive peace' provides important insight. Negative peace is the simple absence of overt conflict. Although not undesirable, negative peace does not imply actual relationship: conflict can be suppressed by the use of power or privilege; it can be silenced by force; conflicting parties can be prohibited from contacting each other. Although these strategies may well diminish the stark destruction of hostility, they do little to address the reasons the conflict arose in the first place. For this reason, negative peace is 'pseudo-peace'. Galtung notes that positive peace is the actual goal of all conflict, and especially that of conflict in a healthy relationship. Disputants do not overlook the causes of conflict, but come to an agreement on how to develop an equitable relationship that satisfies all parties' needs, thus obviating conflict. Positive peace rests on good will, harmony, justice and order, qualities supported by positive psychology.

16.8 Positive Conflict Transformation and Peace-Building

Relational and collective conflict transformation and positive peace-building are undertakings with concurrent and integrative pathways. Peace-building is a long-term, creative, growth task. Conflict resolution is always emotional, personal and costly unless it is accomplished superficially, in which case it is not resolution at all. Peace-building focuses on strengths and positive commitments to overcome, transcend or transform negative events and feelings. Positive peace-building involves any activity which fosters understanding among disputants and can even reconstruct relationships broken by past conflict.

Joseph Bock (2001) outlines four types of peace-building which are used at sequential stages in a conflict. **Promotive peace-building** is quiet, unobtrusive relationship promotion. This may occur, for example, between parties who might commonly be perceived to be enemies such as divorcing couples or gang and community members. Relationship and joint activities are used to indirectly bridge differences and distance. **Preventive peace-building** is somewhat more deliberated and occurs specifically in situations where enmity has begun but constructive dialogue is still feasible. The focus is issue dialogue and relationship exploration in the hope of finding common ground for understanding and action, thus preventing the release of negative feelings. **Pre-emptive peace-building** occurs when a conflict is ripe but has not yet erupted to become overt. Peace and restraint are called for, along with cautions that the issues require attention if conflict is to be warded off. This is immediate, short-term crisis prevention which rises out of a sense that struggle is about to become heated. **Reparative peace-building** occurs at the end point of a destructive conflict and involves rebuilding, repairing and reconciling the brokenness caused by conflict. Reparative peace-building is not always possible if the relationship is sufficiently damaged to inhibit repair.

Deeply positive conflict process is built on virtues, strengths and a commitment to positive feelings and correlated with safety, prosperity, wellbeing and health. Positive peace-building therefore goes much further than the simple cessation of conflict to emphasize the creation of relationships characterized by cooperation, friendly interactions and generosity of spirit.

If conflict can be constructive or even catalytic, then the task is not how to rid ourselves of conflict, but 'what personal abilities, strengths and potentials within our nature can we draw on to create the good life' – in other words, positive dynamics (Wylie 2003:51). Here, practical work in positive psychology effectively explores ways to reinforce the individual and collective resilience required to persist with conflict until it reaches actual resolution.

16.9   Positive Emotional Skills

Barbara Fredrickson (2001) observes that positive emotions serve not only to build relationship but also to improve an individual's social resources. Positive emotions work as a buffer against negativity, shoring up resilience and expanding strategies for coping with difficult challenges. As the repertoire of potential solutions increases, so does the capacity for problem-solving. This theory would predict that as conflicts are constructively resolved, individuals and relationships become stronger so that future arguments are more quickly and satisfactorily resolved, and individuals are able to meet their needs well (also Rummel 1991).

Naomi Greenspan (2004) distinguishes two elemental forms of emotion, which she calls light emotions – pleasant, subjectively desirable feelings such as gratitude, joy and faith – and more negative dark emotions – subjectively unpleasant, painful feelings such as grief, fear or despair which signal vulnerability. To be healthy, we need to experience an authentic mixture of both light and dark. Either excessive darkness (pain) or excessive lightness (happiness) leads to perceptual distortion. If we are unable to tolerate both light and dark emotions, we suppress or deny them, and they are transformed into toxic emotions, expressed in reactivity, pathology and collective destructiveness. The toxic process poisons individual and collective wellbeing and also contributes to the likelihood of conflict. Greenspan suggests that we must relearn to accept all feelings, in both light and dark manifestations, to restore wholeness of being and understand ourselves and our world. Greenspan's approach would encourage all conflict participants to be authentic emotionally, trusting their inherent wisdom to guide actions toward constructive patterns. Balanced feelings can without doubt guide, heal and transform. Her practical 'Three Skills' – attend with mindfulness to all feelings, befriend them and surrender the dark manifestations – are useful when learning how to process conflict constructively. The positive, lighter feelings, but the darker ones, each have their own 'reasoning' and are essential to actualization of the goals of conflict.

Greenspan's work focuses the broader foundation of 'emotional intelligence' (EI), the insight articulated by Daniel Goleman (1995). EI describes the ability to identify, assess and manage one's own emotions and those of others. These abilities are manifest in Goleman's four fundamental competencies: self-awareness, social awareness, self-management and relationship management (Goleman 2000). Each of these learned competencies supports healthy relationship functioning, particularly when in conflict. Individuals with high EI show empathic understanding of the deeper, potent content of a dialogue. Given an accurate understanding of the heart of a conflict in the context of a valued relationship, resolution is facilitated through skills based on EI. Individuals with high EI consistently prefer to use collaborative means to reach solutions (Jordan and Troth 2002). In addition to positive receptive and expressive communication skills, key EI abilities that support conflict processing include effective personal stress relief and emotional awareness (Segal 2008). This suite of skills reinforces the insight and patience needed to process conflict carefully without resorting to the use of destructive tactics.

16.10   An Environment Which Cultivates Positive Conflict Resolution

Virtues and inner strengths protect against the subjective negativity of conflict, contributing to both individual and relational resilience. 'Our strengths are our best protections... this buffers us against our weaknesses' (Seligman in Wylie 2003). Signature strengths which support constructive conflict processing are hope and optimism, justice and temperance, wisdom, courage, humanity and transcendence.

These positive character strengths and associated behaviours can be taught and refined through numerous methods (Decety and Meyer 2008; Keysers and Gazzola 2009). No matter where we start, someone will benefit. Martin Seligman (in Wylie 2003) describes the development and intervention challenges:

(a) To teach optimism, gratitude, forgiveness;
(b) To 'develop character, positive emotion and strengths, completely independent of alleviating problems' and
(c) To 'recraft what we are doing to better use our strengths', and to 'help people identify what they are really good at...' (Wylie 2003).

Development and growth take place naturally in both informal and formal settings, and character strengths correlate with age, maturity and experienced challenges. This implies that all conflict can be instructive, though not all lessons learned will be positive. The best learning is connected with real experiences where learners can work through conflict to recognize and appreciate the positive dimensions of a relationship and experience hope about resolution. Positive psychology suggests that optimal learning occurs in a context of enjoyment and success, engagement and meaningful exploration, using varied pedagogic methods. An effective learning environment is integrated and interwoven, offering learners repeating opportunities to explore and experiment with their emotional and conflict experiences, reactions and skills. Learning is enhanced with interest, respect and affection, and students become engaged and active and belong. Facilitators have specific expectations of learners, but also provide an accepting, supportive environment.

16.11   Conclusions

Conflict is an intrinsic part of every relationship, and many aspects have been covered in this chapter. The following common themes have emerged.

Conflict is not necessarily unhealthy or destructive but, under optimal circumstances, the dynamics of conflict can be constructive and catalytic of self-knowledge and strengthened relationship. Conflict does not need to be avoided.

Conflict is normal even in healthy relationships and does not threaten strong relationships. When tolerated and processed openly, conflict can support interpersonal growth.

Specific conflict resolution behaviours occur within the context of a broader interpersonal tone and history and are interpreted in light of that context. This crucially affects the impact of specific behaviour.

Specific patterns can protect against the unpleasant and undesirable aspects of conflict. The positive, active behaviours explored in this chapter are:

- Maintaining a positive, friendly intent.
- Acknowledging that the effects of actions may not be congruent with the intent.
- Communication is helpful when it includes surface talk, authentic mutual disclosure and searching inquiry, but minimizes non-consensual dominance, critical fighting and spiteful interpersonal war.
- Respect for the fragility of trust, along with a commitment to build, sustain and repair trust through trustworthiness.
- A hopeful attitude toward conflict does not attempt to eliminate it through avoidance, self-sacrificial accommodation, coercion or futile compromise, but does maximize collaborative problem-solving which acknowledges the presence of a problem and also works to preserve the relationship.
- A commitment to positive, active peace-building which generates a healthy relationship, uses emotional skill and maturity and relies on personal and group resilience.

Positive virtues or character traits support effective conflict resolution and can be cultivated through informal and formal experimentation, personal reflection and relationship transformation.

Multidisciplinary theory and research evidence confirms that conflict can be healthy and constructive.

Future directions for the Positive Psychology of Conflict Resolution scholarship are merely suggested in this chapter and must be explored elsewhere. These include broadened use of scientific assessment of conflict dynamics, sources and roots of conflict, and also of positively influential resolution and intervention techniques, research on organizational structures which support positive conflict resolution, and developing and testing effective professional practices in the arena of international conflict and diplomacy.

References

Adler, R. B., Rosenfeld, L. B., Proctor, R. F., II, & Winder, C. (2006). *Interplay: The process of interpersonal communication.* Don Mills: Oxford.

Bock, J. G. (2001). *Sharpening conflict management.* Westport: Praeger.

Cassady, J. C., & Eissa, M. A. (Eds.). (2008). *Emotional intelligence: Perspectives on educational and positive psychology.* New York: Peter Lang.

Decety, J., & Meyer, M. (2008). From emotion resonance to empathic understanding: A social developmental neuroscience account. *Development and Psychopathology, 20,* 1053–1080.

Eidelson, R. J., & Eidelson, J. I. (2003). Dangerous ideas: Five beliefs that propel groups toward conflict. *American Psychologist, 58*(3), 182–192.

Fowler, J. H., & Christakis, N. A. (2010). Cooperative behavior cascades in human social networks. *Procedings of the National Academy of Science, 10*(12), 5334–5338.

Frederickson, B. L. (2001). The role of positive emotions in positive psychology. *American Psychologist, 56*(3), 218–226.

Galtung, J. (1990). Cultural violence. *Journal of Peace Research, 27*(3), 291–305.

Gibb, J. R. (1961). Defensive communication. *Journal of Communication, 11*(3), 141–148.

Gilmore, S. K., & Fraleigh, P. W. (1985). *Communication at work*. Eugene: Friendly.

Goleman, D. (1995). *Emotional intelligence*. New York: Bantam.

Goleman, D. (2000). An EI-based theory of performance. In D. Goleman & C. Cherniss (Eds.), *The emotionally intelligent workplace*. San Francisco: Jossey-Bass.

Gottman, J. (1999). *The marriage clinic: A scientifically based marital therapy*. New York: WW Norton.

Greenspan, N. (2004). *Healing through the dark emotions: The wisdom of grief, fear and despair*. Boston: Shambala.

Jordan, P. J., & Troth, A. C. (2002). Emotional intelligence and conflict resolution: Implications for human resource development. *Advances in Developing Human Resources, 4*(1), 62–79.

Keysers, C., & Gazzola, V. (2009). Expanding the mirror: Vicarious activity for actions, emotions and sensations. *Current Opinions in Neurobiology., 19*, 1–6.

Kilmann, R., & Thomas, K. W. (1975). Interpersonal conflict handling behaviour as reflections of Jungian personality dimensions. *Psychological Reports, 37*, 971–980.

LeBon, G. (1896). *The crowd: Study of the popular mind*. Released 1996 by Project Gutenberg.

Lewicki, R. J., & Tomlinson, E. C. (2003). Trust and trust building. In G. Burgess & H. Burgess (Eds.), *Beyond intractability*. Boulder: Conflict Research Consortium. http://www.beyondintractability.org/essay/trust_building/

Lewin, K. (1948). Resolving social conflict: Selected papers on group dynamics. In G. W. Lewin (Ed.), *Resolving social conflict*. New York: Harper and Row.

Miller, S., Wackman, D., Nunnally, E., & Miller, P. (1992). *Connecting*. Evergreen: Interpersonal Communication Programs.

Rahim, M. A., & Magner, N. R. (1995). Confirmatory factor analysis of the styles of handling interpersonal conflict: First order factor model and its invariance across groups. *Journal of Applied Psychology, 80*, 122–132.

Robert, M. (1982). *Managing conflict from the inside out*. Austin: Learning Concepts.

Ross, L. (1977). The intuitive psychologist and his shortcomings: Distortions in the attribution process. In L. Berkowitz (Ed.), *Advances in experimental social psychology* (Vol. 10, pp. 173–220). New York: Academic.

Rummel, R. J. (1991). *The conflict helix: Principles, practices of interpersonal, social and international conflict and cooperation*. New Brunswick: Transaction.

Segal, J. (2008). *The language of emotional intelligence: The five essential tools for building powerful and effective relationships*. New York: McGraw-Hill.

Tannen, D. (1999). *Argument culture*. New York: Random.

Tavris, C., & Aronson, E. (2007). *Mistakes were made, but not by me*. Orlando: Harcourt.

Taylor, S. E. (2006). *Tend and befriend: Biobehavioral bases of affiliation under stress*. Sage: Association for Psychological Science, Current Directions in Psychological Science series.

Walton, R. E. (1969). *Interpersonal peacemaking: Confrontation and third party consultation*. Reading: Addison Wesley.

Walton, R. E. (1987). *Managing conflict: Interpersonal dialogue and peacemaking*. Reading: Addison-Wesley.

Wehr, P. (1979). *Conflict regulation*. Boulder: Westview.

Wilmot, W., & Hocker, J. (2011). *Interpersonal conflict*. New York: McGraw-Hill.

Wylie, M. S. (2003). Why is this man smiling? *Psychotherapy Networker, 27*(1), 46–51.

Zimbardo, P., Johnson, R. L., & McCann, V. (2009). *Psychology: Core concepts*. New York: Pearson.

Lois Edmund is Assistant Professor, Conflict Resolution Studies at Menno Simons College, Winnipeg, Manitoba, and Book Reviews Editor of *Peace Research Journal*. Contact: l.edmund@uwinnipeg.ca

Chapter 17
The Repair and Restoration of Relationships

Peta Blood

17.1 Introduction

Conflict is an inevitable part of life and can occur in any setting. At times conflict can present positive opportunities for growth and learning, whilst at other times it can have destructive outcomes. Recognising the signs of conflict and developing the skills to repair harm in the aftermath of conflict and wrongdoing are essential for families, schools, organisations and communities. Conflict can take an emotional toll on those involved and needs to be managed in a way that the dignity and wellbeing of those involved can be restored. It also requires that the responsible parties take accountability for their part in the incident and ensure that they take action to make amends. Restorative justice offers much hope in this regard.

Restorative justice and the range of restorative practices have been found to effectively manage this process in a way that meets the needs of those involved. Working *restoratively* to resolve conflict means looking at the resultant harm and how to assist those who have been impacted to deal with this. Whilst some models of conflict resolution might seek to put aside emotions in the conflict resolution process, restorative justice seeks to work with the emotional impact. It does this by starting from the premise that people are often significantly affected by what has happened. The venting of emotion in a safe forum can assist those involved to shift from the negative range of affect and operate more in the positive range of emotions. Emotional wellbeing is enhanced through the appropriate expression of emotion, building understanding of what has happened and creating closure in order to move on. As such, restorative practices can operationalise aspects of positive psychology by turning a traumatic event into one for growth and healing. This chapter will

P. Blood (✉)
Restorative Practices International (RPI Circle Speak), Sydney, Australia
e-mail: peta@circlespeak.com.au

S. Roffey (ed.), *Positive Relationships: Evidence Based Practice across the World*,   277
DOI 10.1007/978-94-007-2147-0_17, © Springer Science+Business Media B.V. 2012

outline how restorative practices have been adopted in various settings to make a difference when conflict, crime and wrongdoing have affected others.

17.2   The History of Restorative Justice Developments

Working restoratively is a way of approaching harm, conflict and wrongdoing in schools, families, workplaces and communities. Restorative justice emerged in the 1970s as a response to the failings of the retributive system of justice and rehabilitation models of the day (Lemonne 2003). Primary to this push were the need to prevent the re-victimisation of victims through the judicial process and to involve community in the repair of harm. This contributed to the development of alternate conflict resolution strategies designed to be responsive to the needs of those involved (Lemonne 2003).

Various authors have charted the development of restorative justice and commented on the diverse roots of this work. Hopkins (2009) refers to four strands of practice development that contributed to the gradual emergence of restorative justice around the world. The first of these involved victim-offender mediation initiated by the Mennonites in the mid-1970s, a practice pivotal in the development of the restorative justice movement. Victim-offender mediation offered victims a say in how offenders could take responsibility for their actions and to make amends for what they had done. This gave victims a voice and held offenders to account rather than locking them away from the very people they had harmed. Another strand involved the First Nations people of Canada and the development of sentencing circles. These built on traditional communitarian processes to bring members of the community together with the judiciary to determine the most appropriate sentence for a crime involving one of their own. Sentencing circles enabled those who had a stake in the matter to be involved in determining what needed to happen to repair the harm done by a member of their community.

Circles have since developed to repair harm, reintegrate wrongdoers into community and as part of the judicial process for sentencing and pre-release. In the 1980s, the Maori people of New Zealand were working through a similar process, resulting in the development of Family Group Conferencing (FGC) as the first legislated model to deal with young offending in a restorative manner. Like the First Nations people of Canada, this built on a long tradition of indigenous collaborative problem-solving practices (Hopkins 2009). Since this time, there has been a proliferation of practice emanating from New Zealand, Australia and North America.

The term restorative justice is now used interchangeably with terms such as restorative approaches, restorative measures and restorative practices, dependent on the setting in which it is applied. The term 'restorative practices' was first adopted by Australian practitioners working in schools. This distinguished practice from the justice setting and acknowledged the existence of a range of informal and formal practices. These ranged from a formal conference to deal with suspension and expulsion through to informal restorative conversations to deal with low-level conflict and disruption. Rather than see a restorative approach as just an alternate method of discipline or conflict resolution, practice was diversified to look at ways to strengthen relationships across the school community. Likewise, Canadian practitioners refer to restorative measures in schools, whilst Scottish and British practitioners refer to a range of restorative approaches.

Whilst still an emerging field, there is a diverse range of practice that includes circles, victim-offender mediation and conferencing. Practice varies in terms of who attends, who facilitates the process and the reason that people have been brought together. Restorative justice provides flexibility for adaptation to different contexts and cultural settings. Common names attributed to conferencing include: Family Group Conferencing (FGC), Family Group Decision Making (FGDM) and Community Accountability Conferencing (CAC). Conferences vary in terms of whether they are scripted as in the case of the Australian CAC model and whether participants have private time for deliberation as in the case of FGC and FGDM. Today, FGC is commonly practised in the juvenile justice sector. FGDM is more evident in care and protection and family matters, whilst the scripted model of conferencing is synonymous with the educational sector. Practice has been further developed to include a range of informal to formal practices that are used in schools, workplaces and residential settings. These will be explained in more detail later.

17.3   Definition

Restorative justice offers an alternate response to crime and wrongdoing, starting from the premise that when crime or wrongdoing has occurred, people have been affected and that someone will have obligations to repair that harm (Zehr 2002). Whilst a clear definition of restorative justice is yet to be agreed on, Zehr's (2002) pillars of restorative justice form the elements of most working definitions. These are:

1. Establishing who has been harmed and what their needs are
2. Determining who has an obligation to repair that harm
3. Engaging key stakeholders in the matter

Restorative processes built around these pillars take into account the ripple effect of harm by seeking to involve all who have a stake in the matter. This could be in terms of the impact on them or their loved ones, or that they were somehow involved. In a restorative frame, these people are critical to the process. An example in a school situation occurs when a student is sent from the classroom for disciplinary reasons. Often they are dealt with in isolation and then returned to the classroom. The teacher and other students may still be annoyed with them, whilst others may still expect the errant student to behave in a certain way. In this instance, the teacher and the other students are key stakeholders in the process. Unless they are included or involved in some way, they may maintain their view of the wrongdoer or carry unresolved emotional issues triggered by the incident. For the student at the centre of the issue, they walk back in carrying their feelings about what happened without the opportunity to make amends. The pattern of behaviour is likely to continue.

In a restorative frame, the student would be called to account for their behaviour and be provided with the opportunity to acknowledge the harm, hear how it has affected others and together look at what needs to happen to repair the harm and move forwards. This requires a paradigm shift in the way institutions and communities respond to crime and wrongdoing, or a shift in hearts and minds.

Restorative justice moves from the traditional punitive systems of discipline and justice to one that is responsive to the needs of those involved and less dependent on the state (Lemonne 2003; Zehr 1990). Pranis et al. (2003), in describing the practice of circles, articulate this as shifting from:

1. Coercion to healing
2. Individual to collective
3. State dependence to self-reliance within community
4. Punishment to healing and a renewed sense of justice

Braithwaite (2003) describes this as a victim-centred process focused on the repair of harm, as opposed to the retributive or formal justice system, which is offender oriented and focused on punishment, blame and stigmatisation. In the traditional system, crime and wrongdoing is seen more as an offence against the state as the judicial process seeks to determine what law has been broken, who is to blame and how they will be punished. At sentencing time, the offender is given an opportunity to put forward a case for mitigating the circumstances of their crime and reducing the penalty imposed on them, i.e. 'I was intoxicated at the time and not in control of what I did'.

Despite numerous criminal justice reforms, the victim's voice still struggles to get heard. Helen Garner's (2004) portrayal of the death of Joe Cinque is a case in point. At the centre of the court process are two offenders who were responsible for Joe's premeditated death. Throughout Garner's description of the respective court cases, the question lingers 'But what about the victim, Joe?' Whilst the offenders and the offenders' families have a voice in the process, the victim and the victim's families are absent except on the occasion when their anger, rage and distress spills over into the court. What they desire throughout the case is a chance to say who the victim was to them and for the offenders and the court to hear who they took away. Alternatively, in the documentary *Facing the Demons* (Ziegler 1999), which tracks the family of 18-year-old Michael Marslew (killed in a botched armed robbery on a takeaway food outlet) confronting two of the four offenders responsible for Michael's death, the family thank the offenders for the opportunity to humanise the victim and to say what he meant to them as a coworker, as a friend and as a son. Follow-up interviews with the family and friends show how this had let them get on with their lives. This included the father of Michael going on to work with Karl, one of the offenders, to help young people not get into trouble.

Despite changes and moves to offer more restorative processes, the traditional court system is still impersonal, state oriented and overly offender focused. In many ways, the early kings of England have much to answer for, by taking away the right of communities to deal with wrongdoing within their own community and making it their business to be the punisher, often in barbaric and publicly humiliating ways. Prior to this, if you stole a pig from your neighbour, your community would call on you to repay the neighbour in a way that replaced the food or breeding stock that you stole. In order to do this, you may labour for your neighbour, you may give him an animal of yours or find a way to address that wrong. From a sociological perspective, the responsibility for crime and wrongdoing was taken out of the hands of the very communities affected by that crime and put in the hands of some authoritarian figure or institution. Since this time, we have continued to see the professionalisation of crime and wellbeing as we rely on others to take care of our needs and to deal with society's deviance – a by-product of the industrialised world.

As the Cinque and Marslew cases highlight and Zehr (2002) affirms, crime is a personal violation of people and their rights. When someone's home is broken into, it is a violation of their property and their personal space. Secondary to this, it might be seen as an offence against the good order of the state, there to protect its people. Restorative justice is about taking care of the needs of those involved in crime, conflict and disruption and the roles of those responsible to repair that harm. As Moroney (2010) states, the prison system locks offenders away from society, where they are not forced to face the damage that they have done. Victims and their loved ones and the families of the offenders are left to face the community, often with devastating effects. Restorative justice is inclusive in an effort to address the ripple effect of harm by taking into account that crime often affects many people. More often than not, those who are important in the lives of those directly involved are also affected, even if only out of concern for their loved ones or because they too have been impacted by what has happened. Communities need to pay attention to the needs and concerns of victims and the roles that offenders/wrongdoers have in meeting the needs of those involved (Zehr 2002). To not do this leaves people in precarious places having to deal with the impact on their lives in their own way or to seek professional help.

17.4   How Does Restorative Justice Work?

Whilst debate exists as to what types of interventions constitute effective healing, it is generally accepted that helping those involved to tell their story is a significant part of the process. It allows for the integration of what happened (the version of events) with the impact this has had at an emotive level. As Yoder (2005) indicates 'acknowledging and telling the story counteracts the isolation, silence, fear, shame, or "unspeakable" horror' of the event (p. 53). Restorative practices allow those involved to share their version of what happened and the impact this had on them.

In the aftermath of conflict and trauma, people initially go through a process of trying to make sense of what has happened. Yoder (2005) indicates that this happens automatically as those involved try to come to terms with the preceding event in the immediate aftermath. With time, the process unfolds for those involved making sense of their life or their view of the world and how that has been affected. Conflict itself can result in major upheaval that can have destructive consequences for those involved or constructive consequences when people are able to make sense of what happened, to learn from it and to move on. How the traumatic event is interpreted and integrated is crucial to a person's accurate sense of self and their view of the world. This is no more evident than in the 2010 BP Oil disaster in the Gulf of Mexico where the damage to the environment and to the livelihoods of those working on the coastline is likely to continue for many years to come. The human victims need acknowledgement of the harm done to their livelihoods and to their communities, and they need to see that those responsible are called to account and make amends.

The restorative justice philosophy is about valuing relationships and understanding the needs of those involved. This addresses the emotional or *affective* needs as well as a primal need to belong, which works across cultural boundaries. As Zehr and Mika (2003) state 'restorative justice is a continuum of responses to the range of needs and harms experienced by victims, offenders and the community' (p. 41). The author's own experience of working with those harmed and those affected is that their needs mirror the process that Yoder outlines and that their needs are ultimately similar. In the face of having done harm or been harmed, people need to:

- Have their say
- Be heard
- To understand and be understood
- Make sense of what happened
- Know that what happened was not fair or was not intended
- Have time out/space to reflect (perhaps talk to a trusted other)
- Make amends
- Feel OK with self and OK with others
- Repair relationships

When these needs are met, this helps bring a sense of closure and restore a sense of wellbeing for all involved. In the case of those responsible, this amounts to having a chance to make amends and restore their place in community.

Take for instance a family conflict involving Kathy, who is the victim of childhood abuse. After being steadily groomed by her perpetrator, Kathy went on to marry the offender, not knowing that anything was wrong with the initial covert relationship. After the marriage dissolved a few years later, Kathy realised what had happened to her was abuse and took steps to ensure the offender was appropriately dealt with and punished for his wrongdoing. Whilst sexual abuse is a serious issue, related conflict emerged in Kathy's family as her parents and siblings struggled to manage how they felt about what had happened. There were those that felt that justice had been served and Kathy ought to get over it and not speak about this horrendous shame. Kathy's mother refused to talk about it, whilst her father would get angry if the topic was raised. Her siblings aligned themselves accordingly. Kathy, whilst she felt that justice had been served through the court, needed her family to understand the impact this had had on her and that she was still being punished by her family for having spoken the truth. What is clear is that conflict and trauma can have far reaching impact on others, and they need to be involved in processes to bring about extended healing.

17.5   Affect and Script Psychology (ASP)

The success of restorative justice processes is that they work at a deep level to repair emotional harm. Silvan Tomkins' (1962, 1963) Affect and Script Psychology (ASP) has much to offer in understanding the biological roots of emotions and how restorative justice helps in trauma recovery. This is something that has been understated in the commentary about the effectiveness of restorative justice, despite victim satisfaction being one of the most commonly used measures to determine a successful restorative process. Much of the debate instead focuses on whether restorative justice reduces re-offending, which was not the original intent of the process.

Tomkins described nine core affects or patterns of response that are innate to human beings. These fall on a continuum from positive to negative and include the neutral affect of *surprise-startle*. On the positive end of the continuum is the affect of *enjoyment-joy* and *interest-excitement* which generally feel good. On the negative end of the continuum, we experience six uncomfortable forms of affect on a range from *anger-rage, fear-terror, distress-anguish, disgust, dismell* and *shame-humiliation*. Negative affect feels unbearable, and we are moved to find ways to feel better or to neutralise the pain. The neutral affect of *surprise-startle* is the affect that merely resets the system. When affect is said to be triggered, it is taken to mean that a 'known pattern of biological events' has been set in train (Nathanson 1992: 49). For this to occur, there must be a stimulus that triggers the affect. For example, the little known affect of *dismell* is a sensory smell response triggered by an offensive odour, or, more commonly in the modern world, is seen as the rejection of something without sampling, as in the case of racism. As an affect is triggered, we take notice and start to ascribe feelings or emotions to that sense. When people are affected by conflict and trauma, they may experience any or all negative affects. It can be difficult to work through this. Help may be needed to return to a state of wellbeing and positive affect.

Understanding the biological aspects of emotionality is crucial to understanding the range of affect triggered in situations of conflict and upheaval and how to work with it. Tomkins (1962, 1963) said that learning how to read affect in the faces of others can assist with understanding what is happening for them. This assists us to see a situation from a different perspective and adapt our approach to dealing with it, thereby becoming smarter about conflict management. Roth and Newman (1992) indicate that one of the challenges in working with those who have been traumatised is to help them shift from preoccupation with the trauma to finding an adaptive resolution to the negative affect of 'helplessness, rage, fear, loss, shame, and guilt' (p. 221). Of these affects, shame will be explored in depth to understand what happens for people caught in the conflict cycle and how we can assist those involved to deal effectively with what has happened. As Tomkins (1962, 1963) controversially stated, shame is the negative affect that precedes all other negative affect. In learning more about ASP, it is clear that Tomkins saw shame as a warning sign that something is wrong and that corrective action needs to be taken. At the same time, it is relatively easy to see how offenders carry shame for their actions, how some victims feel shame in terms of what happened and how their loved ones also carry shame about what happened. This is especially so for the families and friends of wrongdoers. Regardless of how people view the significance of Tomkin's work, it is important in understanding how restorative practices work at a deep emotive level.

17.6   Kelly's Blueprint for Healthy Relationships

Human beings have a primary need for healthy attachments with others they can rely on in times of need (Kelly 2009). A sense of secure attachment allows us to function at an optimum level, feel safe and have a positive view of self and others. Shaver and Mikulincer (2009: 447) state: 'This pervasive sense of security based on implicit beliefs that the world is generally safe, that attachment figures are helpful when called upon, and that it is possible to explore the environment curiously and engage effectively and enjoyably with other people. This sense of security is rooted in positive mental representations of self and others'.

In order to maintain healthy relationships, we need to manage our emotional wellbeing. Kelly (2009) describes a central blueprint for relationships in which the following four rules must work in tandem: We need to maximise positive affect, minimise negative affect, minimise the inhibition of our affect and maximise our ability to do all three. The mental and emotional wellbeing of human beings in relationship with each other is maintained when the blueprint is maintained. Kelly (2009) states that: 'When circumstances in our lives hinder our ability to follow these rules and we either have to ignore one of them completely or overemphasize one at the expense of the others, there is significant reduction in the quality of our lives and our relationships' (p. 24).

This can be difficult to achieve when cultural norms dictate how emotion can be expressed, with the minimisation of negative emotion encouraged in some cultures, particularly around death and dying. To express how we feel about the loss of someone or how an event has been triggered can be a shame-evoking experience in itself. I recall a situation in my police forensic career of being ridiculed by another forensic operative, when several colleagues had experienced a stress response in reaction to a series of traumatic incidents and high workload without sufficient support or rest. The same operative managed his own stress through drinking and being difficult to work with. By ridiculing another, he could effectively distance how he felt about his own workload and in some way feel better about himself by denying his own stress levels. By not getting in touch with his own issues, he can feel temporarily better about himself.

17.7   Why Is Shame Important to Understand?

Kaufman (1993) states that 'to feel shame is to feel *seen* in a painfully diminished sense. Shame reveals the inner self, exposing it to view. The self feels exposed both to itself and to anyone else present. ... it is an entirely inner experience' (p. 17). Shame stops someone feeling good about themselves or others. If people do not have the capacity or processes for dealing with their shame and the punishing feelings associated with this, they potentially alienate themselves from others, withdraw, attack themselves or attack others. At its worst, people who experience shame (which we all do) may do all four (Nathanson 1992). When we become aware that we have done something to harm another, we are likely to experience shame and not feel good about ourselves or our actions. Likewise, when we have been harmed by another's actions, we too experience shame, as our relationships with others change and our sense of self-worth is shaken.

Shame is a normal part of the human experience and is innate to human beings (Nathanson 1992). It is difficult to talk about and often a part of an experience that most seek to disown. Shame feels uncomfortable and we will do anything to avoid it. We may run away from these uncomfortable feelings and in turn withdraw from the relationships around us, often at great cost to the self and others, or we may adopt a confrontational style to avoid how bad we feel. Take for example finding out that a partner is unfaithful. Not only can this event derail the relationship but also both parties are likely to feel a sense of shame in the aftermath of this issue being exposed. The partner who had the affair is likely to feel ashamed of what they have done, whilst the other partner is likely to feel confused, angry and that they are somehow to blame – which is one of the shame responses.

If we are unable to deal with the situation effectively, we are likely to try and displace the way we feel. According to Nathanson (1992), we have several possibilities; see the *Compass of Shame* (Fig. 17.1). The four responses include a withdrawal from the situation and the other person, attacking ourselves through negative self-talk or self-harming (such as self-mutilation), attacking others (physically or verbally) or avoiding the situation and its toxic feelings by drinking or refusing to talk about it (a form of denial). Consider potential responses to the issue of infidelity

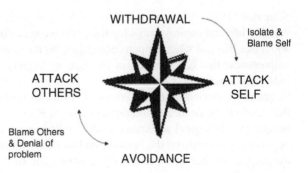

Fig. 17.1 Compass of shame (Adapted from Nathanson 1992)

above. One partner may be outraged that they have been exposed and resort to violent outbursts (attack other), whilst the other may internalise the matter feeling that they are in some way to blame (attack self). At the same time, family members and significant others can be outraged, insist on the relationship dissolving or be in varying stages of disbelief. All are defensive ways of coping with the *shame* that has been triggered.

When we are not managing the shame we feel, there is a tendency for certain poles of the compass to combine. Our response is likely to relate to whether we are more likely to internalise or externalise our reaction to what is happening.

Those that are likely to attack others and adopt a confrontational approach are also likely to avoid the situation and deny that there is a problem or that they were responsible. In another explanation of the power of shame to motivate behaviour, Ahmed and Braithwaite (2004), in discussing bullying behaviour, use the notion of shame *displacement* to explain how, as destructive as it is, it is a protective mechanism for the wrongdoer or person responsible, as they are blaming others and pushing the problem away from themselves. Bullies frequently offer excuses to minimise their role in a shameful situation, denying their responsibility. This might in part explain why studies have found that bullies do not necessarily have the diminished sense of self-esteem that we might imagine.

On the other side is the victim who is typically *internalising* the shame by withdrawing from the situation and berating themselves for being too weak. They internalise the problem and feel they are to blame, which fits with Seligman's (1990) view of pessimism. No one can maintain this state of 'attack self' for lengthy periods of time without the risk of further self-harm or switching poles to attack other. In the school massacres committed by school students, this switch is all too evident. Those responsible for these devastating acts at some stage withdrew or were forced to withdraw from their school community, only to turn and attack others, blaming them for what had happened. What was lacking for these students was a secure attachment or sense of belonging with their peer group, their school community and, in some cases, their families.

17.8 What Can Be Learned from Positive Psychology

Seligman (1990) draws on extensive evidence that suggests there are two ways of viewing life and coping with what happens: we are either optimistic or pessimistic about our life and what happens around us. At the core of pessimism is a sense of helplessness that can develop in the face of tragedy and loss, when nothing an individual does makes a difference. As Roth and Newman (1992) suggest, this is frequently experienced by survivors of sexual and other trauma and is something that needs to be dealt with therapeutically. In Kathy's case, she had sought much needed psychological assistance to deal with her ongoing issues. In the end, the opportunity to confront the person that had taken her innocence from her, to share the impact on her and her family, enabled her to take her power back in the situation. It also enabled her family to deal with the extended impact on them and to reunite the family.

A positive view would say that what hurts us can make us stronger when it is handled effectively. These events can put us in touch with our deeper self and facilitate self-growth (Boniwell 2008), or they can cause us to reconsider the very nature of our purpose on this planet (Roth and Newman 1992). Whilst it is possible that someone may have the resilience to manage this process themselves, others will need to engage in a therapeutic or healing approach. Sullivan and Tifft (2005) indicate that restorative justice and its range of practices foster healing in others. As people 'we develop our potentialities as human beings and enhance our collective wellbeing when our needs are respected, expressed, listened to, defined with care, and ultimately met' (p. 167).

Positive psychology explores mental health, what it is to feel good, what qualifies someone as a good person and what constitutes a group or community's social responsibility (Boniwell 2008). The range of strong negative emotions generated in trauma and conflict get in the way of people feeling good about themselves; they may question their very being and the virtues of the community to which they belong. As Drozdek et al. (2006) indicate, this may result in questioning their very existence. Questioning the self can lead to feelings of inadequacy and self-blame for what has happened and trigger a host of negative emotions, including the affect of shame. These negative emotions can also have a destabilising effect on communities.

17.9   Restorative Practices

A fully restorative process seeks to bring together those responsible, those harmed and those who are significant in the lives of those harmed and responsible, to repair the harm. Each practice in its own right might be completely or partially restorative, dependent on the impact on others and who is involved. For example, mediation around the separation of a couple with children may be partially restorative if it assists the couple to work through their differences, but it does not take into account the impact the separation has on the children and the extended family who are often left reeling in the aftermath of a family break-up. Involving children and others in a family decision-making circle (FGDM) or conference may assist in absolving children of blame for the relationship breakdown and assisting them to stay clear of the conflict (Grych and Fincham 1993). This hopefully prevents an ugly situation developing that can perpetuate throughout the years between fractured families. By involving those who have a stake in the matter, there is an opportunity for all involved to have their say and together work towards the best possible solution. Kathy's case was an example of this. This also aligns with a growing body of research that indicates that families who are more restorative in nature by having firm boundaries and strong support are less likely to have delinquent children (Braithwaite 2003; Coloroso 2009).

Bringing restorative practices into our families, schools, workplaces and communities is a way to transform conflict. In doing so, it is important that we understand what people's needs are and be comfortable in dealing with the range of strong emotions that are triggered. The Truth and Reconciliation Commission (TRC) in South Africa is an example at a community level of an attempt to deal with the human rights violations of the apartheid era. The nation chose not to perpetuate the process of retribution by seeking an alternate way of dealing with the harm and taking responsibility for gross breaches of human rights, largely perpetuated by those carrying out government policy. Whilst the process has its detractors, it is held as an example of a nation taking responsibility for attempting to speak the truth and to start the reconciliation process (Vora and Vora 2004).

By taking a restorative approach to our lives and our interactions with others, we can start transforming our families, schools, workplaces, communities and nations. By working with children to equip them with these same values and the skills to manage repair of relationships, this will flow into families, their relationships with others and their workplaces. Take for example a young man with anger management issues who had been suspended from school many times throughout his schooling. Each time he was suspended, the angrier he would get, and the angrier others would get towards him. Everything changed when a teacher took the time to have a conversation with him and inquire what needed to happen to make a difference. By asking questions such as:

What happened?
What were you thinking at the time?
What have you thought since?
Who has been harmed? How?
What needs to happen to repair the harm?

The young man was able to get in touch with the impact of his action, find a way to discharge his shame and move on, not getting suspended again for his entire schooling. On asking him what had happened, he clearly articulated how someone had shown him how to come back from when he had done the wrong thing. Until this point he didn't know how, which translated into heightened frustration, anger and further incidents of harm. As Kelly (2009) indicates, he overemphasised the negative affect of anger at the expense of feeling good about himself, reducing the quality of his own life and those around him. Without this intervention, he was a likely candidate for violence in community, particularly in relationship with others, as he struggled to control this emotion.

17.10 Role of the Facilitator

The role of a skilled facilitator is central to the success of restorative justice (Latimer et al. 2005). As in the case above, it took not only the willingness of the wrongdoer to look at doing things differently but also the skill of the facilitator (in this case a teacher) who guided the adolescent through the process by asking the right questions.

This included patience and an openness to helping him find a way that worked. It also required ongoing persistence and an intervention plan to change his behaviour over time. In effective processes, preparation is everything, as is the facilitator's ability to trust and manage the group process. Facilitator skills outlined by Hopkins (2004) include the need to:

- Be impartial and non-judgemental
- Respect the perspectives of all involved
- Listen actively and empathically
- Develop rapport amongst participants
- Empower participants to come up with solutions rather than suggesting or imposing ideas
- Use creative questioning
- Above all else, to be warm, compassionate and patient

Applying these skills enables the facilitator to prepare participants so that they can have a challenging conversation, feel free to share their story and express their emotions in a safe way. To facilitate a process where people are not prepared risks further harm. When restorative processes are facilitated well, those involved return to a state of wellbeing, as in Kathy's case. To do this, facilitators need to take a positive psychology approach in being optimistic about outcomes and believing that those involved can take responsibility for their behaviour and be healed in the process. Together they work with the capacity of those involved to find a solution for all and hopefully prevent the reoccurrence of further harm. From a traumatic experience, growth, learning and change can occur. Restorative approaches have been integrated with a range of different approaches, including solution-focused thinking, non-violent communication (NVC) and narrative therapy. The blending of approaches bodes well for a more responsive way of working with conflict and trauma and preventing this from happening. The latter signifies a development in restorative practice, where an emphasis on prevention through the development of healthy connections is as prominent as a behaviour response, particularly in schools and care settings. Working restoratively is an approach to working with others both when things are going well and when they are not going well. As Sullivan and Tifft (2005) suggest, 'how healthy we are, how spiritually grounded we are, how moral we are, can be measured by how much we are committed to meeting the needs of all and to living out relationships in which seeking the equal wellbeing of all is our intention' (p. 169). These are perhaps hard principles to maintain but worthy ones to aspire to.

17.11   From Restorative Justice Practices to Restorative Communities, Cities and States

At the core of this process is the need to build strong, healthy communities that see incidents of crime and wrongdoing as a violation of people and a signal that the community has work to do to repair the harm. Restorative justice is a communitarian process that implies that you are restoring good order. In many cases, the functionality of the community involved is questionable, whether this be whole sections of communities, workplaces, schools or families. Hoyle and Noguera (2008), for example, question the ability of some parents to effectively support their children in restorative approaches either because they are somehow complicit or struggle to deal with their own shame about their parenting ability.

Increasingly, we are seeing examples of whole towns, cities, states, territories, counties or areas moving towards a restorative approach in everything they do, in an effort to transform their communities. This has led to a wave of practice, perhaps better referred to as transformative justice (Hopkins 2009). The city of Hull in the United Kingdom is an example of an economically and socially challenged city working to ensure that all people and services that interact with children and young people work in a restorative way (Mirsky 2009). Initiated in 2007, preliminary findings are encouraging at several levels. Collingwood Primary School reported shifting from a school requiring special measures to an outstanding school within 2 years of implementing a restorative approach (Mirsky 2009). Similarly, in Australia, Charnwood Primary School in the Australian Capital Territory (ACT) went from a school where no one wanted to send their children or to work there to a thriving school within 2 years of implementing a range of measures that included restorative practices. The school was anecdotally credited with contribution to the reduction of crime within the area, because in the view of local police, the young people (many from socially disadvantaged situations) were no longer involved in crime because of what the school were doing. The successful implementation of restorative practice in schools and at a justice level has led to the ACT to adopting a restorative approach to their whole territory (ACT Government 2008).

The city of London in the United Kingdom recently called a meeting of those interested in developing a restorative city, following initiatives supported by the Home Office in 1997 to promote restorative justice in working with young offenders (Hoyle and Noguera 2008). Key providers in the regional area of Wodonga in Victoria, Australia, have united together to improve the outcomes for young people and adolescents with engagement issues in schools. Here, police, community health and schools have come together to use Family Group Conferencing (FGC). This approach offers a 'family-centred, strengths-focused, culturally sensitive and community-based approach to family decision-making and case planning' (Parker 2009). Since its inception, the project has seen overall reductions in truancy, suspension, expulsions and criminal activity.

Combined with the growth of practice in schools across the United Kingdom, Australia, New Zealand, North America and emerging areas in the Asia Rim, it is hoped that the proliferation of practice in educational arenas will see a corresponding reduction in youth offending. Braithwaite (2004) indicates that schools provide an ideal place to start to develop restorative communities, not only from the perspective shown here, but also from the notion of schools as the hub of their communities. Whilst these initiatives take time, it is encouraging that policy makers see this as a positive way forwards, and that 36 years on, restorative practices continue to evolve.

17.12 Conclusion

Conflict is an inevitable part of life. From a positive psychology perspective, the effective management of conflict and traumatic experiences allows us to develop emotional resilience, so that we are better able to manage the ups and downs of life. The blueprint for healthy relationships helps us to understand that any block to feeling good about ourselves will invoke a host of negative emotions and cause disconnect in our community. We need to know how to repair these breaches for our own wellbeing and that of those around us. Restorative practices encourage the appropriate expression of negative emotion by giving those involved and who are affected the chance to have a say and to be heard. When the impact of conflict is expressed, those responsible are more likely to have empathy for the other person, and all parties are more able to move forwards feeling better about themselves and others. At the same time, the communities of care around the central players are more able to accept the decision that has been made and also to move on. This allows for the best chance of the restoration of relationships and an effective outcome for all. The adoption of restorative practices by institutions, families, schools and communities is providing hope that together we can make a difference and transform our communities.

References

Ahmed, E., & Braithwaite, V. (2004). "What, Me Ashamed?" Shame management and school bullying. *Journal of Research in Crime and Delinquency, 41*(3), 269–294.

Australian Capital Territory Government. (2008). *Restorative justice principles in youth settings – final report*. Canberra: ACT Standing Committee on Education, Training and Young People.

Boniwell, I. (2008). *Positive psychology in a nutshell* (2nd ed.). London: Person Well-Being Centre.

Braithwaite, J. (2003). Restorative justice and a better future. In E. McLaughlin, R. Fergusson, G. Hughes, & L. Westmarland (Eds.), *Restorative justice: Critical issues*. Milton Keynes: SAGE Publications in association with The Open University.

Coloroso, B. (2009). *The Bully, the Bullied, and the Bystander: From preschool to high school – How parents and teachers can help break the cycle of violence* (Updated edition). New York: HarperCollins.

Drozdek, B., Turkovic, S., & Wilson, J. P. (2006). Posttraumatic shame and guilt: Culture and the posttraumatic self. In J. P. Wilson (Ed.), *The posttraumatic self: Restoring meaning and wholeness to personality*. New York: Routledge.

Garner, H. (2004). *Joe Cinque's consolation*. Sydney: Picador.

Grych, J. H., & Fincham, F. D. (1993). Children's appraisals of marital conflict: Initial investigations of the cognitive-contextual framework. *Child Development, 64*(1), 215–230.

Hopkins, B. (2004). *Just schools: A whole school approach to restorative justice*. London: Jessica Kingsley Publishers.

Hopkins, B. (2009). *Just care: Restorative justice approaches to working with children in public care*. London: Jessica Kingsley Publishers.

Hoyle, C., & Noguera, S. (2008). Supporting young offenders through restorative justice: Parents as (In)appropriate adults. *British Journal of Community Justice, 6*(3), 67–85.

Kaufman, G. (1993). *The psychology of shame; theory and treatment of shame-based syndromes*. London: Routledge.

Kelly, V. C. (2009). *A primer of affect psychology. Resource document.* Silvan Tomkins Institute. Retrieved May 13, 2010, from http://www.tomkins.org/Affect_Script_Psyc.html

Latimer, J., Dowden, C., & Muise, D. (2005). The effectiveness of restorative justice processes: A meta-analysis. *The Prison Journal, 85*, 127–143.

Lemonne, A. (2003). Alternative conflict resolution and restorative justice: A discussion. In L. Walgrave (Ed.), *Respositioning restorative justice.* Devon: Willan Publishing.

Mirsky, L. (2009). *Hull, UK: Toward a restorative city.* Restorative Practices eforum. http://www.iirp.org/pdf/Hull.pdf

Moroney, S. (2010). Restorative options for an offender's spouse. In J. P. J. Dussich & J. Schellenberg (Eds.), *The promise of restorative justice: New approaches for criminal justice and beyond.* Boulder: Lynne Rienner Publishers.

Nathanson, D. L. (1992). *Shame and pride: Affect, sex, and the birth of the self.* New York: W. W. Norton and Company, Inc.

Parker, R. (2009). Getting tough or getting together: A model of engagement. *Family Relationships Quarterly, 13*, 15–17.

Pranis, K., Stuart, B., & Wedge, M. (2003). *Peacemaking circles: From crime to community.* Saint Paul: Living Justice Press.

Roth, S., & Newman, E. (1992). The role of helplessness in recovery from sexual trauma. *Canadian Journal of Behavioral Science, 24*, 220–232.

Seligman, M. E. P. (1990). *Learned optimism: Optimism is essential for a good and successful life you too can acquire it.* New York: Random House.

Shaver, P. R., & Mikulincer, M. (2009). Adult attachment strategies and the regulation of emotion. In J. J. Gross (Ed.), *Handbook of emotion regulation.* New York: Guilford Press.

Sullivan, D., & Tifft, L. (2005). *Restorative justice: Healing the foundations of our everyday lives* (2nd ed.). Wonsey: Willow Tree Press.

Tomkins, S. S. (1962). *Affect/imagery/consciousness* (Vol. 1: The positive affects). New York: Springer.

Tomkins, S. S. (1963). *Affect/imagery/consciousness* (Vol. 2: The negative affects). New York: Springer.

Vora, J. A., & Vora, E. (2004). The effectiveness of South Africa's truth and reconciliation commission: Perceptions of Xhosa, and English South Africans. *Journal of Black Studies., 34*(3), 301–322.

Yoder, C. (2005). *The little book of trauma healing.* Intercourse: Good Books.

Zehr, H. (1990). *Changing lenses.* Scottdale: Herald Press.

Zehr, H. (2002). *The little book of restorative justice.* Intercourse: Good Books.

Zehr, H., & Mika, H. (2003). Fundamental concepts of restorative justice. In E. McLaughlin, R. Fergusson, G. Hughes, & L. Westmarland (Eds.), *Restorative justice: Critical issues.* Milton Keynes: SAGE Publications in association with The Open University.

Ziegler, A. (1999). *Facing the demons.* Canberra: Ronin Films.

Peta Blood is a leading contributor to the restorative justice movement in Australia and internationally. As a former police officer, she has applied the principles and practices of restorative justice in a range of settings, although for the past 10 years she has focused on the implementation of restorative practices in schools. Peta is a co-founder of Restorative Practices International (RPI), an international association for restorative practitioners.

Contact: e-mail: peta@circlespeak.com.au.

Index

Printed by Printforce, the Netherlands